Bioethics and the Brain

Bioethics and the Brain

Walter Glannon

OXFORD
UNIVERSITY PRESS

2007

OXFORD

UNIVERSITY PRESS

Oxford University Press, Inc., publishes works that further
Oxford University's objective of excellence
in research, scholarship, and education.

Oxford   New York
Auckland   Cape Town   Dar es Salaam   Hong Kong   Karachi
Kuala Lumpur   Madrid   Melbourne   Mexico City   Nairobi
New Delhi   Shanghai   Taipei   Toronto

With offices in
Argentina   Austria   Brazil   Chile   Czech Republic   France   Greece
Guatemala   Hungary   Italy   Japan   Poland   Portugal   Singapore
South Korea   Switzerland   Thailand   Turkey   Ukraine   Vietnam

Published by Oxford University Press, Inc.
198 Madison Avenue, New York, New York 10016

www.oup.com

Oxford is a registered trademark of Oxford University Press

Library of Congress Cataloging-in-Publication Data

Glannon, Walter.
Bioethics and the brain / Walter Glannon.
p. cm.
Includes bibliographical references and index.
ISBN 978-0-19-530778-8

1. Brain—Research—Moral and ethical aspects.   2. Neurosciences—Research—
Moral and ethical aspects.   3. Medical ethics.
4. Bioethics.   I. Title.

' RC343.G53 2006
174.2968—dc22   2006040119

3   5   7   9   8   6   4   2

Printed in the United States of America
on acid-free paper

For Yee-Wah

Preface

This book is an integrated investigation of some of the ethical issues that have emerged and will continue to emerge as a result of our ability to map, monitor, and intervene in the human brain. I focus primarily on the clinical neurosciences of psychiatry, neurology, and neurosurgery, rather than on theoretical neuroscience. Although the ethical issues I examine have important implications for law, social science, and public policy, my main concern is with the philosophical aspects of these issues. These include questions about benefit, harm, and responsibility, as well as related questions about free will, personal identity, and the self. The discussion through all the chapters is informed by the most recent empirical research in clinical neuroscience. I also use examples from prominent contemporary medical and legal cases and examples from literature to introduce, illustrate, and provide a nuanced discussion of the main questions.

I am grateful to the two readers who reviewed the manuscript for Oxford University Press (whom I later learned were Grant Gillett and Erik Parens). They gave me many thoughtful and constructive comments that were extremely helpful in preparing the final version of the manuscript. My editor, Peter Ohlin, was very supportive of the project from the outset. Jeffrey House, also from OUP, was supportive as well and gave me valuable advice at a critical point about how to proceed with the project. Lara Zoble skillfully resolved some difficult editorial problems. I have benefited from the comments of referees for and editors of some of the journals in which parts of the book have been published. David Steinberg helped me to clarify some of the points in the discussion of free will in chapter 3, and Neil Levy gave me very insightful comments on the entire manuscript. I presented some of the material in this book to audiences at a joint meeting of the American Society for Bioethics and Humanities and the Canadian Bioethics Society in Montreal in October 2003 and at the University of Calgary in May 2004. The comments from both audiences have been very helpful. I offered a course on this topic at the University of Calgary in the winter 2006 term. My students in the course, Elske Straver, Jordan Kirkness, Adam Koppany, Heather Chypiska, and

Jonathan Van de Vliert, made me rethink some key questions. I am also grateful to Teresa Yee-Wah Yu for valuable discussion of many of the issues I address. And I thank Judy Illes, both for her pioneering work in the field of neuroethics and for organizing a conference in San Francisco in May 2002, which further stimulated my interest in the subject.

I thank the Johns Hopkins University Press for permission to publish parts of "Depression as a Mind-Body Problem," *Philosophy, Psychiatry and Psychology* 9 (2002): 243–254, "The Psychology and Physiology of Depression," *Philosophy, Psychiatry and Psychology* 9 (2002): 265–269, and "Endophenotypes," *Philosophy, Psychiatry and Psychology* 10 (2003): 277–284. I thank the BMJ Group for permission to publish parts of "Transcendence and Healing," *Journal of Medical Ethics/Medical Humanities* 30 (2004): 70–73, "Medicine through the Novel: *Lying Awake*," *Journal of Medical Ethics/Medical Humanities* 31 (2005): 131–134, and "Psychopharmacology and Memory," *Journal of Medical Ethics* 32 (2006): 161–165. And I thank Blackwell Publishing Ltd. for permission to publish parts of "Neurobiology, Neuroimaging, and Free Will," *Midwest Studies in Philosophy* 29 (2005): 68–82, and "Neuroethics," *Bioethics* 20 (2006): 37–52.

Contents

Bioethics and the Brain

Introduction

Some of the most innovative and exciting work in contemporary medicine is being done in the clinical neurosciences of psychiatry, neurology, and neurosurgery. Advances in these areas during the last 25 years, combined with advances in radiology, have provided new insight into the relation between the human brain and the mind. Neuroimaging—in the form of computed tomography (CT), positron emission tomography (PET), magnetic resonance imaging (MRI), single photon emission computed tomography (SPECT), and functional magnetic resonance imaging (fMRI)—can reveal the neurobiological bases of normal mental activity, as well as psychiatric and neurological disorders. Previously, these bases were inaccessible to purely psychological inquiry and remained elusive. Neurosurgery performed on conscious patients has also yielded a better understanding of the relation between the brain and the mind, as has the ability of psychotropic drugs to alter cognitive and affective mental states.

The significance of these advances is underscored by the fact that psychiatric and neurological disorders affect roughly 400 million people globally. These disorders includes such diseases as schizophrenia, depression, bipolar disorder, and obsessive-compulsive disorder, as well as such diseases as Alzheimer's and Parkinson's. In June 2004, the *Journal of the American Medical Association* published results from the world's largest survey on mental health. From 1 to 5 percent of the populations of most countries surveyed have serious mental illness, much of it untreated or undertreated.[1] More recently, results from a national survey on mental illness published in June 2005 showed that about half of all Americans will have conditions that meet criteria of the *Diagnostic and Statistical Manual of Mental Disorders* (DSM-IV-TR) over the course of their lifetime.[2]

Brain imaging may detect early signs of neuropsychiatric diseases well before their characteristic symptoms appear. This type of imaging may also monitor the effects of drugs used to treat these diseases. Psychosurgery can alleviate and possibly eliminate the symptoms of obsessive-compulsive disorder (OCD), major depressive disorder (MDD), and other severe neuropsychiatric conditions that are refractory to other treatments. Electrical and magnetic stimulation of the cerebral cortex and subcortical regions may relieve these symptoms in a less invasive way. Implanting and stimulating electrodes deep in the brain can enable people with motor control diseases such as Parkinson's to regain some control of their bodily movements. Similar control might be achieved with brain-computer interfaces for motor neuron diseases such as amyotrophic lateral sclerosis (ALS). Antidepressant and antipsychotic drugs may restore or regenerate neuronal connections disrupted or destroyed in depression and schizophrenia. It is now even possible to use psychotropic drugs to enhance normal cognition and mood.

But the ability to measure, intervene in, and alter the neural correlates of the mind raises important ethical questions. These questions are arguably weightier and more momentous than any other set of questions in any other area of bioethics. This is because techniques that target the brain can reveal and directly affect the source of the mind and the deepest aspects of our selves: free will; personhood; personal identity through time; the relation between the mind and the body; the soul. These interrelated philosophical concepts all encompass cognitive, affective, and conative mental capacities, which include beliefs, emotions, desires, and volitions that are generated and sustained by the brain. One's identity as a person, one's experience of agency, and one's general sense of self consist in the unity and integrity of one's mental states. It is because the brain generates and sustains these states that intervening in the brain can affect the nature and content of our minds and thus who we essentially are.

Core Definitions and Questions

Many of the questions that I address fall within the field of neuroethics, which can be defined roughly as the study of ethical issues pertinent to information about the brain.[3] More precisely, neuroethics is a branch of bioethics concerned with ethical issues arising from different measures of and interventions in the brain or central nervous system.[4] It lies at the intersection of the empirical brain sciences, normative ethics, philosophy of mind, law, and the social sciences. The philosophical significance of monitoring and manipulating the brain centers primarily on the overlap of normative ethics and the philosophy of mind.[5] For whether an action benefits or harms one depends on how it affects one's mind. Images of the brain can provide information about the mental capacity and behavior of persons. This information can also provide a basis on which to intervene in the brain to treat neuropsychiatric conditions. These interventions may be direct or indirect, as in the neurological effects of altering certain functions of immune and endocrine systems connected to functions in the central nervous system.

In this book, I explore some of the emerging ethical issues in standard and experimental clinical neuroscience. I examine whether and to what extent the procedures and drugs I have mentioned can benefit or harm us. Actions benefit persons when they are consistent with or satisfy their interests. Actions harm persons when they are inconsistent with or defeat their interests.[6] Whether an action benefits or harms a person will influence the reasons for or against that action, which, in turn, will determine whether the action is obligatory, prohibited, or permissible.[7]

An action is obligatory if it is supported by an ethically decisive reason—that is, the reason for doing the action overrides any opposing reason for not doing it. An action is prohibited (or impermissible) if there is an ethically decisive reason for not doing it. And an action is permissible if there is no ethically decisive reason for or against it. There will be reasons for performing the action, but not decisive or overriding ones.

Because many of the procedures, techniques, and drugs that I discuss are novel or experimental, and because their long-term effects on people are not yet known, it may not be warranted to claim that there are ethically decisive reasons for or against them. Accordingly, many of my claims and arguments on particular issues will appeal to the weaker notion of permissibility, rather than the stronger notions of obligation and prohibition. One notable exception is predictive brain imaging, where there is an obligation for researchers and clinicians to present information about the brain to patients and research subjects in a way that acknowledges the uncertainty about its significance. They also have an obligation to disclose information about any known risks from different interventions in the brain. More generally, the uncertainty about the consequences of these interventions underscores an obligation to conduct studies that can accurately assess their risks and benefits.

Each of us has an interest in being able to deliberate about and choose to perform certain actions. In addition, we have an interest in being able to experience such positive moods as pleasure, joy, and satisfaction. We also have an interest in being able to remember past experiences and to anticipate and plan for the future. These interests presuppose normal cognitive, affective, and conative functions, which rely on normal brain functions. Disorders of belief, mood, and volition resulting from disorders of the brain can harm us by defeating these interests. Neuroimaging, neurosurgery, psychosurgery, psychopharmacology, and electrical and magnetic stimulation of the brain aim to benefit us by correcting or controlling brain disorders and thereby restoring normal mental functions. As noted, psychopharmacology may also be used to raise mental functions and capacities above a normal level.

Yet some of these interventions in the brain may also harm us in unpredictable ways. Thus we need to carefully weigh the ratio of the probable benefits to the probable harms of using them. It is not only the probability of harm that we need to consider but also the magnitude of harm these interventions might entail. The assessment of the benefits and harms of these techniques will influence the reasons for or against permitting them. Obtaining information about or intervening in the brain will be permitted if there is no medically and ethically decisive reason not to perform these actions, and the absence of such a reason will be based on the judgment that the probable benefits outweigh the probable harms. These actions would be impermissible if there were a decisive reason not to perform them. The reason would be based on the judgment that the probable harms outweighed the probable benefits.

The brain remains the most complex and least understood organ in the human body. It is also much more dynamic and sensitive to intervention than any other part of our anatomy and physiology. In the light of this complexity and sensitivity, and of the dependence of the mind on the brain, it is crucial that we carefully assess the short- and long-term effects that imaging, surgery, pharmacology, and stimulation of or for the brain might have on the mind. Does the availability of this technology mean that we should use it? If we answer this question affirmatively, then how should we use it? Should we use brain scans only for diagnostic purposes? Should we use them for predictive purposes as well? For which types of diagnosis would they be indicated and useful? How should researchers and clinicians interpret the information derived from these scans, and how should the information be presented to research subjects and patients? When a psychiatric disorder is refractory to all other treatments, is it permissible to use psychosurgery to control or alleviate its symptoms? What are the long-term effects of psychotropic drugs on the brain and mind? Would it be permissible to use pharmacological agents for the off-label purpose of enhancing cognitive and affective capacities? When does a person die? How does our response to this question influence our judgments about the permissibility or impermissibility of such actions as withdrawing life-support or procuring organs for transplantation at the margin between life and death? This book addresses these and related ethical questions.

Brain and Mind

Neuroscientist V. S. Ramachandran claims that "the boundary between neurology and psychiatry is becoming increasingly blurred, and it's only a matter of time before psychiatry becomes just another branch of neurology."[8] But there are considerable differences between the underlying mechanisms and symptoms of psychiatric and neurological disorders, which should make us resist the temptation to reduce one to the other. Most psychiatric disorders have a distinctive psychopathology. The phenomenological experience of abnormal beliefs, emotions, and volitions differentiates the symptoms of psychiatric disorders from the symptoms commonly associated with neurological disorders. It is estimated that between 40 and 70 percent of people with Parkinson's disease experience cognitive symptoms that progress to dementia. Yet any psychopathology associated with these symptoms is considered secondary to the primary neurodegenerative movement disorder. The neurodegenerative Alzheimer's disease has a definite psychopathology associated with loss of memory and other cognitive functions. But it does not have the same phenomenological effects on cognition, mood, and volition as psychiatric conditions like schizophrenia, depression, and general anxiety disorder. At the very least, these considerations suggest that we should generally characterize the conditions I have mentioned as neuropsychiatric disorders and not reduce them all to neurology.

Neuroscientific research has shown that mental illnesses once thought to be entirely psychogenic have biological causes. Many of these illnesses can be characterized generally as disorders of the mind arising from dysfunction in the brain.[9] Conscious and unconscious beliefs and emotions may play a role in the pathogenesis of major depression and general anxiety disorder. But systems in the brain are involved in the regulation of these mental states. The etiology and symptomatology of mental illnesses include both biological and psychological properties. This does not mean that there is a linear relationship between neurons and normal or abnormal states of mind, or that states of mind are solely a function of events occurring at the neuronal level. Rather, the mind is a reflection of interaction between neurons and the internal environment of the body, which may include immune and endocrine systems in addition to the central nervous system. The mind is also a reflection of interaction between the organism and the external environment. These two types of interaction are not mutually exclusive but interdependent.

Theoretical and clinical neuroscience has put Freud's views on the mind in a new and interesting light. It is widely accepted that Freud believed that mental disorders could be explained in psychoanalytic terms as the result of repressed memories of primitive states in the unconscious mind. Yet Freud was primarily a neurobiologist who took himself to be describing neurobiological forces when discussing the mind. A neurobiological explanation of certain mental phenomena is, in principle, consistent with Freud's psychological explanation. For example, limbic and paralimbic areas of the brain can repress certain negative emotional memories without fully availing themselves of the normatively constrained information in cortical processing. This appears to support Freud's view about the primitive unconscious nature of these mechanisms.[10] Recent fMRI studies have identified a network of brain regions that keeps unwanted memories below the surface of consciousness, which suggests the sort of psychological defense mechanism for memories that Freud proposed.[11]

Neuroscientific research has repudiated behaviorist views of mind championed by psychologists such as J. B. Watson and B. F. Skinner, and philosophers such as Gilbert Ryle. They all essentially held that the brain could be treated as a black box, and that we could understand the nature of mind by ignoring inward experience and instead paying attention to people's outward linguistic and physical behavior. Contrary to what these psychologists and philosophers claimed, looking into the brain may provide us with a better understanding of mind and behavior. Neuroscientist Jean-Pierre Changeux offers one defense of this position: "The development of the neurosciences has brought another way of looking at behavior. The neuronal content of the black box can no longer be ignored. On the contrary, all forms of behavior mobilize distinct sets of nerve cells, and it is at their level that the final explanation of behavior must be sought."[12]

The connections between the brain and the mind have been revealed in many ways. Long before the advent of brain imaging, in the 1880s, the British neurologist David Ferrin and colleagues showed that direct electrical stimulation of the brain could change behavior. This was perhaps the first indication that certain regions of the brain correlated with certain mental states and behavior. Similar insights were obtained by the Canadian neurosurgeon Wilder Penfield, beginning in the 1930s. Penfield would carefully place an electrode on the surface of the exposed temporal lobe of some of his patients undergoing surgery for epilepsy. By eliciting memories of patients' long-forgotten experience through electrical stimulation, Penfield provided evidence that their episodic memories were stored in this region of the brain. Penfield noted: "It is clear that the neuronal action that accompanies each subjective state of consciousness leaves its permanent imprint on the brain."[13] Many patients undergoing brain surgery remain conscious while receiving local anesthesia. Electrically stimulating the surface of the somatosensory cortex, for example, can produce conscious sensations of touch and alter one's orientation in space and time. More recent high-resolution PET and fMRI scans are an extension of the work of Ferrin, Penfield, and others in constructing a more refined map of the structural and functional neural substrate of the mind.

Although the mind has a neurobiological underpinning, the mind is not reducible to the brain. So I do not accept Changeux's reductionist claim that the "final" explanation of human behavior will come from studying neurons alone. There is much more to the human mind and human behavior than the mobilization of distinct sets of nerve cells. The emergence of the mind from the brain cannot be explained entirely in terms of brain function because, qua emergent, the mind consists in qualitatively new properties not exhibited by the physical properties of the brain. These include the property of representing the body and events from the external environment to the brain and making them meaningful to us. How the brain develops depends at least partly on how it responds to the body and to events in the environment. This response depends on beliefs and other mental states relaying information about the environment back to the brain, which cannot be done by neurons alone. It is also questionable whether the first-person phenomenological feel of subjective experience can be entirely captured by third-person descriptions of brain function. The human mind expresses itself through a chain of molecular events and processes. But the mind is more than just a function of molecules.

The Mind–Body Problem

Some of the issues I address are germane to the philosophical mind–body problem. But some qualifications are in order. As it is typically conceived, the mind–body problem involves questions of how consciousness can arise from the brain, and how mental events can causally interact with physical events in the brain if these two types of events are ontologically distinct.[14] Understanding the neurobiological basis of conscious awareness has been the most difficult problem for neuroscientists. Consciousness appears to depend on distributed neural components acting in a functionally integrated way. Interactions of the neocortex, the most recently evolved region of the brain, with the thalamus and the upper midbrain appear to play a central role in these mechanisms.[15] But it is still not known precisely how conscious awareness arises from these mechanisms. This should be described more accurately as the mind–brain problem. I will not discuss this problem at any length here.

Assuming that neuroscientific techniques can reveal or alter the neural correlates of the mind, I focus on how measuring or manipulating these neural correlates can affect our mental states in respects that can benefit or harm us. I also explain how interventions in systems outside the brain can affect the neurobiological basis of the mind. There is holistic interaction between the central nervous system and other bodily systems. So my concern is not so much with the narrower mind–*brain* problem as with the broader mind–*body* problem.[16] Indeed, an explanation of the emergence of the mind requires an even broader framework, one that includes interaction between and among the brain, the body, and the external environment as a tripartite reality. This tripartite structure shapes the human organism and how the brain is inscribed within the patterns of adaptation in which the organism participates.

As components of this tripartite structure, systems of the brain and body should be understood in terms of the adaptive role they play in maintaining homeostasis. This refers to the balance of essential bodily functions through the action of interdependent physiological mechanisms. Through homeostasis, organs and organ systems are neither underactive nor overactive. Maintaining this balance is critical to the survival of the organism. We need to ask *how* processes in the endocrine and immune systems influence, and are influenced by, processes in the central nervous system. More generally, we need to ask *why* these systems interact and why beliefs, emotions, and other mental states emerge from these systemic interactions. Causal questions should be framed by this broader teleological question. Before considering various interventions in the brain, we need to ask why neural events in different brain regions generate mental events, why (in some neuropsychiatric conditions) mental events can causally influence events in the brain and body, and whether these interactions have evolved to serve an adaptive purpose for the organism as a whole. Questions about the relation between the brain and the mind, and how altering one can affect the other, should be raised and discussed within an evolutionary framework.

I avoid using fanciful thought experiments involving brains in vats, zombies, or exotic potions that cause humans to metamorphose into other species. These examples are the stock in trade of some philosophers. Yet many of them are implausible and thus not very helpful in sorting out and critically reflecting on our intuitions about the brain and mind. This is because these examples rest on broadly logical possibility and are not supported by what science has shown to be empirically possible. In many instances, assumptions are made that fall outside the realm of empirical possibility. This can result in question-begging arguments in which the proposition to be proved is assumed in one of the premises. Ethical questions about how neuroimaging, neurosurgery, neurostimulation, and psychopharmacology can benefit or harm us, as well as metaphysical questions about how these techniques might influence our understanding of free will, personal identity, and the self, must be sufficiently scientifically informed. This requires that any philosophical claims or speculation about the types and implications of intervention in the brain be generally consistent with clinical neuroscience and rely on a posteriori rather than a priori arguments.

As the philosopher and psychiatrist Henrik Walter notes, "good philosophy needs a dab of speculation, which, however, should be firmly anchored in historical and empirical knowledge."[17] Further, he says: "We can consider neurophilosophy as a discipline that moves in on the mind–brain problem from two opposite directions. Either we begin on the empirical side and happen upon philosophical questions, or we set out with philosophical puzzles and need empirical findings to solve them."[18] My approach is closer in spirit to the first method Walter describes. After explaining the brain functions that underlie cognitive, affective, and conative mental functions, I describe actual and probable techniques in clinical neuroscience and explore some of the ethical issues they raise.

Ethical Issues in Neuroscience

In chapter 2, I provide a brief guide to the brain and explain how different brain regions regulate different mental functions. I describe the mind as a higher level set of properties that emerge from lower level physical properties in the brain and body. The mind does not become independent of the brain and body once it emerges from them. It interacts with them in a bidirectional way to maintain homeostasis and ensure the survival of the organism. I explain that the biological basis of the mind is not localized in one brain region but is distributed through many regions of the brain. In fact, the mind does not emerge from the central nervous system (CNS) alone, but from the CNS and its interactions with endo-crine, immune, and possibly other systems of the body. Thus, while the mind has a biological basis, it is not entirely *neuro*biological. This distinguishes the mind–body problem in medicine from the mind–body problem in philosophy, which is concerned primarily with the relation of the mind to the brain. In the last section of the chapter, I describe the self as a first-person qualitative experience consisting of a set of mental capacities based on biological functions in the brain and body and the organism's relation to the environment. I explain how dysfunction in certain brain regions can disturb or disrupt different aspects of the self, which can yield insight into the pathophysiology and psychopathology of many neuropsychiatric disorders. This account establishes a framework for the discussion of the different measures of and interventions in the brain in chapters 3–6.

Chapter 3 is an exploration of the ethical implications of diagnostic and pre-dictive neuroimaging. Brain scans may help to confirm diagnoses of neuropsychi-atric disorders by revealing brain abnormalities associated with these disorders. Brain scans can also aid in monitoring the effects of drugs and psychotherapy on affected brain regions. I consider whether brain scans could tell us that violent offenders or psychopaths were able or unable to control their behavior. This leads to the question of what brain scans might indicate about free will and moral and legal responsibility. Brain imaging might also predict whether individuals at high risk of having schizophrenia, Alzheimer's, and other neuropsychiatric diseases would develop them by showing early signs of structural and functional brain abnormal-ities. However, the information researchers and clinicians derive from predictive imaging is fraught with uncertainty. This can affect whether patients and research subjects give valid informed consent to this type of imaging. Predictive neuroim-aging may have positive or negative psychological effects on patients and subjects, depending on how they interpret and respond to what can be ambiguous infor-mation about the brain.

Chapter 4 is an examination of pharmacological and psychological interven-tions in the brain, paying particular attention to psychopharmacology. After pointing out that the long-term effects of psychotropic drugs are unknown, I explore the use of novel therapeutic drugs that target not only the brain but also hormones from the endocrine system that can influence the brain. Some of these drugs hold the promise of preventing or erasing unconscious emotional memories impli-cated in depression, anxiety, and posttraumatic stress disorder (PTSD). But it is possible that using these drugs to cure or control one type of psychopatholgy could cause a different type, such as the elimination of a normal fear response to threatening events. In prescribing or administering these drugs for a therapeutic purpose, we should aim to maintain a healthy balance of bodily systems. I go on to consider the placebo response as a form of therapy and give some examples of situations in which it could be ethical to give a placebo to a patient or research subject. Then I explore the contentious question of whether we could justify forced behavior control of violent offenders and other individuals through pharmacological means.

In the last section of chapter 4, I discuss off-label uses of psychotropic drugs for the nontherapeutic purpose of enhancing cognitive and affective capacities. These uses are examined against the view that there may be evolutionary reasons for limits on memory storage and retrieval and attention, and that these limits may be part of an adaptive purpose. Even if the use of these drugs did not result in any adverse physiological effects, they might exacerbate rather than reduce social inequality. At a deeper level, the prospect of psychopharmacological enhancement raises a question that has both metaphysical and ethical aspects: In what sense would these drugs benefit the people who took them? People benefit from an action when it makes them better off than they were before. But if the drugs caused radical changes in one's psychological properties, to the point of altering one's identity, then it is unclear in what sense someone who took such a drug would be better off.

Chapter 5 examines different forms of neurosurgery, psychosurgery, and neurostimulation for neurological and psychiatric disorders. I consider some of the issues surrounding benefit and risk in surgery to remove brain tumors. I then discuss how the weighing of potential benefit and harm figured in the justification of the high-risk surgery in July 2003 to separate Ladan and Laleh Bijani, the Iranian twins joined at the head since birth. In addition, I discuss the use of fetal and embryonic stem cells for neural tissue transplantation to treat neurodegenerative conditions. Obtaining informed consent from patients can be problematic in neurosurgery and especially psychosurgery. The target of this intervention is the very organ on which the cognitive and affective capacities of reasoning and decision-making necessary for consent depend. Dysfunction in cortical and subcortical regions of the brain, or in pathways linking these regions, can impair or undermine these capacities. I examine the ethical justification for substitute decision-making for ablation of brain regions of affected patients who are unable to consent to such a procedure on their own. I also raise the question of whether psychosurgery, as distinct from psychopharmacology, could ever be justified as a form of behavior control for violent offenders.

This is followed by a discussion of the potential risks and benefits of electrical deep-brain stimulation for motor disorders such as Parkinson's. I go on to examine some of the ethical issues surrounding transcranial magnetic stimulation (TMS), electroconvulsive therapy (ECT), and vagus nerve stimulation (VNS) for cognitive disorders such as OCD, anxiety disorders, and mood disorders such as depression. Then I explore the potential benefits and harms of thought-controlled brain–computer interface systems for conditions such as quadriplegia and ALS and end the chapter by considering the use of deep-brain stimulation for intractable pain and palliative care.

Finally, chapter 6 is a discussion of brain death and its ethical implications for such actions as the withdrawal of life-support and organ procurement. I consider the extent to which the declaration of death is based on biological criteria and whether these criteria are exclusively neurological. There is also analysis of the respects in which the psychological properties that ground one's interests and constitute one's biographical life depend on the physical properties that constitute one's biological life. I assess whole-brain and higher brain criteria of death and how they bear on the question of whether we are essentially persons or human organisms. Discussion of two prominent legal cases will illustrate the divergence of public opinion on these neurological and metaphysical questions. Arguing that only the higher brain criterion of death and the related view that we are essentially persons can explain how we can have moral status, I discuss the ways we can benefit from or be harmed by actions done to our bodies at the margin between life and death.

Conclusion

Neuroscience is the most rapidly advancing area of medicine and biotechnology. Although, in some respects, basic and clinical neuroscience is still an emerging field, brain imaging, psychopharmacology, psychosurgery, and neurostimulation have been used in standard and experimental settings for some time. The ethical implications of these practices are at least as important and worthy of the same attention as stem-cell research, predictive genetic testing and screening, or other contentious issues in bioethics. These include not only traditional bioethical questions about autonomy, informed consent, nonmaleficence, and beneficence but also more fundamental questions involving the intersection of ethics with metaphysics and the philosophy of mind. Acknowledging the differences between actual and possible applications of neuroscientific techniques, we need to identify, respond to, and anticipate the ethical dilemmas that have arisen from these techniques and those that will arise from them in the future. It is because intervening in the brain can affect us so directly and deeply that we should be debating the ethical issues generated by different practices in clinical neuroscience.

Brain, Body, and Self

We need an account of the relationship between the brain and the mind to understand what brain scans can reveal about the neural correlates of our mental states. Such an account is also necessary to understand how surgical, pharmacological, or other interventions in the brain can alter these states. In this chapter, I describe different regions of the brain and how they regulate different bodily functions. I also describe how the brain regulates cognitive, affective, and conative capacities at the level of the mind. These interacting mental capacities are generated and sustained by interacting systems in the brain. Seeing how dysfunction in certain brain regions results in various psychopathologies can yield insight into the normal and abnormal neural correlates of normal and abnormal states of mind.

I present and defend an account of mind as a set of capacities that emerge from functions in the brain and body. These capacities play a role in maintaining internal systemic balance and ensuring the survival of the organism. The biological basis of the mind is not located in one region of the brain but is distributed through many brain regions. Indeed, I show that the biological basis of the mind is not limited to the brain but involves immune and endocrine systems as well. So the mind has more than just a neurobiological underpinning. Interactions between and among the central nervous, immune, and endocrine systems influence, and can be influenced by, our mental states. In psychiatric disorders such as depression and anxiety, pathological mental states can negatively influence these three and possibly other biological systems. I formulate a conception of the self as a function of five basic psychological properties corresponding to different biological functions in the brain and body, as well as their relation to the external environment. Different components of the self can be adversely affected when there is dysfunction in one or more regions of the brain or in systems outside the brain. The issues that I outline will set the stage for discussion of the ethical issues pertinent to measuring and intervening in the brain.

A Short Guide to the Brain

The nervous system consists of the central nervous system (CNS), which includes the brain and spinal cord, and the peripheral nervous system (PNS), which includes nerve fibers outside the skull and spine. The PNS is subdivided into the sensorimotor nervous system and the autonomic nervous system, which is further subdivided into sympathetic and parasympathetic systems.[1] These latter two systems play a critical role in initiating and inhibiting the body's stress response, which I will explain shortly.

There are two types of cells in the brain, glial cells and neurons, which have different functions. Glial cells regulate the transportation of metabolites and protect neurons and their immediate environment. This class of brain cells includes astrocytes, oligodendrocytes, microglia, and Schwann cells. Neurons regulate communication and information processing within the brain. Glia are much more numerous than neurons, outnumbering them by about 9 to 1. Each neuron consists of a cell body and branching fibers called axons and dendrites. Axons carry signals away from the cell, while dendrites carry signals to the cell. Cell bodies, dendrites, and glia make up the gray matter of the brain, and myelinated axons make up the white matter. The white matter is so named because glial cells form white fatty sheets called myelin. The gray matter is so named because of the color of the cell bodies of the neurons and of the surrounding blood vessels. Gray matter constitutes the cortex, while white matter constitutes the nerve cells under the cortex. Synapses are branches of neurons that control the sending and receiving of messages to and from neurons. Glia can influence the formation of synapses and which neuronal connections become stronger or weaker over time. The brain has both excitatory and inhibitory synapses. As the names imply, the first type of synapse makes the neuron more responsive to incoming signals, while the second type of synapse makes the neuron less responsive to these signals (fig. 1).

Neurotransmitters are the chemical vehicles that bridge the synaptic cleft between an axon and a dendrite, or between two axons. They play a critical role in allowing communication between neurons and thereby regulate many brain functions. The main neurotransmitters and hormones with neuromodulating effects are epinephrine (adrenaline), norepinephrine (noradrenaline), cortisol, acetylcholine, dopamine, and serotonin. The major excitatory neurotransmitter glutamate and the major inhibitory neurotransmitter gamma-aminobutyric acid (GABA) together also act as modulators of neuronal activity. Epinephrine, norepinephrine, and dopamine are collectively called catecholamines, and their effects are called adrenergic. Cortisol is the most potent of hormones called glucocorticoids. The effects of acetylcholine are called cholinergic, and those of serotonin are called serotonergic. This classification will be helpful when we consider the effects of drugs that excite or inhibit hormones and neurotransmitters in chapter 4.

Serotonin, norepinephrine, and dopamine are involved in the regulation of mood. This is due primarily to their activity in neurons and neuronal receptors in the limbic system and prefrontal cortex. Disturbances in dopamine transmitter systems have been implicated in addictive behavior. Dopamine also plays a role in cognition and motor functioning. Excess dopamine has been associated with some

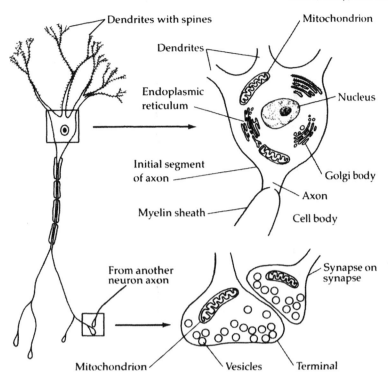

FIGURE 1. Major parts of a neuron. The cell body contains all the same organelles as other cells. The initial segment of the axon where it leaves the cell body is naked – not covered with myelin. Mitochondria are present in the cell body, the fibers, and the terminals; the terminals also contain small, round vesicles believed to contain neurotransmitter chemicals. Synaptic connections from the fibers of other neurons cover the cell body and dendrites, and in many neurons the synapses on dendrites can be seen as little spines. The axon itself has no synapses on it except sometimes at its synaptic terminals, where other neuron axon terminals may form "synapses on synapses." From *The Brain: An Introduction to Neuro-science* by Richard F. Thompson. © 1985 by W. H. Freeman and Company. Used with permission.

of the symptoms of schizophrenia and attention deficit/hyperactivity disorder (ADHD). Too much dopamine impairs the cognitive ability to "gate" or filter out irrelevant information from the environment and to sustain attention to immediate tasks. It can cause the brain to become overwhelmed with excessive information, especially in schizophrenia. A reduction of dopamine-producing neurons in the substantia nigra region and nigrostriatal pathway of the basal ganglia has been implicated as a cause of the motor disorder in Parkinson's disease. As is the case with other neurotransmitters and hormones, too much or too little dopamine can lead to various neuropsychiatric disorders.

Acetylcholine plays an important role in the pathway between the hippo-campus and prefrontal cortex that regulates the formation, storage, and retrieval of certain types of memory. The loss of cholinergic neurons in these areas has been associated with the dementia that characterizes Alzheimer's and some other neurological diseases. A mood disorder such as depression mainly involves low levels of serotonin due to abnormalities in the way this neurotransmitter is taken up into the synaptic cleft, the space between two cells at their contact point. It may also be due to reduction in the number of neurons or receptors for serotonin, norepinephrine, or dopamine. Selective serotonin reuptake inhibitors (SSRIs) and other psychotropic drugs are designed to modulate synaptic uptake of the relevant neurotransmitters and restore them to normal levels. As with other mental disorders, the causes and effects of an abnormally functioning serotonin system in depression are distributed through several brain regions at cortical and subcortical levels. In this particular mood disorder, the most affected regions are the limbic system and prefrontal cortex.

Consider the main structural and functional features of the various regions and systems of the brain. Working from the bottom up, the brainstem and spinal cord control such functions as heartbeat, respiration, and reflexes. One important part of this region is the ascending reticular formation. This contains a number of neuron groups and fiber tracts that run the full length of the lower brainstem (medulla, pons, and midbrain). These groups modulate the activity of neurons throughout the central nervous system, carrying information to the cerebellum, hypothalamus, limbic system, and cerebral cortex. The neurons and fibers in the reticular formation are involved in regulating the sleep-wake cycle and levels of arousal while we are awake. The more active the reticular formation is, the more able we are to focus attention on events external to us. Destruction of or damage to the neurons and fibers in this structure results in coma, which I will discuss among other brain states in chapter 6.

The basal ganglia and cerebellum are located above the brainstem and co-ordinate movement by interpreting and coordinating sensory information from other areas of the brain. Neurodegeneration in these regions can cause impairment or loss of motor control, which occurs in Parkinson's disease. Hemorrhagic (too much blood caused by a ruptured artery) and ischemic (too little blood caused by a clot blocking an artery) strokes in these regions, as well as in the thalamus, can also result in motor and sensory deficits. Moreover, abnormal neuronal development in the basal ganglia, cerebellum, hippocampus, and frontal cortex has been identified as a cause of the cognitive, motor, and affective symptoms of schizophrenia. From its position above the brainstem, the thalamus filters information from the sensory organs. Located just below the thalamus on either side of the third ventricle is the hypothalamus, which plays a critical role in the control of such bodily functions as temperature, sex, thirst, and hunger. It is also a major player in the body's stress response, acting in concert with the pituitary gland, which is attached to it (fig. 2).

The highest and most recently evolved region of the brain is the cerebral cortex, which is divided into frontal, temporal, parietal, and occipital lobes in each of the cerebral hemispheres. The frontal lobes regulate conscious thought and executive functions such as planning and decision-making. They also regulate the mental properties associated with personality. A particular frontal region, the prefrontal cortex, is largely responsible for cognitive control. This consists in the

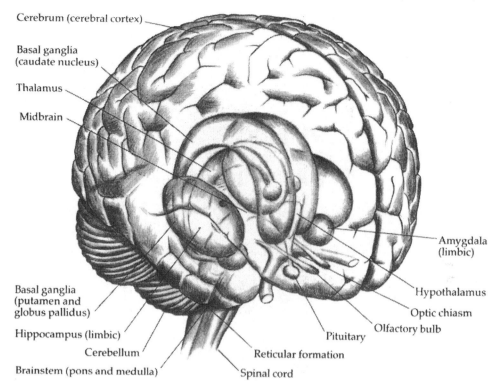

Cerebrum (cerebral cortex)

Basal ganglia
(caudate nucleus)

Thalamus

Midbrain

Amygdala
(limbic)

Basal ganglia
(putamen and
globus pallidus)

Hippocampus (limbic)

Cerebellum

Brainstem (pons and medulla)

Hypothalamus

Optic chiasm

Olfactory bulb

Pituitary

Reticular formation

Spinal cord

FIGURE 2. The human brain. Many structures are buried within the vast forebrain or cerebrum, covered by the cerebral cortex. Some of these in the forebrain are the basal ganglia (caudate, putamen, and globus pallidus), the thalamus, the hypothalamus, the midbrain, the brain stem (pons and medulla), and the cerebellum. The pituitary gland is just below the hypothalamus and connected to it, but the pineal gland is entirely outside the brain. Other structures shown include the partial crossing of the optic nerves from the eyes (optic chiasm) and the olfactory bulb. The spinal cord is the downward continuation of the nervous system from the brain. After W. J. H. Nauta and M. Feirtag, "The Organization of the Brain." In *The Brain* [a *Scientific American* book], San Francisco: W.H. Freeman and Company, 1979. *The Brain: An Introduction to Neuroscience* by Richard F. Thompson. © 1985 by W. H. Freeman and Company. Used with permission.

ability to coordinate thought and action in relation to short- and long-term goals. Various subsections of the prefrontal cortex collectively sustain our mental capacity to control our motivational states and behavior. The temporal lobe contains the primary auditory cortex and, in collaboration with the prefrontal cortex, is involved in learning and memory. The parietal lobes are located in the middle of the cortex. They regulate the processing of language, tactile information, and orientation to space and time, which is controlled by the somatosensory area. Just in front of this area is the motor (precentral) cortex, which controls movement. At the back of the brain, the occipital lobes contain the visual cortex, which initiates the processing of sensory information and regulates vision (fig. 3).

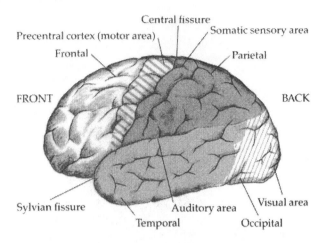

FIGURE 3. Major subdivisions of the cerebral cortex. The central fissure separates the frontal and parietal lobes or areas, and the Sylvian fissure separates the temporal lobe from the rest of the cortex. The occipital lobe is at the back end of the brain. After R. F. Thompson, *Introduction to Physiological Psychology*, New York: Harper & Row, 1975. *The Brain: An Introduction to Neuroscience* by Richard F. Thompson. © 1985 by W. H. Freeman and Company. Used with permission.

Perhaps the most significant feature of the brain is its *plasticity*.[2] This refers to the ability of nerve cells to modify their activity in response to changes in the brain, body, and external environment. The brain has the capacity to rewire itself in such a way as to allow intact regions to take over motor, cognitive, and other tasks ordinarily controlled by other regions that have become dysfunctional. This ensures that the functions critical to the survival of the organism are carried out. In this respect, the brain is the most adaptive organ in the human body. For example, in people who are blind because of damage to the visual cortex in the occipital lobe, the auditory cortex in the temporal lobe can play a greater role in regulating one's orientation in space. Furthermore, damage to the parietal lobe resulting from a stroke can impair one's linguistic ability. But new neuronal connections can form in the temporal and frontal lobes, enabling one to regain some language skills. In addition, lesions from infections such as bacterial meningitis or encephalitis, or from tumors, in the frontal lobe can impair one's ability to plan and make decisions. But new neuronal connections may form between other brain regions and the cerebellum. The new connections may enable the cerebellum to take over some of the task of mediating the cognitive and affective processing necessary for executive functions.

The limbic system controls much of the emotional processing in the brain. "Limbic" derives from the Latin word "limbus," which means "margin" or "rim." The limbic system is the rim of the cerebral cortex on the medial surface of the hemisphere that encircles the diencephalon. It consists of both cortical and subcortical structures, including the anterior and posterior cingulate gyri, amygdala, hippocampus, nucleus accumbens, and locus ceruleus. The anterior cingulate plays an important role in mediating cognitive and affective processing when we deliberate and make decisions. In a different set of functions, the nucleus accumbens regulates the dopamine reward system, dysregulation of which can lead to addictive behavior.

The most critical component of the limbic system is the amygdala, a subcortical structure located deep within the temporal lobe that regulates primitive emotions such as fear. The amygdala projects to the hypothalamus as well as to the frontal lobes. Through its interaction with the hypothalamus, the amygdala plays a crucial role in the stress response and in maintaining homeostasis. Through its interaction with the hippocampus, the amygdala regulates emotional memory. The amygdala can also influence planning, decision-making, and other cognitive functions by projecting to the prefrontal cortex. This last type of interaction is one example of the constant flow of information processing between different circuits in higher and lower regions of the brain. These systems regulate each other in virtue of a complex bidirectional network of feed-forward and feedback loops, ensuring that no system becomes dysregulated and that systemic balance is maintained within the brain (fig. 4).

It will be helpful to describe the body's response to external stimuli to clarify this point.[3] Information about stimuli reaches the amygdala by either of two sensory pathways. The sensory thalamus may send the information directly to the amygdala via a "low road" that elicits an emotional response to the stimulus. It bypasses the sensory cortex and occurs outside of our conscious awareness. Alternatively, the information may go from the sensory thalamus to the sensory cortex

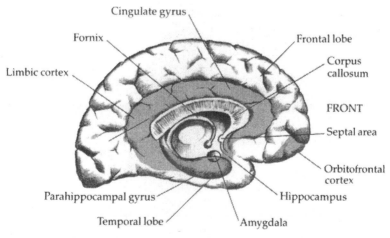

FIGURE 4. Limbic system. The view of the midline, or medial, wall of the brain. The major parts are the hippocampus and the amygdala, which are buried in the depths of the temporal lobe, the septal area, and several regions of cerebral cortex surrounding the corpus callosum: the cingulate gyrus, the parahippocampal gyrus, and the orbitofrontal cortex. The fornix is a large bundle of nerve fibers interconnecting portions of the limbic system (e.g., hippocampus and septal area). After E. R. Kandel and J. H. Schwartz, *Principles of Neural Science*, New York: Elsevier / North-Holland, 1981. *The Brain: An Introduction to Neuroscience* by Richard F. Thompson. © 1985 by W. H. Freeman and Company. Used with permission.

and then to the amygdala. This "high road" provides a more accurate representation of the stimulus to the brain.[4] The first pathway involves a quicker response to the stimulus, a feature of the organism's more primitive reaction to events that may pose a threat to its survival. Not all perceptions or beliefs along the second pathway and the high road of the sensory cortex are within our conscious awareness. Some of these mental states are unconscious and, together with unconscious emotional memories in the amygdala, enable us to have appropriate conditioned responses to threatening events. In this regard, unconscious mental states are more critical to our survival than conscious mental states. Beliefs and emotions become conscious only when they become part of our working memory.

What I have just described is central to the body's stress response. More accurately, there are two related stress responses. These involve two overlapping systems: the hypothalamic-pituitary-adrenal (HPA) system; and the sympathetic-adrenal-medulla (SAM) system. In a stress response characterized by fear, the amygdala activates the hypothalamus to secrete corticotropin-releasing factor (CRF), which then causes the pituitary to release adrenocorticotropin hormone (ACTH). This, in turn, causes the release of glucocorticoids, specifically cortisol, from the adrenal cortex. Cortisol influences the pituitary and the hypothalamus through positive feed-forward or negative feedback loops, causing the pituitary to increase or decrease further production of ACTH. This depends on the level of cortisol in the body. Ordinarily, when a stimulus is no longer perceived or experienced as a stressor or threat, cortisol production decreases, and the HPA system returns to its normal state.

A different pathway is activated in a stress response characterized by effort. The sympathetic arm of the autonomic nervous system signals the adrenal medulla to release adrenaline into the blood stream and to organs such as the heart and lungs to prepare the body for "fight or flight" against or from a threat. When this heightened sense of awareness has passed, the parasympathetic nervous system acts as a negative feedback mechanism stopping the release of adrenaline. While the HPA system is activated in fearful or threatening situations, the SAM system is activated in situations requiring effort. In fact, both systems are involved in the fight-or-flight response, since fear-inducing stimuli can initiate effort to confront or avoid an actual or perceived threat.

These regulatory mechanisms can become dysregulated in situations of chronic stress, constant fear, or trauma, when the body fails to shut off or reduce the flow of cortisol or adrenaline. If the stress response becomes chronic, excess cortisol can induce the locus ceruleus to release noradrenaline, which further activates the amygdala and hypothalamus to produce more CRF and prolong the stress response. Interacting systems in the brain and body that are designed to be part of an adaptive response to a threat become part of a maladaptive response to the environment. Some forms of major depression, general anxiety disorder, and post-traumatic stress disorder appear to have this general type of etiology. Hypersecretion of cortisol (in depression) and adrenaline (in PTSD and anxiety) can disrupt fear-regulating negative feedback loops in the brain. Excessive fear and other negative emotions become firmly embedded as unconscious memories in the amygdala. When triggered by a certain stimulus, these memories can repeatedly generate a heightened stress response that is out of proportion to the actual nature of external events. This process all too often results in the psychopathology that characterizes these psychiatric disorders.

A stress response gone awry can also have pathophysiological effects on endocrine, immune, and other systems in addition to the CNS. There is a delicate balance between and among stress-related hormones such as CRF, ACTH, cortisol, and adrenaline that is maintained by a complex regulatory network. Too much or too little of these hormones or of neurotransmitters can impair this regulation and balance and disrupt the normal interaction between the CNS and other systems of the body.[5] Both psychological and physiological aspects of the stress response can do this. For example, negative emotions such as fear or anxiety can disrupt the hypothalamus and its connection to the enteric nervous system in the gut, producing an excess of serotonin that can result in irritable bowel syndrome. These emotions can also trigger or increase the release of inflammatory cytokines from the immune system when the airway is exposed to an allergen in an asthmatic attack. Figure 5 illustrates how the mental disorder of depression can have adverse effects on multiple bodily systems.

The point of these examples is to show the importance of balanced mechanisms between cortical and subcortical regions of the brain, and the adaptive role these mechanisms play in maintaining homeostasis and the health and survival of human organisms. Equally important, these examples also show how systems outside the brain can modulate the mechanisms of the central nervous system in ways that can alter our mental states. The discussion of surgical, pharmacological, and other interventions to treat mental disorders or enhance normal mental functions in chapters 4 and 5 will require asking how these interventions might affect regulatory mechanisms and the systemic balance within the brain and body. Although altering "soft-wired" neural circuits in the cortex can directly affect the conscious mental states that make us persons, altering "hard-wired" neural circuits in subcortical areas can affect unconscious emotions and beliefs figuring in fear and other conditioned responses that are necessary for our survival as organisms. Because subcortical circuits are more fundamental to survival than cortical circuits, and because the first type function outside of our conscious awareness and control, there are strong medical and ethical reasons to be particularly cautious when intervening in these areas of the brain.

Still, conscious and unconscious states of mind are interacting and mutually influencing. This is because of the interaction between the higher and lower brain systems that underlie these mental states. Altering mental states at one level by altering the corresponding systems in the brain can positively or negatively affect mental states at the other level, and vice versa. The bidirectional pathway between the prefrontal cortex and the limbic system is especially significant for the ethical implications of the measures of and interventions in the brain that I will discuss in the next four chapters. The interaction of these brain regions forms much of the neurobiological underpinning of our beliefs, emotions, intentions, decisions, and actions.

Although I have mentioned different aspects of the mind, I have not yet given an adequate account of the mind. Nor have I given an adequate account of the

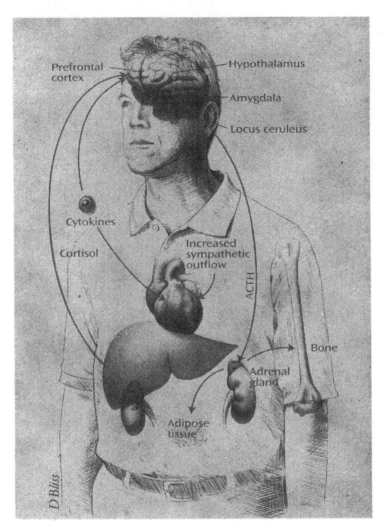

FIGURE 5. Depression: a disease of the mind, brain, and body. "Depression is one of the most prevalent diseases in the world today. Ten percent of the U.S. adult population suffers with the illness every year, with many persons receiving either no or inadequate treatment. Psychiatrists know depression is an illness that affects the mind and mood of a sufferer, altering that person's core experience of others and the world around them. But now, research convincingly shows that significant morbidity and mortality are associated with the primary manifestations of depression beyond that occasioned by the disturbed effect. Patients with major depression have a doubling of mortality at any age, independent of suicide, smoking, or other risk factors for poor health. There is emerging evidence that depression patients have a significant loss of cells in the prefrontal cortex, a brain area important in discerning reward versus punishment, in shifting mood from one state to another, and in exerting cortical restraint on the amygdala fear system through the hypothalamic-pituitary-adrenal (HPA) axis and the sympathetic nervous system. An increase in cortisol and nor-epinephrine secretion represents a highly adverse biochemical environment, a condition that is likely to contribute to many different adverse outcomes, including increased visceral

relationship between the mind and the brain. Since the principal ethical concern about neuroimaging and surgical or pharmacological intervention in the brain is how these techniques can affect the mind, we need a more detailed description of what the mind is and of the mind's connection to the brain. My aim is not to try to defend a single "correct" theory of mind with "knockdown" philosophical arguments, but instead to present a plausible account of mind that is consistent with the findings of the clinical neurosciences.

An Account of Mind

The mind consists of conscious beliefs, desires, feelings, and intentions. It also consists of unconscious beliefs and emotions, such as fear, that are involved in our conditioned responses to external events and other stimuli. These mental states and their associated properties emerge when the brain reaches a certain level of complexity. Properties of the mind are qualitatively distinct from properties of the brain, since by definition emergent properties are not possessed by their component parts. Because emergence is a process, the mind should also be characterized as a process, or a set of properties, rather than a thing. As noted in chapter 1, the mind is not reducible to the brain because the intentionality of the mind is not solely a property of neurons and other physical features of the brain. "Intentionality" refers to the directedness of beliefs and other mental states to the body and the environment. It is the process through which the mind represents the body and environment to the brain and the organism as a whole. While the brain itself cannot have beliefs or other mental states, our capacity to have mental states necessarily depends on functions of interacting subcortical and cortical regions. Our mental states contribute to the plasticity of the brain and to the patterns of relatedness in the holistic interaction between human organisms and the external environment.

It is important to emphasize that the mind and brain are not distinct and independent substances. Rather, they are higher level and lower level aspects of a single entity, a human organism. Mind and brain collaborate to maintain equilibrium between bodily systems and thereby enhance the ability of the organism to survive. The mind represents events in the external environment to the body and

---

fat, insulin resistance, increased inflammation, enhanced blood coagulation, deficient fibrinolysis, decreased bone formation, and increased bone resorption. These changes support the concept of depression as a systemic disease that may have primary medical manifestations. Moreover, depression has adverse effects on comorbid medical diagnosis as well, such as coronary artery disease, diabetes, and osteoporosis. Indeed, emerging data have shown that prospective treatment of depression in patients who have experienced myocardial infarction increases chances of a good medical outcome and survival. Thus, detection of depression in all ill persons is critical, and the pursuit of new and more effective treatments for depression will increase psychological, psychiatric, and medical health worldwide." —Philip W. Gold and Dennis S. Charney, *Diseases of the Mind and Brain: Depression: A Disease of the Mind, Brain, and Body, Am J Psychiatry,* Nov 2002; 159: 1826. Reprinted with permission from the *American Journal of Psychiatry* (Copyright 2002). American Psychiatric Association.

brain as something with which the organism is fully engaged. This cannot be done by neurons, synapses, and neurotransmitters alone but through the coordinated activity of lower-level neural networks and higher-level mental states. In this regard, the mind functions as a more highly refined sensory-processing system than the subcortical and cortical brain systems from which it emerges. The mind enables the organism to distinguish benign, advantageous, and threatening events and to make them meaningful to it. While the brain generates and sustains the mind, the mind influences the brain and body in its role as a sensory processing system. The earlier descriptions of adaptive and maladaptive stress responses are an illustration of this fact.

We may gain a better understanding of the relation between the brain and the mind by thinking of it as analogous in some respects to the relation between the innate and adaptive arms of the human immune system.[6] Innate immunity is biologically older and more primitive than adaptive immunity. As the body's first line of defense against pathogens, the innate arm becomes fully mobilized when presented with any antigenic stimulus and requires no prior acquaintance with it. The adaptive arm works together with the innate arm to recognize and eliminate pathogens from the body. Adaptive immunity has emerged over time as a more specific response to an antigenic stimulus, given its capacity to develop a memory of that stimulus. Adaptive immunity is divided into two components, the cellular response and the humoral response. The first involves sensitized T cells that react to cells infected by an invader, while the second involves the production of antibodies in response to a specific antigen. Interconnected immune functions work in concert through finely tuned checks and balances to mount a defense against pathogens. These mechanisms help to maintain appropriate cellular and humoral responses to threatening microorganisms. A hyperactive response from either of these branches can disrupt the critical mechanisms and result in autoimmune disease. Regulatory T cells are particularly important in maintaining this balance. Helper T cells arouse killer T cells to fight pathogens. Regulatory T cells suppress or limit the activity of killer T cells if they threaten to spiral out of control and destroy the body's own tissues.

The mind is to the brain as adaptive immunity is to innate immunity. Our mental states have emerged from the cerebral cortex as a more specific response to external stimuli than the more basic response of the subcortical brain. At a more primitive level, just as an inadequate innate immune response to a pathogen can lead to a fatal infection, an inadequate response from the thalamus-amygdala pathway to an external threat can result in the demise of the organism. At a more advanced level, just as dysregulated killer T cells of the adaptive immune system can destroy the body's own tissues, a dysregulated set of beliefs and emotions can disrupt the HPA axis and result in destructive physiological and psychological responses. The adaptive immune system is the body's refined internal sensory system; the mind is the body's refined external sensory system. Beliefs ordinarily function like regulatory T cells in ensuring that the brain and body do not over-react to stimuli. When beliefs fail to do this and instead represent benign stimuli as threats to the brain and body, they can disrupt normal functions in the central nervous and other systems. An essential function of the mind that is designed to be

adaptive in responding to stimuli can become maladaptive and lead to physiological and psychological disorders.

In fact, the mind and immune system can interact with the central nervous
and endocrine systems in ways that can influence the functions of the entire
organism. The idea that all of these systems interact, and that altering one system
can alter the others, is the principle behind the field of psychoneuroimmunology.[7]
In the next section, I will explain how activation of certain immune molecules can
alter the CNS and consequently the nature and content of one's mental state.
Before doing that, however, let's first assess the plausibility of the emergent account
of mind against some alternative accounts.

According to substance dualism, mind and body are ontologically distinct
immaterial and material substances. The most prominent exponent of this theory,
René Descartes, claimed that although mind and body causally interact through
the pineal gland in the brain, the relation between the mind and the body/brain is
contingent rather than necessary. It is possible for the mind to exist and function
independently of the brain and body.[8] But any plausible account of the mind holds
that mental states are necessarily generated and sustained by the brain, and substance dualism cannot explain how mental states can exist independently of the
brain. Nor does Descartes explain how the pineal gland mediates mind–brain
interaction. In the 1970s, philosopher of science Karl Popper and neurophysiologist
John Eccles proposed a different version of dualist interactionism.[9] They argued
that the nonphysical mind could influence the physical brain through finely balanced interactions taking place at synapses. But they offered no satisfactory explanation of how this interaction might work.

Few philosophers and even fewer neuroscientists accept substance dualism.
Instead, some defend reductive materialism. This theory says that consciousness
and other forms of mentality are not simply caused by neural processes or states.
Mental states *just are* neural states.[10] This strong form of materialism is reductive
because it says that the nature and content of mental states can be explained
entirely in terms of the material structures and functions of the brain. Some would
go so far as to say that this theory explains away all mental phenomena.

The content of our mental states involves features of the social and natural
environment to which these states are directed. Moreover, the brain functions that
generate and sustain states of mind can change in response to the external world,
given the property of plasticity and the holistic interaction between the organism
and the environment. For these reasons, it is questionable whether the mind could
be explained entirely in terms of the physical features of the brain. It is also questionable whether the first-person subjective phenomenology of experience could be
captured by third-person objective physical explanations of brain structure and
function alone. The qualitative experience of pain underscores the inadequacy of
reductive materialism. There is something it is *like* to feel pain that cannot be
explained entirely in terms of neurobiology. Neuropsychiatrist Todd Feinberg explains this phenomenon as follows: "From the outside, we cannot ultimately reduce
the experience of 'pain' to the neural state that creates it because there is nothing
material from the outside perspective to reduce.... Our visions, our minds, our
pains, are personal and have no material existence for anyone but ourselves."[11]

Similarly, the feeling of being depressed cannot be captured by explaining the condition in terms of synapses, neurotransmitters, and receptors in certain types of neurons. The mind is not reducible to the brain because appeal to the brain itself cannot entirely explain these external and internal features of the mind.

This position seems to introduce another version of dualism: property dualism. The distinction is not between mental and physical substances, but between mental and physical properties related contingently rather than necessarily. It still leaves us with the problem of explaining how the mind can interact with the brain if it is ontologically distinct from it. The nonreducibility of the mental to the physical appears to entail epiphenomenalism, the view that the physical can causally affect the mental, but not the other way around. The upshot of this view is that the mind plays no causal role in our behavior. Philosopher Jaegwon Kim spells out the problem of the explanatory exclusion of the mental: "If mental properties are physically irreducible and remain outside the physical domain, then, given that the physical domain is causally closed, how can they exercise causal powers, or enjoy any kind of causal relevance, in the physical domain?"[12]

The theory most often invoked to solve this problem is supervenience, which holds that there is a one-way dependency relation of higher level mental properties on lower level physical properties. Every mental property has a physical base in the brain that guarantees its instantiation. If a person experiences pain, then the mental property of having this experience is an instantiation of some underlying physical property in the brain and nervous system that regulate it.[13] But there are at least two problems with supervenience. It is too general a theory to explain the complexity behind the emergence of mental properties and mental states from integrated physical systems in the brain. In addition, supervenience fails to acknowledge that there is a two-way dependency relation of mind on brain and brain on mind. Both criticisms are important for understanding the neural correlates of normal and abnormal states of mind. They are also important for understanding how different interventions in the brain can influence and alter our cognitive, affective, and volitional states.

The conscious mental state of fear, for example, is often generated by the perception of an event or environmental cue as a stressor. Belief and fear emerge from the activity of populations of neurons in many different brain regions. Whether and to what extent these neurons are activated is regulated by feedback loops between the sensory thalamus and the amygdala, on one level, and the sensory cortex and the amygdala, on another level. Furthermore, the phenomenological quality of these mental states depends partly on the activity of neural pathways connecting the hippocampus, brainstem, and hypothalamus.[14] In addition, the decision to perform a certain bodily movement on the basis of belief and fear depends on the coordinated neural activity of the parietal cortex, prefrontal cortex, and cerebellum. All of these brain regions underlie the mental process that extends from the initial sensory perception to action. This suggests that there is no one-to-one causal relation between a particular brain state or event and a particular mental state or event. There are no neuron-by-neuron catalogues that directly relate the first type of state or event to the second. Instead, mental states and events emerge from a process involving multiple neuronal pathways that interact in cortical and subcortical regions of the brain. To invoke supervenience and claim that every mental property depends on a physical base in the brain that guarantees its instantiation fails to capture all of the components of this process. One might claim that mental states are supervenient on widely distributed neural networks. But this would not offer a very helpful model of how these networks interact. Nor would such a claim acknowledge the interdependence of brain and mind and the influence of the environment on the brain-mind relation.

Most theories of mind tend to locate the physical basis of the mind in the cerebral cortex. Yet the model I have presented indicates that the physical basis of the mind is not localized in this one brain region but is distributed through many brain regions. Localized views rest on cognitive science models of the mind. As neuroscientist Joseph LeDoux points out, these models are inadequate because they leave emotion and conation (desire, motivation, volition) out of their account of the human mind.[15] By focusing on the cerebral cortex, they largely ignore limbic structures, the cerebellum, and other systems that interact with the cortex in sustaining a tripartite set of cognitive, affective, and conative capacities. Cognitive science models also pay insufficient attention to an important feature of brain plasticity. Each person's brain and mental states are unique because no two people's brains, and no two organisms, respond to the environment in the same way.

On the account of mind that I am defending, mental states emerge as higher level properties from lower level physical properties in the brain. In addition to these physical properties, the emergence of mental states depends on interaction between the organism and the environment. It is in virtue of this holistic loop that we are able to construct the self, to make ourselves in our own image.

A particular version of emergentism provides the most accurate explanation of the relation between the brain and the mind. To borrow Todd Feinberg's terminology, there are two distinct types of hierarchy that can explain how mentality emerges from the brain: nested and nonnested. In a *nonnested hierarchy*, although successive levels of physical properties in the brain causally interact, each emerging level becomes independent of the others. Once it emerges at the top of the hierarchy, the mind becomes independent of the lower physical levels that generated it.[16] This nonnested account can be called "emergent dualism." It holds that, beyond a certain point of complexity in the brain, mental properties become independent of the physical properties from which they emerge. In a *nested hierarchy*, the properties associated with lower physical levels in the brain are intertwined with, or nested within, the properties associated with the higher emergent mental level. By holding that higher level and lower level properties are interdependent, the nested hierarchy version of emergentism avoids the main problem with property dualism.[17] It does not have to explain how mental properties can be self-sustaining and can interact with physical properties of the brain if they are only contingently related to and conceptually independent from them. Because the nested hierarchy view considers mental properties and brain properties to be interdependent aspects of a single entity, it can be called "emergent monism."

This position is consistent with what philosopher John Searle calls "biological naturalism."[18] The conscious and unconscious beliefs, desires, and emotions that constitute the mind are in certain respects biological phenomena. Yet in other respects they have subjective features that resist a reductive explanation in terms of physical features of the brain. The mind is an emergent feature of the brain in the same way that digestion is an emergent feature of the stomach, or that liquidity is an emergent feature of the system of molecules that constitutes our blood. Mind and brain are not independent entities, but two interdependent aspects of one biological system. There is both brain–mind and mind–brain causality. The biological system at issue is the human organism, which is situated within and is in constant interaction with the external environment.

A critical notion in the nested hierarchy account of mind is *constraint*. As Feinberg defines it, constraint refers to the control a higher level of a hierarchy exerts over a lower level of a hierarchy. Following Feinberg, we can explain mental constraint of brain systems by thinking of the mind and brain as analogous to higher level and lower level properties of the human lung. At a higher level, the lung displays emergent features not possessed by and thus not reducible to the mitochondria in its cells. If the lung did not breathe, the body would not have oxygen, and if it did not have oxygen, the mitochondria would not be able to carry on cellular respiration. "In this manner, the higher-level property of breathing constrains the activity of the mitochondria. When the system is considered as a whole, the mitochondria contribute to the emergence of the lung. And the lung in turn constrains the mitochondria."[19]

Similarly, the higher level properties of the mind constrain the lower level properties of the brain and central nervous system. Mental states like beliefs and emotions are adaptive when they enable the organism to discriminate between threatening and benign stimuli by processing sensory information accurately and efficiently. When this occurs, the mind constrains brain and bodily systems so that they are neither over- nor understimulated in response to external events. In particular, beliefs that accurately represent events to the organism enable the cortex to constrain the amygdala fear system through the HPA axis and the sympathetic nervous system. At the same time, the neural correlates of our mental states are adaptive when they modulate these states in virtue of their normal biological function. In this way, the brain ensures that the mind accurately represents the external world to the organism. When the relevant neural correlates become dysregulated, they can lead to delusions, hallucinations, excessive fear, or other pathological mental states that are out of line with actual states of affairs. Dysfunctional neurological and psychological states can become maladaptive and result in neuropsychiatric and physical diseases. Another example of how the mind might constrain the brain is the use of functional magnetic imaging to control chronic pain. In one study, patients with chronic pain were asked to try to increase and decrease their pain while watching images showing activation of the areas of the brain involved in pain perception. The idea was that the response by patients to the images in terms of their thoughts might modulate their experience of pain. If effective, this type of experiment could demonstrate that one's mental states could influence the brain and thereby reduce pain.[20]

Unlike supervenience, constraint in a nested hierarchy model of mind operates in two directions: from mind to brain, and from brain to mind. This extends Feinberg's definition to include both higher and lower levels of activity. The bidirectional property of constraint is an adaptive property because it promotes the health and survival of the organism by promoting systemic balance between the mind and the body. A causal explanation of how mind and brain interact should be framed by a more general teleological explanation of why this interaction serves the needs of the organism as a whole.

Although the brain is the main biological source of the mind, it is not the only biological source. I have described how certain abnormal endocrine functions can adversely affect the brain and result in pathological states of mind. In some of these cases, certain functions of the immune system can play an equally deleterious role. We need to give a more detailed analysis of how endocrine and immune systems interact with the central nervous system and in turn influence the mind. I will analyze these interactions with a view to considering how intervening in these systems may benefit or harm us.

Why We Are Not Just Our Brains

Who we are as persons is determined by the nature and content of our mental states. The fact that these states necessarily depend on the brain explains why mapping or manipulating the brain can have such far-reaching metaphysical and ethical implications. Regarding the question of the biological basis of our psychological properties, the brain is often contrasted with genes. Some Mendelian high-penetrance single-gene diseases directly affect brain function and cause severe neurological disorders with devastating physical and psychological symptoms. Penetrance refers to the probability of a gene or genetic mutation manifesting in particular phenotypic traits associated with disease or behavior. One recent study has suggested that psychopathic traits in children are due largely to a genetic component.[21] But genetic penetrance is highly variable. Generally, genes do not determine but only shape the broad outline of one's thought and behavior. There is a genetic component in schizophrenia and some forms of depression; but genes are not the only causal factor in the development of these disorders. Genes are just one component of complex casual pathways that underlie normal and abnormal states of mind.

How genes affect the neural mechanisms underlying our behavioral traits depends on how genes are influenced by other internal biological factors and the external environment. These epigenetic factors can influence whether or to what extent genes are expressed, how genes shape brain structure and function, and how they shape mental traits.[22] Our brains are more directly involved in regulating our thought and behavior than our genes. Some would say that we are not our genes. But we *are* our brains. LeDoux expresses this view in saying that "the essence of who we are is encoded in our brains."[23] Yet this account is misleading and inaccurate because it ignores the respects in which bodily systems other than the CNS can influence our mental states. The biological basis of our mental states involves more than just our brains. Four examples support this claim.

First, chronic hypersecretion of cortisol from the adrenal cortex may lead to degeneration of neurons in the hippocampus.[24] This is one region of the brain playing a critical role in episodic and possibly other forms of memory, which can be described roughly as an unconscious or conscious belief about the past.[25]

Specifically, the hippocampus is involved in the encoding, storage, and retrieval of episodic memory of events that we have experienced. Unlike other types of memory, episodic memory has a subjective, autobiographical quality.[26] Through what is known as consolidation, immediate or short-term memories are converted into more enduring long-term memories. This is made possible by the process of long-term potentiation (LTP), where repeated stimulation of sets of neurons strengthens communication across synapses. A reduction in hippocampal neurons can result in the gradual erosion of episodic memory. In some respects, this effect is similar to the retrograde amnesia caused by damage to the hippocampus and other regions of the medial temporal lobes that regulate memory. Retrograde amnesia is characterized by an inability to recall memories of experiences, facts, or events. It is distinct from anterograde amnesia, which is characterized by an inability to form new memories.

For many philosophers, personal identity is defined in terms of continuity of psychological properties.[27] These properties include the capacity to be consciously aware of oneself in the present, to recall the past, and to anticipate the future. One persists through time as the same individual in virtue of these and other psychological relations. Because the capacity to remember past experience is a necessary component of psychological continuity, loss of episodic memory can disrupt these psychological relations and therefore disrupt one's experience of persisting through time. Increased cortisol over time might also result in loss of neurons in the prefrontal cortex, which regulates reasoning and other aspects of agency that we associate with personhood. A hormone secreted by the adrenal glands, a source outside the brain, can have deleterious effects on regions of the brain that ground mental states that are critical to personhood and personal identity.

Second, infectious agents such as viruses and psychological stress can activate the immune system and cause it to release cytokines. These are molecules that function as messengers of the immune system and are secreted by lymphoid cells in response to stimulation. Cytokines generally are immunomodulatory in the sense that they amplify some immune responses and inhibit others. Inflammatory cytokines such as interleukin 1 (IL-1), interleukin 6 (IL-6), and tumor necrosis factor-alpha (TNFα) secreted in response to infection or stress can penetrate the blood–brain barrier. They may also be released by neurons. This class of cytokines can disrupt the HPA axis, leading to dysregulation of the inhibitory mechanisms involving CRF, ACTH, and cortisol that maintain the balance between interacting nervous and endocrine systems.[28]

The relationship between psychological stress, hormones, and cytokine activation is complex and not fully understood. Yet some studies have shown a correlation between high levels of inflammatory cytokines and low levels of neurotransmitters such as serotonin and dopamine in some regions of the brain. These studies suggest that cytokines can be psychoactive and may be implicated in some psychiatric disorders.[29] Cytokines activated in response to infections can result in psychopathological symptoms similar to those associated with cytokines activated in response to stress-related psychiatric disorders. They can induce a syndrome of what Hans Selye and others have called "sickness behavior," which includes symptoms of anhedonia, fatigue, disruption of sleep-wake cycles, and cognitive dysfunction. In animal models, blocking these cytokines has diminished or eliminated symptoms of sickness behavior induced by infection or cytokine administration.[30] In humans, these symptoms may be adaptive if, by forcing the body to rest, they both enable the immune system to neutralize the pathogen causing the infection and allow bodily systems to regain homeostasis. But it is unclear how such symptoms could be adaptive if they persist for too long and become pathological, as in many cases of major depression.[31]

Third, autoimmunity may also play a role in psychiatric disorders. The immune system can release autoantibodies in response to an infection. These can alter the function of melanocortin peptides, which carry messages between nerve cells in the brain and regulate the neurological bases of appetite control and the stress response. Anorexia nervosa and bulimia are two psychiatric disorders that have been associated with these immune mechanisms.[32] The general upshot is that a certain class of cytokines, and possibly also autoantibodies, can have a negative effect on cognition, mood, and volition. In this respect, the immune system can influence the nature and content of some of the mental states that make us the persons we are.

A fourth example of how systems outside the brain can influence the brain and our mental states is the effect of adrenaline on unconscious emotional memory. Adrenaline is secreted by the adrenal medulla and promotes consolidation of memories of fearful events in the amygdala. This is an adaptive mechanism when it enables us to form a memory of a threatening event and to avoid or respond appropriately to events like it in the future. But hypersecretion of adrenaline in response to a traumatic event can lead to the consolidation of memories that can cause dysregulation of our normal response to fear-inducing stimuli. This can result in the heightened maladaptive fear response characteristic of PTSD. In this type of psychopathology, fear dominates one's emotional life and can adversely affect the content of one's desires, beliefs, intentions, and emotions in addition to fear. It can also adversely affect the emotional content of one's episodic memories.

The four examples I have presented involve maladaptive responses of systems outside the CNS that can adversely affect the mind and result in different types of psychopathology. They are all instances of interaction among body, brain, and mind. This is not to suggest that endocrine and immune systems have only negative effects on the central nervous system, brain, and the mental states they generate and sustain. Psychopathology occurs only when these systems are not functioning properly. Most of the time, the normal functioning of endocrine and immune systems modulates normal brain and body functions in an adaptive way that promotes the health and survival of the organism. Normal brain and mental functions presuppose normal functions of these other systems. Learning and memory, for example, depend on hormones circulating throughout the body and brain. It is not just direct surgical or pharmacological interventions in the central nervous system that can affect the brain and the mind. Interventions in the endocrine and immune systems can also modulate brain functions and mental capacities in both beneficial and harmful ways and therefore can have significant neuroethical implications.

The Self

According to the *Oxford English Dictionary*, a "person" is a "self-conscious or rational being." It defines "consciousness" as the property of being "awake and aware of one's surroundings and identity." These definitions are similar to the one given by the contemporary philosopher Derek Parfit, who says that "to be a person, a being must be self-conscious, aware of its identity and continued existence over time."[33] The last part of this definition refers not only to the synchronic concept of personhood but also to the diachronic concept of personal identity. It is traceable to the seventeenth-century British philosopher John Locke. Some philosophers use "personal identity" and "self" interchangeably. Others distinguish these two concepts. Those who draw the distinction describe personal identity in terms of a unity relation among psychological properties, and the self in terms of a broader range of psychological and physical properties. The self consists not only of conscious awareness of one's persistence through time but also the phenomenological experience of agency and embodiment. Personhood and personal identity are components of the self, which is a richer and more complex notion.

The Western concept of the self can be traced to Hellenistic philosophy, wherein the Stoics refined the Platonic term for "imagination" (*phantasia*) to mean a collection of individual imaginations (*phantasiai*). Stoic philosophers tried to explain how individuals could recognize multiple experiences as their *own* and form a concept of an inner subjective unity. The concept of the self developed further through modern philosophy, and has become most commonly understood in terms of the first-person perspective of a thinking subject. For Descartes, in particular, the first-person perspective of the self characterized the subjective experience of mental states as private and not publicly accessible. Generally, neuropsychiatric disorders can be described as conditions that adversely affect the phenomenological quality of this first-person experience and disturb or disrupt the integrity of the self.[34]

I will adopt the second, richer, concept of the self. This requires an account of how the psychological capacities that constitute our selves correlate with neuronal mechanisms in the brain. As part of this account, I will show how abnormalities in these mechanisms can result in neuropsychiatric disorders that can disturb, disrupt, or shatter the self. Although the self can be characterized as a psychoneuroimmunological concept consisting of integrated properties of the mind, brain, and body, brain dysfunction alone can undermine the integrity of the self. I will also consider how interventions in the brains of individuals with these disorders can alter or restore the self, and whether this should be the purpose of these interventions.

Ramachandran maintains that there are four defining characteristics of the self.[35] These four characteristics all involve first-person conscious awareness. First, we have a sense of continuity, of persisting through time from the present to the future. Second, we have a sense of coherence or unity. In Ramachandran's words, "in spite of the diversity of sensory experiences, memories, beliefs and thoughts, you experience yourself as one person, as a unity."[36] Third is a sense of embodiment, an awareness of oneself as anchored to one's body. Fourth is a sense of agency, of free will, the sense of being in control of one's behavior and one's destiny.

Antonio Damasio offers a more complex concept of the self, a hierarchical model that has both nonconscious and conscious levels.[37] At the most fundamental level is the "proto self," consisting of systems in the hypothalamus and brainstem that represent the state of the organism and are critical to maintaining homeostasis. At a higher level is the "core self," consisting of systems in the cingulate gyrus and thalamus that are necessary for basic consciousness in the here-and-now. At the highest level is the "autobiographical self," which involves what Damasio calls "extended consciousness" and emerges from systems in the hippocampus and areas of the cortex. Here the notion of the self extends from the remembered past to the anticipated future. Although the proto self and core self are necessary for the emergence of the autobiographical self, only this last level aligns with Ramachandran's model and our commonsense intuitions about the self.

Ramachandran's model is incomplete because it leaves out a critical fifth component of the self: the ability to perceive and respond appropriately to the external world. Many of our conscious mental states are outwardly directed and include the awareness of being situated in the social and natural environment. Events in the external environment figure in the content of one's mental states, which represent these events to the brain and organism and make them meaningful to one. The brain, the body, and the external context constitute a tripartite reality that shapes the human organism and the self. So we should conceive of the self as consisting of five components: unity; continuity; embodiment; agency; and relatedness to the external world.

Our understanding of the self as a feature of the human mind has come largely through ascertaining that dysfunction in certain regions of the brain can cause different types of psychopathology. Imaging and other techniques enable us to map the neural correlates of both normal and abnormal mental states. Damasio explains how amnesic and agnosia (inability to recognize objects by use of the senses) syndromes are disorders of extended consciousness that can disrupt the autobiographical self by disrupting psychological unity and continuity.[38] Retrograde amnesia is perhaps the most devastating neurological disorder for the self because of its effects on the episodic memory linking our awareness of the present with our awareness of the past.

Ramachandran describes an even more intriguing array of neurological disorders. For example, in Capgras syndrome, individuals may identify a family member or close friend as an impostor pretending to be the real person. This is probably due to dysfunction in the pathway between the limbic system regulating emotion and the prefrontal cortex regulating cognition, as well as dysfunction in the pathway connecting the visual cortex with the limbic system. An individual with Capgras perceives the known person but fails to identify the person as who he or she really is because the individual's perception lacks the emotional hue ordinarily associated with it.[39]

Schizophrenia also involves brain dysfunction that interferes with the ability to respond appropriately to the natural and social environment. This disorder involves abnormalities in dopamine and serotonin neurotransmitter systems. In full-blown schizophrenia, delusions and hallucinations are associated with dysfunction in the prefrontal cortex, hippocampus, and basal ganglia, due to the abnormal development of gray matter in these regions. When the normal neural networks underlying cognition are severely disrupted, the schizophrenic cannot tell the difference between his or her own internally generated images and images from the external world.

Although the neural mechanisms are still not completely understood, the inability or difficulty of many autistic individuals to communicate and interact with others may be traceable to abnormalities in pathways between the limbic area and the prefrontal cortex. The symptoms manifest in varying degrees, but a general disconnection between cognition and emotion seems to lie behind autism. This is similar in some respects to what occurs in Capgras. Postmortem studies of the brains of individuals with autism have shown a decreased number of neurons in limbic regions such as the amygdala, hippocampus, and anterior cingulate.[40] Autism may also involve dysfunctional mirror neuron systems. These systems fire in response to chains of actions linked to intentions. They are distributed through the premotor cortex, posterior parietal lobe, superior temporal sulcus, and insula. Mirror neurons regulate the ability to understand others' intentions and to grasp the social meaning of their behavior. This occurs through direct simulation rather than through cognition.[41] Like schizophrenia, autism involves abnormalities in dopamine and serotonin systems and probably arises from mutations in multiple genes.

But autism is unique in several respects. In addition to their difficulty in understanding another person's perspective, some individuals with autism have impaired concept formation and inferential reasoning. They can focus on the details of parts but not on the general patterns of wholes. Although this may be described as a type of psychopathology, the ability to see parts or details normally denied to conscious awareness could also explain some forms of genius. Autistic disorders fall along a neuropsychiatric spectrum that may include severe mental impairment at one end and creative genius at the other.[42]

Asperger's syndrome is an autistic spectrum disorder (ASD) notable for discrepancy between cognitive abilities and affective disabilities in people. This combination makes the syndrome appear to be the opposite of Williams-Beuren syndrome, another neurodevelopmental disorder in which individuals are excessively social but typically have cognitive retardation. Asperger's may also involve discrepancy between a cognitive ability and a cognitive disability in the same person. Some mental traits may fall on the high-function end of the spectrum, while others may fall on the low-function end. For someone with an extraordinary cognitive trait, a diagnosis of Asperger's might not be considered a disability. On the contrary, one might consider it an intellectual gift.

It is believed that the Indian mathematician Srinivasa Ramanujan (1887–1920) and the Austrian philosopher Ludwig Wittgenstein (1889–1951) had some form of ASD. Temple Grandin is arguably the world's most accomplished and well-known adult with autism. Currently a professor of animal science at Colorado State University, she has authored numerous articles in scientific journals and livestock periodicals, as well as several books. She is a noted designer of livestock handling facilities. Those who would point out that these individuals have had a cognitive or affective disability would have to acknowledge that someone with a negative mental trait or traits has contributed greatly to mathematics, philosophy, and animal welfare. The three gifted individuals I have mentioned may not be as rare as one might think. It is estimated that the incidence of savant ability in children with autism may be as high as 10 percent. In the United States, autistic spectrum disorders may affect as many as 2–6 per 1,000 children.

These are examples of "neurodiversity," which recognizes that many people have a mix of neurological abilities and disabilities and celebrates differences in people's neurological traits. Nevertheless, in ASD and the other neurological and psychiatric disorders I have described, there is an abnormal relation between the subject and the external world. It is caused by dysfunction in the brain's ability to interpret the physical and social environment. This abnormality can alter or preclude the unity and integrity of the self, given that external events influence the content of the psychological properties that constitute the self. Although moderate forms of ASD may involve unique mental ability, people with this condition may have increasing difficulty in life as they age and social interactions become more complicated. Psychotherapeutic and pharmacological interventions have been used to try to raise abnormal components of the self in autism to normal functioning. Intensive interventions early in life have been effective in mild to moderate forms of autism. Overall, though, treatment has not been very effective in ameliorating the symptoms of moderately severe to severe forms of ASD.

Unlike psychiatric or neurological disorders such as schizophrenia or Alzheimer's, autistic spectrum disorders affect people from an early age. For people with schizophrenia or Alzheimer's, there is a disruption of the unity and continuity of mental states before and after the onset of symptoms. In this regard, there is a fracturing of the self. In contrast, autistic spectrum and other early-onset neurodevelopmental conditions do not involve a fractured or disrupted self. They consist of a cluster of psychological properties that fall outside the range of what many would consider normal mental functioning and a normal self.

The relevant comparison is not between different earlier and later phases of a person's psychological life, as in schizophrenia. Rather, the relevant comparison is between the mental life of someone with Asperger's, for instance, and someone whose mental life meets the five conditions of selfhood. In schizophrenia, the onset of cognitive and affective symptoms causes a disruption of both the unity and continuity of psychological properties. It is in this sense that the condition causes a fractured self. With autism, when the psychological properties associated with moderate forms of the disorder are present from an early age, and when these properties do not change substantially over time, the condition could meet most of Ramachandran's criteria of selfhood. In severe forms of the disorder, however, the symptoms would preclude meeting several or more of these criteria.

These considerations raise the question of what constitutes normal mental functioning. Very generally, we should say that normal mental functioning consists in the cognitive and affective capacity to interact with others and to perform ordinary tasks of daily life. Mental capacities fall along a spectrum that extends from normal to pathological. Many people have a combination of mental ability and disability. Some have a combination of exceptional mental ability and severe disability. Others may have traits that could be characterized as borderline pathological. Although there may be considerable variation of traits and abilities, many would agree that normal mental traits fall in a broad middle range of the spectrum.

Still, it is not clear when conditions with traits falling outside this middle range should be considered mental illnesses or pathologies. And even if a mental trait were considered an illness or pathology, this by itself would not tell us whether it should be treated. An answer to the diagnostic question would not necessarily provide an answer to the ethical question. The second question would hinge on whether it would be in one's best interests to be treated for a trait involving not only deleterious but desirable aspects as well. It would depend on whether the individual believed that any gain in controlling symptoms of a psychopathology would come at the expense of losing his or her outstanding attributes. Provided that the individual had the capacity to discuss treatment options with a physician and to understand the probable consequences of accepting or refusing cognitive or pharmacological therapy, the decision about whether to be treated ultimately would be his or hers to make. One could refuse treatment despite any difficulties in performing certain cognitive tasks or in interacting with others. As in any condition that is treatable with therapeutic interventions, patient autonomy is the default position. Exceptions to this position are when one lacks the capacity to understand reasons for or against treatment for a condition, and when an untreated condition poses a significant risk of harm to oneself and others. In these instances, a physician caring for the patient would be obligated to treat and could override a patient's refusal.

The embodiment condition of selfhood presupposes the capacity to feel pain and other sensations in the body, which are regulated by nerve endings and channels carrying signals to the brain. How we perceive the body and the external world is regulated by the somatosensory and vestibular systems in the brain. The first of these systems controls our orientation in space and time, while the second provides visual and gravitational stability. Some patients who have had strokes develop paralysis on one side of the body and a condition called anosognosia. They cannot recognize a paralyzed arm as their own because of damage to the parietal cortex and somatosensory system that regulate this type of recognition. A patient receiving a regional anesthetic to block pain sensation in one part of the body may perceive that part of the body as disconnected from the rest of the body and from his or her self. I may perceive my anesthetized arm as belonging not to *me* but to *someone else*. This is only an illusion due to the temporary effects of the anesthetic. Once these effects wear off, the perceived disconnection between the mind and the body ends as well. The patient again correctly experiences all of his or her body parts as connected and feels whole again. The dualistic illusion of mind separated from body gives way to the monistic reality of mind and body as an integrated unity.

"Near-death" experiences might appear to challenge the embodiment condition of selfhood. Some people have described the sensation of viewing their own bodies from above, as though they could exist in a disembodied state. If this were true, then it might support mind–body dualism and repudiate monism on the ground that the self could be separated from the body. But stimulation of electrodes implanted in the juncture of the right temporal lobe and parietal lobe to treat epilepsy has shown that out-of-body experiences (OBEs) can be artificially induced by electrical stimulation of this juncture, as well as the right angular gyrus.[43] This suggests that an OBE, the experience of dissociation of self from the body, may be a symptom of a neurological disorder. It may be a condition resulting from the brain's failure to integrate somatosensory and vestibular information, which is critical to the mind's representation of the body. Damage at the juncture of the temporal and parietal lobes and the right angular gyrus, or the misfiring of neurons in these areas, can alter somatosensory and vestibular systems and distort a person's perception of his or her own body. One sees one's body occupying positions that do not coincide with the position in which one ordinarily feels it. Thus OBEs may be nothing more than somatosensory illusions undermining one's cognitive ability to perceive oneself as essentially attached to one's body. This is an adaptive ability, since the capacity to feel pain and other body-related sensations enables one to avoid certain types of injury to the organism in which one's mind is embodied. The deformities in the limbs of people with Hansen's disease (leprosy), resulting from the inability to feel pain because of damaged nerve endings, are one example of this.

Yet other studies suggest that OBEs may be adaptive. They may be part of a coping mechanism that insulates some people against PTSD and other psychiatric illnesses. In one study, imaging of a subgroup of people with near-death experiences showed activity in the left temporal lobe similar to epileptic seizures that appeared to protect them from developing PTSD and related disorders.[44] These conclusions are preliminary and speculative. Nevertheless, they raise the possibility that certain brain mechanisms and corresponding mental states usually considered abnormal could be part of an adaptive purpose. They also raise the more ethically controversial possibility of manipulating the brain to produce these mental states. I will address this technique in the last section of chapter 5.

The agency component of the self can be impaired or undermined by the anhedonia symptomatic of major depression, the fear-induced inability to execute intentions in anxiety disorders, and the inability to stop the repetitive behaviors in obsessive-compulsive disorder. The inability of some individuals to control impulses may also impair or undermine agency. Brain imaging studies suggest that this lack of control may be due to damage to the frontal lobes, a hyperactive amygdala, or both. Both PET and fMRI scans show that some individuals with these disorders have overactive or underactive metabolism in the orbitofrontal cortex and ventromedial frontal cortex. I will discuss what brain scans revealing these abnormalities might mean for free will and moral responsibility in the next chapter.

All of the neuropsychiatric disorders that I have described show that different brain pathologies can alter or fracture one or more of the five components of the self. Interventions in the brain should restore dysfunctional regions to normal function so that one's experience of agency, unity, continuity, and embodiment and one's ability to relate to the external world can be restored to normal as well. Pharmacological, surgical, psychological, and other interventions can benefit us by repairing fractured neurological components of our selves. Maintaining all five components of the self in healthy order is crucial to one's integrity as a person and having a life free of pain and suffering. Each of these mental capacities is generated and sustained by multiple brain regions and interconnected neural pathways.

Unfortunately, sometimes an intervention to restore the normal neurobiological underpinning of one of these mental properties may damage another.

Repairing a fracture in one neural correlate of one component of the self can result in new fractures in other correlates and components. For example, psychosurgery to treat a disorder of agency, such as cingulotomy for OCD, may inadvertently damage the ventromedial temporal lobe. This can result in retrograde amnesia and disrupt one's experience of psychological unity and continuity through time. Neural stem cells implanted in the hippocampus or prefrontal cortex to generate new neural connections in people with cognitive deficits from strokes or lesions could proliferate uncontrollably or integrate improperly into the intended brain circuits. They could result in brain tumors, or they could overactivate circuits in the temporal lobe, leading to epileptic seizures. A procedure that could benefit one in one respect might harm one in others. This weighing of potential benefits and harms in deciding whether to intervene in the brain is difficult because of the complex interactions between cortical and subcortical regions of the brain. There is still much we do not know about these interactions and how they regulate motor, cognitive, affective, and volitional functions. Our incomplete knowledge of these interactions provides a compelling reason to proceed cautiously with any sort of intervention in the brain.

Philosophers such as Harry Frankfurt have argued that our selves should be "authentic." That is, the psychological properties that constitute our selves should be properties we would choose to have after a period of critical reflection and with which we would identify as our own. Frankfurt holds that when this occurs, the agent *decisively* identifies with general second-order desires, and these are in conformity with particular first-order desires. General desires about the type of behavior one would like to display influence and align with the particular desires that lead to particular actions. When there is conformity between second- and first-order desires, one's identification with one's mental states is wholehearted and complete, and the person has an authentic self.[45] Presumably, this would rule out mental capacities generated through artificial means such as cognition- or mood-enhancing drugs. It would also rule out mental states caused by brain dysfunction. If these were not the sorts of mental states that one would repeatedly choose to have, then they would be inauthentic because they would not be one's own. They would be alien to us because their source would be a brain dysfunction that would preclude one's ability to control the conscious process of reflection, choice, and identification.

But suppose that a person identifies with a certain type of mental state generated by an abnormality in the brain. This state reinforces rather than interferes with a more general set of beliefs that he or she would repeatedly choose to have. The conscious state of identification itself is not caused by any brain dysfunction. Would this person lack an authentic self?

Consider Sister John of the Cross, the fictional character in Mark Salzman's novel *Lying Awake*.[46] Thirteen years after entering a Carmelite convent, her prayers, hymns, and other daily activities have become arduous and devoid of meaning. Her life in the convent has become a spiritual desert. She begins to have ecstatic mystical visions and believes that they are the consequence of her faith and God's response to her prayers. Yet when she is examined for severe migraine headaches, the medical diagnosis is that she has a meningioma, a benign tumor of the tissue lining the outer surface of the brain. The tumor is pressing on Sister John's temporal lobe. Her mystical visions are due to seizures caused by electrical dysfunction in this region of the brain related to the tumor. The association between this type of religiosity and temporal lobe epilepsy has been well documented, most notably by neurologist Norman Geschwind in articles published in the 1960s and 1970s.[47] Hippocrates is known to have called temporal lobe epilepsy "the sacred disease" for the same reason. This is not to suggest that all mystical experience is caused by brain dysfunction, since it does not always involve a feeling of disembodiment and may be achieved through such mental exercises as meditation.

In Sister John's case, though, her mystical experience *is* based on brain pathology. This leads to a sense of disillusion that her experience is the result of a neuropsychiatric illness rather than a gift of divine grace. If she has surgery to remove the tumor, her spiritual ecstasy will vanish, and she will return to the spiritual desert and emptiness she experienced before the onset of her symptoms. The narrator captures the character's dilemma in the following passage:

> Sister John thought: I can't bear the thought of going back to where I was before. I prayed and scrubbed and went through the motions with no feeling of love, only a will to keep busy. If the surgery were to take my dream away, everything I've gone through up to now would seem meaningless. I wouldn't even be able to draw inspiration from the memory of it.[48]

Her reluctance to give up her mystical experience is influenced by Dostoevsky's thoughts about his similar experience during epileptic seizures. She cites him through the words of his main character in the novel *Demons*:

> There are moments, and it is only a matter of five or six seconds, when you feel the presence of the eternal harmony. A terrible thing is the frightful clearness with which it manifests itself and the rapture with which it fills you. If this state were to last more than five seconds, the soul could not endure and it would have to disappear. During these five seconds I live a whole human existence, and for that I would give my whole life and not think that I was paying too dearly.[49]

Sister John then asks herself: "If Dostoevsky had been given the option of treatment, would he have taken it? *Should* he have?"[50]

This character identifies with her mystical experience, even though it is caused by a brain tumor. Is the self she wants an authentic one, a self she would repeatedly choose to have, regardless of the consequences? Would she refuse the surgery in order to retain this self? A quick intuitive response to these questions is that she would not. Although it is a benign tumor, an untreated meningioma would cause more severe seizures and other more serious neurological problems as it penetrated deeper into the temporal lobe and infiltrated other brain structures. In addition to the medical concern, the disconnection between Sister John's mystical states of mind and the external world seems to violate all five conditions of normal selfhood. She realizes the harm that will befall her without removal of the tumor and consents to the surgery. It is a choice that she would prefer not to make, since in either case the consequences are not desirable for her. Yet her choice would also be supported by the realization that her mystical states are really part of a pathological self, alien to her because they are the result of an abnormality in her brain. They are not mental states she would repeatedly choose to have. A normal, healthy self presupposes that one's mental states are generated and sustained by normally functioning brain states.

Even if Sister John believed that the benefits of her mystical experience outweighed any harm from the tumor responsible for it, she probably would not be able to appreciate this experience beyond a certain point. Because seizures overly stimulate excitatory brain circuits, they can disrupt the delicate balance between excitatory and inhibitory functions of neurons and neurotransmitters. Refusing to treat the underlying cause of the seizures would only increase their frequency. This would result in damage to other areas of her brain, leading to cognitive, affective, and psychomotor deterioration. Eventually, she would fall into a coma and die.

In fact, when she first sees the neurologist, Dr. Sheppard, she already has had several heart attacks, chronic nausea, and even a three-day coma. Given the severity of her condition, Dr. Sheppard has a duty of nonmaleficence to Sister John. He is minimally obligated to prevent further harm by persuading her that the surgery would be in her all-things-considered best interests. She has the autonomous right to participate in the discussion with the clinician regarding whether or not to have the surgery. She also has a prima facie right to refuse the surgery. But if her condition undermined her decisional capacity and was an imminent threat to her life, then Dr. Sheppard could override her refusal once her condition began to compromise her capacity for reasoning and decision-making. Patients can refuse treatment for a life-threatening medical condition only if they are competent enough to understand the consequences of forgoing it. At some point, Sister John likely would have lost this competence, after which she would not be able to decide whether to have or forgo the surgery.

An actual case presents a similar set of ethical issues surrounding a neuropsychiatric condition with both salutary and pathological aspects. London resident Tommy McHugh suffered a cerebral hemorrhage that altered his personality. Before this event, he had been a heroin addict and had been incarcerated several times for violent offenses. Prior to the hemorrhage, he had no interest in art; but following the hemorrhage he developed a compulsive interest in painting, sculpting, and writing. American neurologist Bruce Miller, who has studied this case, speculates that damage to the frontal and temporal lobes on the left side of Tommy McHugh's brain may have caused him to become compulsively interested in art.[51] As the brain's executive center, the frontal lobe is critical for inhibition of impulses. Damage to this region can weaken inhibition and unleash creative potential by freeing activity in other regions of the brain, especially the occipital lobe, where the formation of primitive images occurs. Miller has also noted that artistic creativity may appear as a consequence of cognitive pathology in some people with Alzheimer's and frontotemporal dementia.[52] Artistic creativity may increase as the disease progresses and cognitive capacities decrease. Such creativity may be explained by the fact that visuospatial deficits in Alzheimer's lead to less precision and attention to spatial relationships. Tommy McHugh came to identify with his condition and artistic interest, claiming that his life was "100 percent better" than before. Yet his new compulsive interest was the result of a cerebral vascular accident and could be accurately described as a psychopathology. McHugh had scores in the normal range for IQ, but had difficulty in switching trains of thought and in other cognitive tasks.

For a neurological disorder that cannot be treated, the fact that a patient with the disorder is content with his life, no longer engages in criminal activity, and is productive in a creative way should be welcomed. But the fact remains that his artistic urge is a compulsion and thus a type of psychopathology. So we should qualify any description of his new passion as a mental ability. Or at least we should describe this mental ability as inextricably linked to a mental disability. In such cases, the cognitive disability often results in problems with concentration that prevent the person from doing any sustained and coherent artistic work. The cases in which brain injury results in work of outstanding artistic merit are more the exception than the rule. In the rare cases where brain injury results in a new or enhanced artistic ability, the injury is usually mild, and the differences in brain and mental functions before and after the event are subtle.

Besides, one could question whether Tommy McHugh's true self was the one associated with the psychological properties he had before or after the hemorrhage. The mere fact that his mood and self-esteem improved following the hemorrhage does not mean that the cerebral vascular accident somehow restored the psychological properties of a creative person, the real "Tommy," who existed before his life of heroin addiction and criminal offenses. It would strain the limits of plausibility to make such a claim. Even if Tommy's artistic creativity was described positively as an attribute, it would not mean that he had developed a new self. His creativity would be only one component of a larger set of components that collectively constitute his self. Still, this does not address the question of whether someone with this or a similar neuropsychiatric condition should be treated.

Suppose that the brain damage from Tommy McHugh's cerebral hemorrhage could be repaired. Neurogenesis in the affected regions through stem cell therapy or neural tissue transplantation theoretically could restore normal brain function. Suppose, further, that the restoration would mean that the patient would lose his creative passion. A neurologist or neurosurgeon would have to weigh the potential medical benefits and risks of treatment against the medical risks of leaving it untreated. In doing this, the practitioner would also weigh the benefits of a creative passion with which the patient had come to identify against the risks associated with difficulties in planning, decision-making, and other cognitive tasks.

If this patient retained enough mental capacity to know what was in his best interests and that treatment was contrary to these interests, then his doctors would have to respect and not override his refusal of treatment. Granted, his creativity is a compulsion and therefore a type of psychopathology. Moreover, others might believe that he would be better off without the cognitive disability than with it. Yet, unless his compulsion and disability undermined his capacity to understand what was in his best interests, and unless the untreated condition entailed a significant risk of harm to himself or others, he could not be treated against his will. There might be prima facie reasons for pharmacological or surgical intervention to regulate his cognitive functions. But the patient could reject these reasons and insist that he would be better off without any intervention. Similar remarks apply to creative writers with hypergraphia. They may rationally believe that the loss of their creative urge from drug treatment would not be worth any gain in or restoration of cognitive ability. Provided that they were competent enough to know the consequences of refusing medical treatment, they could refuse it.

These considerations raise more general ethical questions. Do psychiatrists, neurologists, and neurosurgeons have an obligation only to manage symptoms by regulating or restoring normal brain function in their patients? Or do they also have an obligation to restore the patient's normal self, the functional set of integrated psychological properties the person had before the onset of a neuropsychiatric illness and psychopathology? Strictly speaking, medical professionals are obligated only to try to achieve the first goal, since only it is specified as one of the basic goals of medicine.[53] In most cases, achieving the first goal will entail achieving the second. One will be a by-product of and consistent with the other. In the case of Sister John, surgical resection of the meningioma restores her normal neurological function and all the normal psychological components of her self. But the physiological integrity of the brain may not map so easily onto the psychological integrity of the self in other cases. This is especially so in mild to moderate psychiatric conditions, which can be illustrated by a hypothetical case.

Suppose that a successful artist sees a psychiatrist because he has been experiencing low mood. The psychiatrist diagnoses the artist as having dysthymia, a mild form of depression. This is a legitimate psychiatric diagnosis. As noted in the discussion of autistic spectrum disorders, just because a condition meets diagnostic criteria for a mental illness does not mean that it should be treated. The artist would like the psychiatrist to help him regulate his mood. He is ambivalent, though, because his moods have strongly influenced his painting, and he fears that antidepressant medication will adversely affect the quality of his work. He takes great pride in and derives much satisfaction and meaning from his painting, which has enriched his life. Yet the diagnosis tells him that the emotions that inspire his creative work are the result of a psychiatric disorder. Unlike Sister John's meningioma, not treating the artist's condition would not entail a significant risk of harm to him. In addition, forgoing pharmacological treatment for dysthymia does not entail the same risk of suicide as it does for major depression and bipolar disorder (10–20 percent among the U.S. population).

Many artists throughout history have identified with the creativity associated with bipolar disorder, temporal lobe epilepsy, and other neuropsychiatric disorders. The hypergraphia of prolific writers such as Dostoevsky, as well as the exceptional creativity of artists such as Van Gogh and composers like Schumann, may be attributed to hyperactivity in certain brain circuits. In the passage I cited from *Demons*, Dostoevsky vicariously suggested that the experience of eternal harmony from his epilepsy was worth any cost to him. But the risks of not treating epilepsy are obvious. In bipolar disorder, the potential harmful consequences of both manic (impaired, impulsive judgment) and depressive (suicidal thoughts) phases of this condition are significant enough that failure to intervene with lithium or other similarly effective drugs would be difficult to justify. Indeed, one could argue that lithium would not diminish one's creativity but would enhance it by allowing one to be more organized, focused, and productive. Treatment may not always be in the best interests of people with bipolar disorder, however. In moderate forms of this condition, an affected but still mentally competent individual may rationally decide that any benefit of pharmacological intervention would not be worth the cost of losing certain abilities. I will present a case in chapter 4 (*Starson v. Swayze*) to support this point.

When people's artistic creativity or other talents are associated with a neuropsychiatric disorder and psychopathology, they may insist that life for them would be worse if controlling the disorder came at the expense of their creativity. But if such a person were under the care of a physician, the person's decision to refuse treatment for this reason could be overridden by the physician. A refusal could be overridden if the physician judged that the disorder posed a significant risk of harm to the patient or to others, and the patient was incapable of understanding the reasons for treatment. During a manic phase, someone with bipolar disorder might agree with Dostoevsky and believe that he or she had a choice between retaining elevated mood and creativity and losing them through treatment. Yet the compulsive nature of hypergraphia or some other creative urge might suggest that such a person would not have the cognitive control to rationally consider the consequences of not having treatment. If the symptoms of the disorder were severe and impaired or undermined the person's decisional capacity, then any choice in the matter would not be his or hers to make. Still, symptoms of neuropsychiatric disorders fall along a spectrum. Unless one's symptoms fall at the severe end of the spectrum and interfere with one's ability to reason, the autonomous right to refuse treatment should be upheld.

In the hypothetical case of dysthymia, only a low-grade psychiatric condition underlies a self that has a unique set of affective properties with which the artist identifies. Even the psychiatrist might be ambivalent about treatment, because there is no great difference between this patient's symptoms and the normal baseline for mood. Dysthymia could be described as a minor deviation from a functional neurological baseline and thus not a condition absolutely requiring a therapeutic intervention. In addition, this condition does not involve a radical disruption of mental states, where these states become substantially different from how they were at an earlier time. Instead, there is a gradual change in the qualitative aspects of the artist's mental states. It is a change to which he adjusts in a positive way and that he considers to be not alien but essential to his true self. Should the psychiatrist focus on the underlying biochemical dysfunction in the patient's brain and prescribe medication to treat it? Or should the psychiatrist not prescribe medication and not alter an aspect of the artist's self that appears to be full of meaning and purpose?

Assuming that the condition is not likely to harm the artist or others and does not undermine or impair his mental competence, the artist would have the autonomy to decide for or against treatment. Yet the fact that he has asked the psychiatrist for help gives some weight to the psychiatrist's professional judgment in discussing with him whether or not to treat his condition. The psychiatrist's discussion will be informed by the psychiatrist's professional obligation to prevent harm to his or her patients. Given the trust that exists between doctor and patient in this case, the psychiatrist may influence the patient's deliberation about his options. The psychiatrist might argue that, although this patient's psychiatric condition has had some positive effects on him, its negative effects on his self and life might be greater in the long term. On balance, the artist would be better off if all aspects of his self were in line with normal brain functions. This could justify cognitive-behavioral therapy or antidepressant therapy. Maintaining a normal functioning brain will have salutary effects on the mind and body and will generate a self with which most of us would want to identify in all of its components. This may or may not promote artistic creativity. But insofar as the patient is competent enough to know what is in his best interests, the decision about treatment should be his alone.

It is possible that an aberrant cause of brain and mental behavior may result in an unusual connection between different cognitive or affective contents that may be beneficial to a person. This connection may lead to insight about reality that would not be open to other persons who did not have the relevant affliction. In some cases of depression, for instance, such an experience may lead a person to have a more realistic appraisal of the world.[54] But these cases are the exception rather than the rule, and this insight would more likely occur in mild to moderate forms of the disorder. In general, when one has a mental disorder, every attempt should be made to regulate or restore the kind of neurobiological functioning that will enable one to decisively identify with certain desires, beliefs, emotions, and intentions. Medical interventions that can do this will uphold one's autonomy and enable one to act and shape one's self and life story with integrity.

Conclusion

Cortical and subcortical regions of the brain interact in complex ways to generate and sustain the conscious and unconscious properties of the human mind. Immune and endocrine systems can also influence the central nervous system and, in turn, the nature and content of our mental states. Dysfunction in any of these systems can result in various psychopathologies symptomatic of psychiatric disorders. Degeneration of structures or functions in the central nervous system alone may also result in neurological disorders that may impair or undermine one's cognitive capacities and one's ability to control one's bodily movements. All of these neuropsychiatric disorders can adversely affect the physical and psychological capacities that make us the persons we are and that constitute our selves. Neuroimaging, psychopharmacology, psychosurgery, and neurostimulation hold the prospect of prevention and more effective treatment and control of these disorders. They may also enable us to enhance normal brain functions.

The relation between the brain/body and mind that I have laid out in this chapter will serve as a framework for discussion of ethical questions about mapping, monitoring, and altering the brain in the chapters that follow. These questions pertain to the ways in which measures of and interventions in the brain can benefit or harm us, whether we are capable of knowing their risks, and the conditions that must be in place for us to consent to them. All of these factors will influence our judgments about when or whether different clinical neuroscientific techniques are permissible. Ultimately, our concern with how these actions can affect our brains is grounded in our concern with how they can affect our minds.

Neuroimaging

The ability to see images of the structural and functional landscape of the brain has been perhaps the most significant achievement in neuroscience. These images have enabled researchers to identify neural correlates of normal and abnormal states of mind. Especially fascinating has been the use of high-resolution, real-time functional brain scans. Brain scans can display the indirect effects of neural activity on local blood volume, flow, and oxygen saturation. These images can identify regions that are metabolically overactive or underactive and can help to explain physiological and psychological characteristics of neurological and psychiatric disorders. Brain imaging may enable clinicians to confirm a diagnosis of these disorders. In addition, it may enable them to track the progression of neuropsychiatric conditions and monitor the effects of drugs to treat them. Imaging might also be able to detect subtle brain abnormalities long before the appearance of symptoms associated with diseases of the brain and mind. In this regard, neuroimaging might predict who would develop these diseases.

But predictive neuroimaging is fraught with uncertainty. It cannot determine that an asymptomatic individual with anomalous brain features will in fact develop a neuropsychiatric disease. Because of this uncertainty, there is potential harm as well as potential benefit in using brain scans for predictive purposes. Similar concern surrounds diagnostic imaging, especially if it is used for nonmedical purposes. There is considerable ambiguity regarding the significance of the information derived from brain imaging. Parties both inside and outside the health care system may have access to this information and interpret it in different ways. Information about the brain may be used to form judgments about whether or to what extent people can control their behavior, which could have significant ethical and legal implications. Given the magnitude of these implications, ethical questions about brain imaging need to be raised and discussed within a broad professional and public framework.[1]

In this chapter, I describe different forms of brain imaging, laying out their design and limitations. Then I explain the ways brain scans can help to diagnose mental disorders, as well as to monitor the progression of these disorders and the effects of treatment for them. A discussion of more ethically controversial uses of diagnostic imaging will follow. This will include what brain scans might tell us about the neurobiological basis of free will and how they might influence our judgments about moral and legal responsibility. I go on to consider ethical issues surrounding predictive imaging, focusing on problems with obtaining informed consent from patients and research subjects. This discussion will also include consideration of the potential benefit and harm of having advance information associated with a neurological or psychiatric disease that one may or may not develop. In exploring the promises and pitfalls of neuroimaging, I underscore the importance of the ethical obligation of researchers, clinicians, and others to exercise great care in obtaining, interpreting, and explaining information about the human brain.

Brain Imaging Techniques

The oldest and clinically most common imaging modality is computed tomography, which was introduced in the 1970s. CT scans provide three-dimensional x-rays displaying different anatomical structures of the brain. Positron emission tomography scans produce images of the functions of different areas of the brain. In a PET scan, a radioactive tracer is injected into the blood stream and follows the blood to the brain. Detectors that are sensitive to the tracer are placed around the skull. When an area of the brain is engaged in neural activity, more blood will flow to that area. The PET detector can sense the increased blood supply because more of the radioactive tracer will be concentrated in that area of the brain. Like PET, single photon emission computed tomography (SPECT) is a type of functional imaging. SPECT uses gamma rays and provides temporal and spatial information about the brain by measuring changes in a radioactive isotope injected into the brain. Yet the images produced by SPECT have poorer resolution and are less detailed than PET images. The newest and technologically most advanced form of imaging is functional magnetic resonance imaging. This technique can simultaneously register structural and real-time functional information about the brain. It is distinct from the more standard magnetic resonance imaging, which maps anatomical structures of the brain rather than brain activity.[2] Still, the spatial and temporal resolution of fMRI is a persistent limitation because it can only capture brain processes of relatively short duration.

PET and fMRI scans are the most helpful in measuring actual brain function and changes in neural activity. Positron emission tomography scans measure changes in glucose metabolism in brain cells, as well as changes in blood flow to various regions of the brain. The more active a region is, the more the neurons need glucose. This will result in increased blood flow and the emission of more positrons in creating an image. Positron emission tomography scans are especially useful because they can measure both cortical and subcortical brain functions. For example, these scans can show depletion of dopaminergic neurons in the substantia nigra region in the brains of patients with Parkinson's disease. Functional MRI is based on the difference between the magnetic properties of oxygenated (aortic) and deoxygenated (venous) blood. The difference between these two types of properties produces the contrast resulting in the image. Although early forms of fMRI used an injected contrast agent, current forms are noninvasive because the tracer is the magnetic properties of the blood itself. This imaging modality is superior to PET because it has more refined spatial and temporal resolution. Actual changes in metabolism and blood flow in the prefrontal cortex can be measured while subjects are performing cognitive tasks requiring attention and vigilance. Functional MRI can also reveal activity in the neural substrate underlying one's affective states. Some studies using this technique involved subjects who became emotionally charged when shown photos of certain events. Their emotions correlated with increased activity in the amygdala and other limbic structures.[3] Especially significant is the ability of fMRI to measure activity in both the prefrontal cortex and limbic system and elucidate the interaction between these areas in sustaining the interacting cognitive and emotional processing that grounds reasoning and decision-making.

Although the development and use of brain imaging has increased our understanding of the neural substrate of many of our psychological traits, it is still limited, in at least five respects. First, there is not yet a reference data base of brain imaging from the general population that is large enough to be used for determining whether every image can confirm a diagnosis or predict a clinically important outcome. Scans would have to be taken from thousands of people over many years to achieve this goal.[4] Second, a particular mental state may depend on activation of some brain areas and inhibition of others. While a substantial degree of metabolic under- or overactivation of an area of the brain may correlate with a psychopathology, it is unclear whether metabolic activity slightly less or greater than normal for the general population would have any clinical significance. Third, because cognitive and affective capacities are based on the activity of many circuits distributed through many brain regions, an image of activity in one region may lead to too narrow an interpretation of the neurological or psychological significance of that image. Fourth, although imaging can show correlations between normal and abnormal brain states and mental states, it cannot provide a causal explanation of the etiology and pathogenesis of neurological and psychiatric diseases. Fifth, imaging cannot capture the adaptive interaction of an organism with the external environment. Brain states function not only by obeying internal constraints and regularities but also in virtue of their dynamic interaction with the external world. Because imaging provides at most correlations rather than causal connections between brain states and mental states, it would be misleading to describe imaging as a form of mind reading.

These limitations notwithstanding, with increased resolution brain scans may become more helpful in the diagnosis and prediction of many mental disorders. They may also tell us something about the brain's role in regulating human behavior. In the next three sections, I will explore some of the ethical implications of using brain scans for diagnostic and predictive purposes.

Diagnostic Neuroimaging

The main purpose of CT, MRI, SPECT, PET, and fMRI scans is to confirm a medical diagnosis of a neurological or psychiatric disorder based on behavioral symptoms and established clinical criteria. Higher resolution forms of this technology can be especially helpful in understanding neurological diseases. As noted, PET scans can reveal depletion of dopaminergic neurons in the substantia nigra region of the basal ganglia and could confirm a diagnosis of Parkinson's disease. Similar scans can reveal amyloid plaques and neurofibrillary tangles in certain regions of the brain and could confirm a diagnosis of Alzheimer's disease. These scans can also show depletion of neurons in the hippocampus and pre-frontal cortex, which are additional anatomical properties of this neurodegenerative disease.

Another possible clinical use of imaging would be to elucidate the pathology of attention deficit/hyperactivity disorder. Single photon emission computed to-mography scans have shown structural abnormalities in the form of reduced brain volume in the right frontal lobe and caudate nucleus of children and adults with this disorder.[5] These regions are part of a distributed neuronal system that sustains attention and behavioral inhibition. Functional MRI could also be helpful in understanding and treating major depressive disorder. This imaging technique can show low glucose metabolism in the prefrontal cortex and anterior cingulate, which is one marker of MDD. Equally significant is the ability of these scans to measure the brain's response to different antidepressants. More refined images of metabo-lism in the affected brain regions could enable psychiatrists to administer anti-depressants that target serotonergic, noradrenergic, and dopaminergic receptors in these regions. This could at once relieve depressive symptoms and minimize ad-verse side effects of the drugs. Studies have demonstrated that changes in brain function over time can be tracked with brain scans after administering antide-pressant medication for both OCD and MDD.[6]

Functional magnetic resonance imaging can also depict changes in brain metabolism following cognitive-behavioral therapy (CBT) to treat depression.[7] Im-aging of patients undergoing CBT has shown that it can modulate some neuronal functions in cortical and limbic regions. The prefrontal cortex, hippocampus, and dorsal cingulate are particularly responsive to CBT. Imaging following antide-pressant drug therapy shows that deeper regions of the brain are more responsive to this modality than shallower regions. Drug therapy appears to reach deeper regions of the brain than CBT. Combining different imaging studies can confirm the efficacy of combined talk and drug therapy for MDD. In general, CBT appears to have a "top-down" effect on the brain, correcting negative habits of thought due to dysfunctional cognitive and emotional processing projecting from the prefrontal cortex to other regions. Drug therapy appears to have a "bottom-up" effect, modulating the functioning of subcortical regions projecting to the cortex. In addition, imaging can show brain mechanisms at work when people deliberately try to forget an event. A recent study has shown that, when subjects are engaged in this cognitive task, there is increased activity in the prefrontal cortex and decreased activity in the hippocampus. This activity underlies the process whereby the mind and brain attempt to eliminate episodic memory from working memory.[8] By using neuroimaging to identify how affected brain regions respond to pharmacological and psychological interventions, these interventions can be tailored to produce maximal benefit and minimal harm for patients.

Earlier, I noted that one of the limitations of neuroimaging is its inability to provide a causal explanation of the pathogenesis of neuropsychiatric diseases. Yet one promising strategy for achieving this goal is to combine imaging with genetics. In chapter 2, I claimed that genes do not determine but only shape the broad outline of our mental and behavioral functions. Nevertheless, they do play a role in these functions, and, in conjunction with brain scans, can shed light on the neurobiological basis of our thoughts, choices, and actions. This could result in more accurate early diagnosis and prediction of these diseases, which could lead to more effective treatment and possible prevention of them. Most psychiatric disorders have a genetic component. One particularly exciting development in this regard has been the use of neuroimaging as one component of endophenotype analysis of genetically complex psychiatric diseases. Thirty years ago, Irving Gottesman and James Shields defined "endophenotypes" as "internal phenotypes discoverable by a biochemical test or microscopic examination."[9] More recently, Gottesman and Todd Gould have defined endophenotypes as "measurable components unseen by the unaided eye along the pathway between disease and distal genotype."[10] Endophenotypes can be characterized as biological markers indicating actual signs of or susceptibility to psychiatric disease. These markers may be neurochemical, endocrinological, neuroanatomical, or neuropsychological. The rationale for endophenotype analysis is that it may enable researchers to gain a better understanding of the biological mechanisms underlying psychiatric disease.

The most clinically significant endophenotypes for mental illness are structural and functional abnormalities in regions of the brain regulating cognition and emotion. Some of the brain scanning techniques I have described can identify these biological markers. Once they have been identified, researchers can find the genetic correlates of these markers, extend genetic analysis to healthy siblings of affected individuals, and thereby tease apart all the biological components of psychiatric diseases. Genetic linkage studies involving monozygotic and dizygotic twins support the view that particular genetic mutations are causally relevant to the pathogenesis of schizophrenia, bipolar disorder, depression, and ADHD.[11]

Genetics can also help in the treatment of psychiatric diseases through its role in drug therapy. *Pharmacogenomics* refers to the role of inheritance in individual variation in drug response and aims to tailor drug treatment according to individual genotype. *Proteomics* refers to the study of the structures and functions of the proteins for which genes code. These two closely related fields have been recognized as important steps toward the goal of personalized medicine. Differences in drug response are due to sequence variants in genes coding for the transport proteins that regulate the absorption, distribution, and excretion of drugs. It is estimated that genetics can account for 20 to 95 percent of the variability in drug response across people.[12] Many drugs fail to control the symptoms and progression of diseases because they fail to target the critical gene, protein, and peptide sequences regulating cell metabolism. In schizophrenia, newer generation drugs like risperidone have fewer side effects than older generation drugs like haloperidol. Still, in many cases, even the newer drugs fail to restore patients' cognitive functioning to the point where they can have normal lives. This problem is probably due to the failure of existing antipsychotic drugs to target dopaminergic and cholinergic receptors in a way that can control psychotic and other cognitive symptoms. The inability of dopamine antagonists to target the critical neuronal receptors can also result in adverse side effects, such as the movement disorder tardive dyskinesia.

Of all psychiatric diseases, schizophrenia has the strongest genetic component. The dysbindin-1 gene, which codes for a protein that is expressed in neurons in many areas of mouse and human brains, has been implicated in this disease. But the precise causal role of this gene, or of other genes, in schizophrenia is still not known. Maternal genetic mutations are not the only culprit. Children fathered by older men with no family history of the disease may be at increased risk of schizophrenia because of accumulated genetic mutations in sperm. If researchers could ascertain how the relevant genes influenced drug response in patients, then they might be able to target genes coding for the proteins regulating dopamine and acetylcholine in the prefrontal cortex, basal ganglia, hippocampus, and other brain regions affected in schizophrenia. Because gene sequences and their effects on neuronal receptors vary across persons, the combination of genetic analysis and brain imaging to monitor the drugs' effects could result in customized pharmacological intervention that would be more effective and safer. This might involve patient-specific dosing of a combination of dopamine antagonists and cholinergic agonists.

Genetic differences extend across ethnic boundaries and can affect the brain's response to psychotropic drugs. For example, Asian patients metabolize haloperidol more slowly than Caucasians. Asian patients are also more likely to develop severe side effects when treated with antipsychotic drugs. Children metabolize psychotropic and other drugs very differently from adults. Some children are fast metabolizers, while others break down the drugs so slowly that they can build up in their bodies and brains and cause adverse effects. These differences are likely due to the ways in which genes control the activity of enzymes that regulate drug metabolism. Both PET and fMRI scans can be a helpful diagnostic and therapeutic tool because they can monitor differences in drug activity in the brain across diverse patient populations.

Research suggests that there is a genetic component in major depression, and at least several genes have been implicated in the disorder. In particular, people with the shorter allele of the 5-HTT serotonin transporter gene may be more susceptible to depression. The belief is that this allele predisposes them to perceive events as more stressful than do other people who do not have it.[13] In studies, subjects with the shorter allele displayed more intense activity in the amygdala measured by fMRI imaging when shown pictures of frightful events. Expression of the allele can interfere with normal serotonin transmission and trigger processes that disrupt fear-regulating feedback loops in the brain. Why some antidepressant drugs can modulate these processes and control psychological symptoms in some patients but not others is not fully understood. Nor is it clear why some patients experience more side effects than others who take these drugs. These problems beset not only older generation drugs like tricyclics and monoamine oxidase inhibitors but also newer generation selective SSRIs and serotonin-norepinephrine reuptake inhibitors (SNRIs). Antidepressant treatment could be more effective if drugs were tailored to interact more precisely with genes coding for the proteins regulating serotonergic and adrenergic receptors in the prefrontal cortex, anterior cingulate, and amygdala. Both PET and fMRI scans could monitor the effects of antidepressant drugs in the critical regions of the brain. Unlike the current trial-and-error approach to drug therapy for depression, therapy could be tailored to each patient's unique brain circuitry and biochemistry. The combination of targeted therapy and neuroimaging could greatly reduce the risk of adverse side effects and increase the benefits of the drugs.

Another area where brain imaging may be helpful is in pain control. As described in the previous chapter, real-time fMRI has been used to enable patients in chronic pain to modulate their experience of pain. By seeing images of activated areas of their brains involved in pain perception, patients can interact with the images and use their thoughts to influence the brain in a way that might attenuate pain. This would provide not just a diagnostic aid but a therapeutic one as well.

There is still considerable uncertainty with respect to what brain scans mean for the pathophysiology of neuropsychiatric diseases. By itself, brain imaging is of limited diagnostic value. As a diagnostic tool, imaging should complement rather than replace established clinical criteria. Nevertheless, the discussion thus far has shown the potential therapeutic value of neuroimaging in diagnosing and treating mental illness. There are other possible uses of diagnostic neuroimaging that are more ethically controversial.

Implications for Free Will and Moral Responsibility

Suppose one person kills another in a fit of rage and is charged with second-degree murder. The offender claims that his action resulted from a violent impulse he could not control. Prosecution and defense agree that a brain scan could test the veracity of his claim. He undergoes a PET scan, which shows abnormally low metabolic activity in and blood flow to the prefrontal cortex and abnormally high metabolic activity in and blood flow to the amygdala. This combination of brain features has been associated with uncontrollable impulses. The prefrontal cortex regulates executive functions involving decisions and actions and is crucial for rational planning and impulse control. The amygdala regulates emotional processing in the limbic system, which projects to the anterior cingulate and prefrontal cortex and can interact with these regions in influencing executive functions. The offender and his lawyer argue that the brain dysfunction undermined his capacity for moral reasoning, impulse control, and thus his ability to control his behavior. To act freely and be morally and legally responsible for one's behavior, one must have the capacity to control it. Because the offender lacked this capacity when he acted, he could not be responsible for killing his victim. He lacked free will and therefore should be exonerated because of his brain abnormality.

Or suppose that a different individual performs a similar act. His act results not from a violent impulse but instead from a lack of empathy for his victim and an inability to feel remorse or act in accord with social norms. An MRI brain scan shows an abnormally small amygdala, a feature that has been associated with psychopathy. He and his lawyer also argue that his brain abnormality and psychopathy are beyond his control and that he, too, lacked free will and should be excused from responsibility for his action.

Would either of these defenses be convincing in a court of law? How do these hypothetical cases test our intuitions about free will and moral responsibility for one's motivational states and actions? To respond to these questions, we need to consider what neuroimaging studies might indicate about the neurobiological basis of behavior. Although it is not always clear why certain neural structures and systems are dysfunctional, brain imaging may yield insight into why dysfunction at the neuronal level can give rise to disturbances at the mental and behavioral level.

Psychopathy is a disorder characterized by diminished capacity for empathy and remorse, and poor behavior controls.[14] Many violent offenders are also unable to control impulses. But their lack of impulse control is much greater than that of psychopaths. Nor do they appear to have the same type of emotional impairment as psychopaths. Brain scans of psychopaths and violent offenders have indicated differences in the brain dysfunction underlying the behavior of these two groups.

Neuroimaging studies of violent offenders conducted independently by Adrian Raine and Richard Davidson have shown hyperactivity in the amygdala and diminished activity in the prefrontal cortex of these individuals when compared with the same brain regions of normal subjects.[15] In contrast, individuals with psychopathy have shown a smaller and less active amygdala, though they often have a hyperactive anterior cingulate, which ordinarily regulates cognitive and affective processing in deliberation and decision-making. The combination of these features in these regions of the limbic system may suppress positive emotions such as empathy.[16] Some studies of individuals with psychopathy have shown intact frontal lobe functioning.[17] Others have had contrary indications. For example, Antonio Damasio and his colleagues found that lesions in the orbitofrontal cortex (OFC) correlated with impulsive and antisocial behavior.[18] Despite seeming cognitively intact, individuals with damage to this region of the brain appear to be unable to conform to social norms when they act. Adults and children with this damage presented with a syndrome resembling psychopathy. Those who have this syndrome display an inability to resolve cognitive conflicts and appear unable to exercise the cognitive and affective control required for moral judgment. More recently, James Blair has obtained similar results from imaging studies on a similar group of subjects.[19]

The OFC receives extensive projections from and sends extensive projections to the amygdala and anterior cingulate. Decreased volume and metabolic activity in the amygdala and increased metabolic activity in the anterior cingulate cortex might explain the emotional deficiency of psychopaths and their impaired ability to make rational and moral choices between different courses of action. The emotion of regret is critical to this counterfactual reasoning and is strongly associated with the feeling of responsibility. The OFC is one of the neurobiological bases of the interaction between cognition and emotion, modulating our capacity to experience regret and responsibility. Damage to the OFC can impair or undermine this combined emotional and cognitive capacity, suggesting that patients with orbitofrontal cortical lesions may not be morally responsible for their behavior.

Damage to the ventromedial frontal cortex can result in a similar type of psychopathology. Neuroimaging of individuals displaying inappropriate social behavior has shown decreased activity in this particular region of the cortex and increased activity in the anterior cingulate. Through its interaction with the anterior cingulate, the ventromedial cortex regulates the emotions that color decision-making. This was the main area involved in the radical behavioral transformation of both Phineas Gage and Damasio's patient "Elliot." In the first case, a metal projectile penetrated Gage's skull and resulted in extensive damage to the ventromedial cortex of his brain as a consequence of an explosion during construction on the Rutland & Burlington Railroad in Vermont in 1848. In the second case, ventromedial damage to the patient's brain was caused by a meningioma. Both Gage and "Elliot" lost their capacity to restrain their impulses, conform to social norms of behavior, and rationally deliberate and plan for the future. To the extent that factors beyond their control caused them to lose this capacity, they were not responsible for their actions. The neurobiological basis of their capacity to reason was so damaged, and their capacity to make decisions was so flawed, that they were no longer able to function effectively as social beings. The lives of both of these patients following brain damage were equally tragic.[20]

At the other extreme from those with violent impulses are people with anhedonia. This is a symptom of many forms of major depression, as well as a subclass of schizophrenia. Individuals lose interest in many activities and cannot motivate themselves to initiate or complete plans of action. Neuroimaging of patients with these disorders has shown reduced activity in the left dorsolateral prefrontal cortex. Some depressed and schizophrenic individuals with damage to this brain region have exhibited a hypovolitional syndrome consisting in drive reduction and impeded initiative.[21] On this basis, one might be inclined to characterize this part of the cortex as the center of willed action.

Brain scans of individuals with obsessive-compulsive disorder exhibit very different neurobiological images. Studies using fMRI have shown reduced metabolic activity in the ventromedial cortex and increased activity in subcortical motor regions. These are manifestations of dysfunction of the orbitofrontal-subcortical circuit, whose component structures include the OFC, caudate nucleus, globus pallidus, and thalamus. Patients with OCD feel that they must do certain things, or that they must think certain thoughts, though they claim that they do not want to and often desperately try to fight these mental states. One hypothesis is that a "worry input" in the frontal lobes projects to the basal ganglia via the ventromedial cortex. The ganglia's reduced filter function impairs the sensory filtering function of the thalamus, producing an abnormality that projects to other brain regions.[22] Another hypothesis is that the obsessions and compulsions are due to a dysfunctional cingulate, which disrupts normal cognitive and affective processing. This is the rationale for the surgical procedure of cingulotomy to treat OCD when it is refractory to all other interventions. It involves altering the main pathway between the limbic system and the prefrontal cortex. The more general point is that OCD impairs the cognitive and emotional processing necessary to choose and act freely.

Executive functions such as reasoning, initiative, and decision-making depend on the interaction of cognitive, conative, and affective processing, which is sustained by interacting cortical-limbic pathways. Each of these pathways modulates the other in a balanced system of positive feed-forward and negative feedback loops. Damage to particular structures of the brain can disrupt this balance and may cause a person to lose control over his or her motivational states and actions. If dysfunction in neural pathways results in impeded initiative and impaired reasoning and decision-making, and these mental capacities are necessary for behavior control, then, arguably, individuals with this type of dysfunction cannot control their behavior. Furthermore, if control of one's behavior is necessary for free will and moral responsibility, then many people with these and other psychiatric disorders would seem to lack free will and not be morally responsible for their actions.

But we need a clear definition of free will to test the plausibility of these claims and arguments. It is also necessary to test the claims and arguments in the two hypothetical cases I presented at the beginning of this section. The will can be defined as a set of conative, cognitive, and affective capacities. The will is free when these capacities enable us to control our behavior by guiding attention, thought, and action in accord with intentions and goals. Responsibility for behavior presupposes free will, which in turn presupposes the requisite guidance control. Given structural and functional abnormalities in the prefrontal cortex and amygdala, the violent offender and the psychopath presumably lacked control over their emotions and impulses and could not be responsible for their actions. In many cases, however, brain abnormalities alone will not explain violent, irrational, or otherwise socially inappropriate behavior. If this is correct, then brain imaging showing a brain abnormality by itself will not be enough to conclude that a person cannot control his or her thoughts and actions and cannot be responsible for them.

Philosophers debating free will can be divided roughly into two groups. "Incompatibilists" generally argue that free will requires the ability to do otherwise, which presupposes that alternative possibilities of action are open to us when we act. These alternative possibilities are incompatible with causal determinism, the theory that natural laws and events in the past jointly determine a unique causal chain into the future. This means that any action one performs at a particular time is the only action one could have performed at that time. Many incompatibilists also argue that free will requires that each of us must be the author and source of his or her actions, which cannot be the case if causal determinism is true. The conviction that alternative possibilities are open to us when we act, and that each of us is the author and source of his or her actions, suggests that causal determinism is false.[23] This is the "libertarian" version of incompatibilism, as distinct from the "hard determinist" version of incompatibilism, which says that we do not have free will because causal determinism is true.

In contrast, most "compatibilists" argue that free will does not require traditionally conceived alternative possibilities of choice and action. Compatibilists generally hold that one acts freely and responsibly when one chooses and acts in accord with one's autonomous motivational states in the absence of coercion, compulsion, or constraint. These motivational states are autonomous, in the sense that one generates them on one's own and consciously identifies with them after a period of critical reflection. Any alternative possibilities are internal rather than external to the agent. They are a function of different combinations of desires, beliefs, intentions, decisions, and the actions to which they lead, rather than possible states of affairs that an agent actualizes by acting. In these respects, free will and responsibility are compatible with causal determinism.[24]

This conception of free will is consistent with the evolutionary account of freedom recently defended by Daniel Dennett. He claims that as humans evolved, they developed the ability to speculate about the future, to consider possible threats that jeopardize their interests and plans, and to choose and act in ways that enable them to avoid these threats. Dennett calls this "evitability," and it confers an evolutionary advantage on humans by enhancing their survival.[25] On this view, the idea of being able to do otherwise is not understood in terms of alternative possibilities as external states of affairs. Instead, it is understood in terms of the mental capacity to deliberate, choose, and act in different ways. As such, it is perfectly compatible with causal determinism.

Neuroscientist Benjamin Libet has published results from experiments showing that the conscious intention to act is preceded by the activity of certain event-related potentials (ERPs) in certain regions of the brain.[26] Our conscious intention to act lags 300–500 milliseconds behind the unconscious brain events that lead to intentions. If free will requires that every event in the pathway leading to action be under our conscious control, then these experiments seem to suggest that the idea of conscious free will is an illusion.[27] Libet's experiments and results appear to threaten the libertarian conception of free will, which says that nothing outside of our conscious motivational states can influence our choices and actions without undermining our agency. Having free will and being responsible for our actions means having contra-causal freedom, the freedom to originate actions that are uncaused by prior events and influences. This is what makes one the author and source of one's actions. Not all libertarians would make this claim. Libertarians who focus on the source of our actions might argue that incompatibilist conditions of free will can be satisfied by undetermined unconscious events. Still, this does not resolve the question of how one can control one's thought and behavior if events in the brain and mind occur outside of one's conscious awareness.

The libertarian requirement for free will seems too strong. It is quite plausible to assume that we can be genuine authors of our actions if we are not impeded in consciously deliberating, choosing, and acting. If our motivational states are not compelled, coerced, or manipulated by artificial means, and if we have the capacity to reflect on, identify with, and execute these mental states in choices and actions, then we can act freely. This is a sufficiently causally robust sense of agency for us to be responsible for our actions. It is only when unconscious brain events interfere with these conscious capacities that the will might not be free. From the mere fact that a brain event precedes a mental event, it does not follow that the first impedes or forces the second.

As Stephen Morse points out, Libet's studies do not imply "that conscious intentionality does no causal work. They simply demonstrate that unconscious brain events precede conscious experience, but this seems precisely what one would expect of the mind-brain. It does not mean that intentionality plays no causal role. Indeed, Libet concedes that people can 'veto' the act, which is another form of mental act that plays a causal role."[28] Furthermore, the claim that all of our intentions and actions arise from unconscious brain events cannot explain the phenomenon of making up or changing one's mind. These events cannot explain why a person chooses and acts in a certain way when faced with two possible courses of action at the same time. Appeal to ERPs or other physical properties of the brain will not explain why a person makes one choice and performs one action rather than the other.

Libet's experiments involve an uncritical acceptance of the timing of brain events and mental events. It is assumed that each type of event occurs at a discrete measurable moment. Yet both types may involve a more extended temporal process. Libet's experiments also suggest that the causal pathway in human agency always goes from unconscious brain events to conscious mental events. But the etiology of depression, anxiety, and other mental illnesses indicates that the causal pathway can go in two directions. Conscious negative beliefs and feelings can cause dysfunction in unconscious brain states and events, which in turn may interfere with our ability to form and execute intentions in actions. In addition, Libet does not offer an explanation for how a mental act can "veto" an unconscious brain event.

Even if unconscious brain events always preceded conscious mental events, this would not threaten our control of our behavior or imply that we were not free and responsible agents. The discussion of the body's response to stimuli in chapter 2 supports this point. Recall the more primitive thalamic-amygdala and more advanced thalamic-cortical-amygdala sensory pathways in this response. The second as well as the first pathway can operate outside of one's conscious awareness. The mere fact that sensory processing occurs outside of one's awareness does not mean that one has no control of the conscious processing of desires, beliefs, intentions, and decisions that result in one's actions. In fact, our capacity for conscious beliefs enables us to discriminate between benign and threatening stimuli and thereby constrain unconscious brain processes. This capacity ensures that unconscious processes in our brains and bodies align with the actual nature of events in the external world.

It is only when brain dysfunction causes an abnormality in conscious sensory processing and decision-making that there might be mild, moderate, or severe impairment of control of our motivational states and behavior. In particular, it is only when abnormal neuronal mechanisms cause us to have exaggerated, blunted, or no responses to fear-inducing and other stimuli that these mechanisms can diminish or undermine our conscious control of our thoughts and actions. When these and other responses of the brain and mind are proportional to the actual nature of events in the social and natural environment, and when they do not impair or undermine our capacity to execute our motivational states in actions, there is no threat to our control of our behavior.

The weaker, compatibilist, sense of free will that I have described and defended can be traced to Aristotle. In the *Nicomachean Ethics*, Aristotle presents the default assumption that a person acts freely (voluntarily) and can be morally responsible for his or her behavior, barring evidence of compulsion, coercion, or ignorance of the circumstances of action.[29] The first two of these conditions can be described as metaphysical, or freedom-relevant, conditions, while the third can be described as a knowledge-relevant, or epistemic, condition. On the Aristotelian model, free will in the broad sense requires that all of these negative conditions be met. Each condition is necessary but not sufficient for the default assumption. All of them are jointly necessary and sufficient for the freedom of thought and action required for a person to act freely and responsibly. A more recent formulation of this conception is that free will consists in the capacity to respond to reasons for or against certain actions. These reasons are moral rather than prudential, in the sense that they involve social expectations about what we should or should not do in performing actions that can affect others. Reasons-responsiveness is an extension of Aristotle's view, because the capacity to respond appropriately to reasons presupposes the capacity for beliefs about the circumstances of action. Reasons-responsiveness also presupposes the capacity to voluntarily have and respond to desires, beliefs, emotions, and intentions and to voluntarily execute these motivational states in choices and actions.[30]

These conative, cognitive, and affective mental states are jointly necessary for a person to be morally responsible for his or her behavior. A person can be excused from responsibility for his or her behavior when any of the three conditions described by Aristotle is present. In any of these instances, the person lacks the requisite responsiveness to reasons to be responsible and can be excused. The impulsive actions of a violent offender or psychopath, the compulsive behavior of a person with OCD, and the delusional thoughts of a schizophrenic would appear to meet Aristotle's freedom-relevant and knowledge-relevant excusing conditions. Scans—PET, MRI, or fMRI—showing structural and functional brain abnormalities correlating with these disorders would appear to confirm that lack of control of thought and behavior, hence lack of free will, was due to something gone awry in the brain. Framed in this way, free will pertains not to the traditional notion of causal determinism and what natural laws and past events allow us to do. Rather it pertains to what we can do given the relation between the brain and the mind.

I am defending a capacity-theoretic conception of free will and responsibility. To act freely and be responsible for one's actions, one need only possess the relevant mental capacities. One need not exercise them in every instance. Yet free will is not an all-or-nothing capacity. It is a capacity that comes in degrees along a spectrum of control.[31] At one end of the spectrum, persons are in complete control of their behavior and are completely responsible for what they do or fail to do. At the other end of the spectrum, persons have no control of their behavior and should be completely excused from responsibility for what they do or fail to do. But many cases of criminal or otherwise harmful behavior fall in a gray area between the two ends. Just as there are degrees of responsiveness to reasons and degrees of control of behavior, so, too, there are degrees of free will and responsibility for behavior.

Some philosophers and neuroscientists invoke quantum theory to explain how events in the brain can occur in a nondeterministic way. They argue that this theory is necessary to explain how human agents can have free will. But we do not need to appeal to quantum theory to explain why people can or cannot control their behavior. Indeed, doing so will tell us little about whether people have the sort of control in question. When we want to know whether a person can restrain his or her violent impulses, can conform to social norms, or can recall performing a certain action, we need to know about the macro-level structures and functions of the brain systems that underlie these capacities. Whether micro-level neural events operate according to quantum theory will not shed much light on the practical and normative senses of free will we use to frame the debate on whether people can control their behavior and can be responsible for it.

There are important differences between moral responsibility and legal liability. In particular, strict liability has no equivalent in the moral domain. In most cases, though, moral and legal conceptions of responsibility presuppose certain mental capacities. The Model Penal Code version of the Not Guilty by Reason of Insanity (NGRI) defense has cognitive and volitional components in its mitigating and excusing conditions.[32] According to the first component, one is not guilty if one suffers from a mental illness causing one to be ignorant of what one is doing, or of not knowing the difference between right and wrong. According to the second component, one is not guilty if one suffers from a mental illness causing one to lose control of one's impulses. These legal judgments about guilt are practically equivalent to moral judgments about responsibility, and therefore we can use them interchangeably.

Different people may possess the cognitive, affective, and conative (volitional) capacities to control behavior in varying degrees. There are no problems in making this claim at either end of the spectrum. When there are no abnormalities in neuronal processing, Aristotle's default conditions can be met, and we can assume that one can control one's motivational states and behavior. In most cases, severe neurobiological abnormalities seem to violate the default conditions and provide strong reasons for saying that one could not control one's motivational states and behavior. The claim that a person with schizophrenia and severe impairment of cognitive, affective, and volitional capacities cannot control his or her behavior could be supported by correlations between these impairments and abnormalities in the basal ganglia, prefrontal cortex, and hippocampus. Similarly, the claim that a person with severe obsessive-compulsive disorder cannot control his or her behavior could be supported by correlations between the observable symptoms and abnormalities in the relevant cortical-limbic pathways. The question of behavior control in these cases could be analyzed further by contrasting brain images of individuals with these disorders with images of individuals who have no mental impairments and normal brain structure and function.

Still, the hard cases are those that fall between the middle and the abnormal end of the spectrum. An adolescent or adult with ADHD may have difficulty controlling his or her impulses and attending to cognitive tasks. These behavioral features may correspond to neuroimaging showing low levels of dopamine in the cerebellum and temporal lobes, which are indicators of the disorder. But there may be considerable variation in the ability of different people with the same disorder to control their thoughts and actions. It is not clear that these differences in behavior control will be solely a function of subtle differences in the activity of dopaminergic or other classes of neurons in the relevant brain regions.

In October 2004, the United States Supreme Court began reviewing the case of Christopher Simmons (*Roper v. Simmons*). Legally, the case raises the question of the constitutionality of the death penalty for young offenders. At a deeper level, it raises questions about how features of the adolescent brain influence our judgments about free will and moral responsibility for individuals in this age group. In 1993, the 17-year-old Simmons and a friend robbed a woman, tied her up with an electrical cable and duct tape, and threw her over a bridge into a river. Simmons was convicted of murder and sentenced to death by a Missouri court in 1994. But the Missouri Supreme Court dropped the death sentence in 2003, resentencing him to life in prison without parole. The state of Missouri then appealed to have the death penalty reinstated. In a 5-to-4 decision on March 1, 2005, the U.S. Supreme Court ruled that imposing the death penalty on convicted murderers who were younger than 18 at the time of their crimes is unconstitutional.

One of the arguments against execution in this case was that, when Simmons committed the crime, the frontal lobe of his brain was not yet mature. Presumably, this made him incapable of rational and moral decision-making and unable to restrain his violent impulses. Because the frontal lobe is critical to impulse control, reasoning, and decision-making, and because Simmons's frontal lobe was not yet fully developed, he was not capable of controlling his behavior at the time of his action and therefore was not responsible for his crime.[33] This would seem to be enough to excuse him and overturn his conviction. At most, it would justify life in prison—not the death penalty.

Structural MRI studies of the brains of children and adolescents show that the frontal lobe develops last of all brain regions. It does not mature until around 21 years of age.[34] These and other studies generally indicate that the brain regions of a child or adolescent function in a more localized way, with more activity in limbic areas than in the cortex. In contrast, adults have more distributive and collaborative interactions among different brain regions. While these interactions in the adult brain promote greater impulse control, immature development of these interactions makes impulse control more difficult for children and adolescents. In addition, adults have more experience confronting situations requiring rational deliberation, which can promote more effective regulation of behavior. Adults also have greater capacity to look further into the future and reason about the foreseeable consequences of their actions. Mature frontal lobes are necessary to regulate behavior in these respects.

But an immature brain alone cannot explain why Simmons committed murder or excuse him from moral and legal responsibility for his act. If all adolescents have immature frontal lobes, and not all adolescents commit violent acts, then simply saying that Simmons's frontal lobes were not fully developed does not provide a convincing reason to excuse him. If a comparison between Simmons's brain at 17 and the brains of others from the same age group could be made, then there might be some basis on which to argue that he lacked the capacity to control his impulse to kill. But the data required to make such a comparison could only be derived from longitudinal imaging studies involving a large number of subjects. These studies have not yet been conducted, and so the data are not yet available. Even if the data were available, they would not be conclusive. In addition to immature frontal lobes, social factors would have to be considered for a causal explanation of an offender's behavior. In the light of this, it is unclear to what extent earlier images of Simmons's brain structure and function at age 17 could have helped the U.S. Supreme Court justices to decide whether or not he had the capacity to control his behavior at the time of the crime. Unless we could conclusively show and agree on how much frontal lobe volume and function is necessary for any person to control his or her behavior, it is unclear to what extent brain imaging could help to answer the moral and legal question of Simmons's culpability.

In psychopaths, extensive damage to or reduction in volume of the amygdala may explain their abnormal reaction to fear-inducing stimuli. On this basis, one might argue that a psychopath was unable to conform to social norms when he or she acted. But it seems plausible that at least some psychopaths are capable of understanding what it means to harm others.[35] This might be enough to influence their motivational states and provide some restraint on their irrational, immoral, or illegal behavior. We could distinguish between individuals who cannot moderate their impulses and act in accord with social norms and those who have the capacity to do this but fail to exercise it. It is not clear how brain scans showing differences in amygdaloid volume, or scans showing differences in blood flow and metabolic activity in the OFC or anterior cingulate gyrus, could explain why one person could and another person could not act rationally and morally. Nor is it clear that the differences in the brain images of the two individuals alone could justify responsibility in one case and exoneration in the other.

A person's ability to consciously form motivational states and to restrain or execute them in action is influenced by the brain. But it can be influenced by factors in the social and natural environment as well. Social expectations can color our perception of the choices and actions that are open to us. Obstacles in the physical space in which we live or physical disabilities can limit the available options we can pursue. Contextual cues about the availability of a substance may play as much of a role in addiction as an abnormal mesolimbic dopamine system. Some people may put more mental effort than others into exercising their capacity to control their behavior. Just because one displays weakness of will does not mean that one lacks the capacity for control and thus lacks free will altogether. In addition, brain scans alone cannot explain the phenomenology of free will, or why we *feel* in control (or out of control) of our actions. This feeling can also influence one's perception of the courses of action that are open to one when one deliberates and makes decisions.

Many people with structural and functional brain abnormalities are not violent and do not display psychopathic behavior. So it is implausible to claim that brain abnormalities detected by neuroimaging always cause these types of behavior. Except in cases of severe dysfunction in regions of the brain directly regulating the capacity for moral reasoning and choice, how much control one has over one's behavior, and whether or to what extent one is responsible for it, will not be determined by measuring brain structure or function alone.

Regions other than the OFC may play a role in the cognitive and affective processing necessary for reasoning and decision-making. Focusing on this region alone may be an oversimplified way of explaining the link between the brain and behavior. An abnormality in this region does not necessarily mean that the balance between cognitive and emotional processing has been entirely disrupted. The parietal cortex, which regulates our orientation in space and time, may also play a role in maintaining this balance.[36] Moreover, while the cerebellum mainly regulates physical balance and coordination, it may also play a role in attention and thus may be another region of the brain involved in thought and behavior. Reasoning and executive functions depend on complex neuronal systems distributed through multiple regions of the cortex, and may involve subcortical regions as well. There are strong links between the executive center in the prefrontal cortex and the parietal cortex, as well as links between these regions and the cingulate gyrus in the limbic system and the cerebellum and basal ganglia in the motor system. So it is misleading to think that the ability to control behavior is confined to the frontal area.

There is no locus of free will in the brain. Dysfunction in one brain region that underlies our capacity for reasoning and choice does not necessarily imply that other regions are also dysfunctional. Nor does it imply that one regional dysfunction alone can undermine the relevant mental capacities. There are redundancies in the brain. Some systems can compensate for others that have been damaged and can perform the same tasks. This is one example of brain plasticity. Indeed, in some cases, plasticity occurs to such a degree that a person's capacity to control thought and behavior can remain intact despite extensive damage to brain regions that in most cases would undermine this capacity.

Todd Feinberg describes the case of a patient that supports this point. "Sonia" was a 32-year-old college graduate and executive secretary who was referred for a neurological exam because of mild paranoia.[37] Although her exam was normal, the neurologist noticed that her head was unusually large and ordered a CT scan. Surprisingly, the scan showed that more than three-quarters of her cerebral cortex was missing. All that remained was a band of cortex around the outside of her brain. Her fluid-filled lateral ventricles were abnormally large, a condition known as hydrocephalus. When this condition develops suddenly in an adult and is not surgically corrected, the patient falls into a coma. As Feinberg explains, this patient most likely survived with so many of her mental functions intact because the condition was present from birth, and her nervous system was able to accommodate itself gradually to the increased pressure. This patient's brain was remarkably able to adjust to damage that might have severely impaired another person's cognitive, emotional, and volitional capacities. A brain scan showing extensive damage to one or more regions of the brain underlying the conscious mind by itself does not prove that a person cannot control his or her behavior.

All of the hypothetical and actual cases I have presented and discussed thus far involve metaphysical criteria of free will and responsibility falling under the broadly construed category of compulsion. The epistemic condition of free will and responsibility requires the capacity to be cognizant or not ignorant of the circumstances of action. Because one's present actions can be part of a causal sequence traceable to earlier actions, the relevant epistemic capacity also includes the capacity to recall having performed actions at earlier times. If one's failure to perform an action at a later time results in harm to another, and the failure to act is causally linked to forgetting having performed an action at an earlier time, then one could be responsible for the harmful consequence on grounds of negligence. One would be responsible for both an omission and the harmful consequence of that omission. But that would depend on whether the person was cognitively able to recall the earlier action. Would a brain scan enable us to distinguish between a memory lapse caused by brain damage or dysfunction beyond one's cognitive control, and a lapse due to one's failure to exercise the capacity to recall the event? Would a brain scan help us to decide whether a person was responsible for an omission?

We need to distinguish five different types of memory.[38] *Procedural memory* involves the capacity to perform motor skills, such as driving a car or riding a bicycle. It is characterized as nondeclarative memory because it involves the unconscious capacity of remembering or knowing *how* to do things. The striatum and cerebellum regulate procedural memory. Procedural memory is distinct from unconscious *emotional memory* of fearful or threatening events. This is the most primitive memory system and the most critical for human survival. Through its interaction with the hippocampus, the amygdala regulates emotional memory. *Semantic memory* involves conceptual and factual knowledge and consists in remembering or knowing *that* something is the case. *Episodic memory* involves the capacity to recall events that we have personally experienced and consists in remembering or knowing *when* an event occurred. Episodic memory and semantic memory are characterized as types of declarative memory because they both involve the ability to consciously recall facts or events. *Working memory* is a type of short-term declarative memory. It is an active system for temporarily storing and manipulating information needed for the execution of complex cognitive tasks, such as deliberating, making decisions, and foreseeing consequences of decisions and actions. The prefrontal cortex regulates working memory by retrieving episodic and semantic memories from the hippocampus and other sites in the temporal lobes. These memories are permanently stored in different parts of the cerebral cortex. Given that our ability to deliberate and make decisions is based on the capacity to recall facts and events, long- and short-term declarative memory systems are interconnected.

Consider the case of Carrie Engholm, a hospital administrator, who drove to work one morning with her young son and daughter in the back of her van.[39] She was not accustomed to taking her daughter. After dropping off her son at day care, she drove to work, forgetting that her daughter was in the van. Unfortunately, her daughter was found dead from hyperthermia later on that day, on which the temperature had risen to over 100 degrees Fahrenheit. Was Carrie responsible for not remembering? Was she responsible for not paying attention to the act of putting her daughter in the van and forgetting it? When she was initially charged with recklessness and brought to court, the judge in the case ruled that she was not guilty. He reasoned that forgetting is an involuntary process. But would it have been reasonable to charge her with negligence, for failing to exercise her capacity to remember? Did she have or exercise the relevant control over her memory lapse? An fMRI scan can show that a particular region of the hippocampus, the parahippocampal gyrus, is activated when people are asked to recall events. This is the main region in which episodic memories are encoded for storage and from which they are retrieved by the prefrontal cortex in working memory. Damage to this region could impair one's ability to recall that a particular event occurred, or when it occurred. Would an fMRI scan of Carrie's parahippocampal gyrus have answered this question? What does this imply for the ethics of memory?

There are several complicating factors that make the question much less straightforward than it might appear at first blush. First, long-term episodic and semantic memory may influence, or be influenced by, short-term working memory. Carrie quite possibly was suffering from information overload at the critical time, with too many cognitive tasks to plan and execute. This could have led to a temporary retrieval block of her episodic memory of putting her daughter in the van. Such a block might have been caused by dysfunction in either the anterior cingulate or the prefrontal cortex, both of which project to the parahippocampal gyrus.[40] Nevertheless, a scan of these regions would not be very helpful after the fact, since they likely would not be activated to the same degree as they would be when one was trying to recall an event. Second, it is unlikely that an imaging device showing increased or decreased activity in these regions would be able to tell us whether she failed or was unable to retrieve the memory, or whether she even could have formed a memory of the event. As I have described it, the issue here is different from the distinction between true and false memories that has figured prominently in court cases involving charges of rape and incest. Third, and perhaps most important, data that would allow one to draw these critical distinctions would only be available from group studies. One would have to average data derived from imaging across many people before a particular image, or set of images, of a person could have any statistical significance.

There is one scenario in which a brain scan might support an argument for the claim that Carrie Engholm was not responsible for her omission. Her failure to remember leaving her daughter in the van may have been one example in a pattern of similar behavior over a period of time. On the basis of this behavior, a scan showing significant damage to her medial temporal lobes would suggest that it was causing anterograde amnesia. This damage would have prevented her from forming new memories and might have explained her inability to recall the critical event. The combination of the brain scan and her pattern of behavior might indicate that she could not be responsible for forgetting something she could not have remembered.

As this technique becomes refined, and databases of patient populations are formed, neuroimaging may eventually be able to help in ascertaining whether one could have remembered an event and prevented harm by responding appropriately to it. This might enable us to refine our criteria of responsibility for omissions. But presently imaging cannot determine whether one has formed and stored a memory of a particular event, or whether one can retrieve it.

To convincingly argue that a person has no control over his or her mental states and actions because of a brain abnormality, one would have to establish a causal connection between that abnormality and those states and actions. Brain scans can show correlations between structural and functional features of the brain and human behavior. But correlation is not necessarily the same as causation. An association of a brain event or set of brain events with an action does not imply that the action directly results from that brain event or set of events. This is one of the main shortcomings of using brain imaging as a technique to assess whether people have free will and can be responsible for their behavior. Imaging data could measure only the statistical likelihood of controllable or uncontrollable behavior over a population. It could not predict how an individual would behave in a particular circumstance. Nor is it clear whether a brain image from an fMRI scan could measure the exercise of free will at specific times, or only independent neurological events and processes that underlie it. Brain-based measures of psychological traits have an illusory accuracy and objectivity. A PET or fMRI scan showing abnormal activity in a region of the brain is not necessarily diagnostic, because it can be modulated by the experimental tasks taken by the researcher to mimic actual functions of the scanner. There is also the potential for bias in the design of functional imaging experiments using brain-damaged patients. What the researcher hopes to find as a result of doing the experiment may strongly influence the way he or she designs and conducts it. This can also influence how data from experiments are analyzed.

The researcher is not the only individual who might have a biased view of brain images. More troublesome is the potential bias of third parties in interpreting these images. If this bias could be eliminated from the design and interpretation of neuroimaging, and the technique could be refined, then we might have a more accurate picture of how the brain influences the mind and behavior. But, as cognitive neuroscientist Martha Farah points out, "for now . . . this is not the case, and there is the risk that juries, judges, parole boards, the immigration service and so on will weigh such measures too heavily in their decision-making." [41] There is considerable potential for abuse of information derived from scans and harm to people who undergo them. One area of potential abuse is forensic brain imaging for assessing criminal liability.

"Brain fingerprinting" has been used in criminal investigations in Iowa and Missouri and might seem superior to polygraph measures. [42] Polygraph machines have an estimated accuracy of around 85 percent in correlating physiological reactions with the falsity of a speaker's testimony. American courts have generally rejected polygraph evidence, on the ground that it is not reliable enough to influence or support judgments about liability. This position has been firmly upheld by a 2003 report by the National Academy of Sciences, which concluded that there is little scientific evidence that polygraphs can identify dishonest responses with any certainty. [43] A polygraph measures physiological responses such as heart rate, sweating, breathing, and other processes that are only indirectly related to brain function. A more advanced technique for detecting deceit in the brain is the use of electrodes to measure ERPs. These brain events were mentioned in Libet's discussion and can indicate the electrical activity of neurons in response to a stimulus, such as a word or image. One type of ERP is the P300 response, which occurs about 300 milliseconds before a mental event and is supposed to be beyond a subject's conscious control. But subjects can imagine certain events during each stimulus and thereby manipulate their responses in ways that can render the test useless.

Some might be inclined to think that neuroimaging could detect lying because it can directly measure brain function. Brain regions activated by lying could be displayed through fMRI. But this work is very preliminary and is still considered a research tool. [44] Because of its illusory accuracy, diagnostic neuroimaging for brain fingerprinting would be even more controversial than polygraphs in trying to measure the truthfulness of a witness' testimony, or in depicting a criminal's state of mind. Technology has a seductive appeal to the general public. In the courtroom, juries are far less likely to question the results of a "scientific" test than the testimony of a witness. Yet, there is no reason to think that brain imaging could provide an accurate picture of a person's state of mind. Moreover, it is questionable whether defendant or nondefendant witnesses could be compelled to undergo brain scans, or whether they could decline by invoking their privilege of non-incrimination, as guaranteed by the Fifth Amendment. Most states have banned the polygraph as evidence in courts of law. For the reasons I have just cited, the use of current neuroimaging for this purpose should be banned as well.

Even if functional neuroimaging were developed to the point where it could accurately measure the brain processes associated with desires, beliefs, intentions, and decisions, it would not provide simple answers to normative questions such as whether or to what degree people can act freely and can be responsible for their behavior. The thoughts of Donald Kennedy, editor-in-chief of *Science*, offer intuitive support for this view:

> As we learn more about the neurobiology of choice and decision, will we reach a point at which we feel less free? Perhaps more important for society, will we eventually know enough to change our view about individual responsibility for antisocial acts? There are those who worry about this. I am not among them, only because it seems so unlikely to me that our knowledge of the brain will deepen enough to fuse it with the mind.[45]

One of the principal reasons why we should not worry too much about neurobiology in the context of free will is that judgments about individual responsibility will always be influenced by social norms. This point follows from what may be the strongest reason for questioning the use of neuroimaging to make ethical or legal judgments about people's behavior. It involves a move from empirical claims about the brain to normative claims about how people ought to behave. Free will and responsibility fundamentally are not empirical but normative notions reflecting social conventions and expectations about how people can or should act. Besides, the examples I have presented show that in most cases empirical measures of brain structure and function alone will not tell us whether a person had or lacked the requisite control of his or her mental states presupposed by free agency and responsibility. Our behavior is not all hardwired in the brain. We hold persons, not their brains, responsible for their behavior because persons are not reducible to their brains.

This does not suggest that persons and brains are independent entities. Persons are constituted by but are not identical to their brains. We hold persons responsible on the basis of the mental states that issue in their actions, and these states are generated and sustained by the brain. But the content of these mental states, the external events to which they are directed, cannot be explained entirely by reference to their neural correlates. The reasons we adduce for holding persons responsible for actions and omissions may very well be influenced, but are not determined, by what we know about the brain. Although our understanding of free will and responsibility may become better informed by brain science, normative claims and judgments cannot be reduced to empirical ones. It is not neuroscientists but society that will decide how empirical information about the brain influences our judgments about what constitutes free will and when people can be held responsible for their behavior. Morality is not just a function of neurobiology.

In the future, higher resolution brain scans may enable researchers to more precisely identify features of the brain involved in the regulation of reasoning and executing intentions in actions. They may also enable researchers to distinguish between true and false memories, determine whether people can form and retrieve memories, and discern whether people are lying or telling the truth. Ideally, the combination of this technology and established clinical criteria will contribute to a clearer understanding of the difference between full responsibility on the one hand and excuse or mitigation on the other. If brain scans could enable us to move from a correlation to a causal connection between the brain and the mind, then the information derived from functional neuroimaging could be a helpful diagnostic and forensic tool indeed.

Yet brain imaging cannot capture the influence of environmental factors on the mind. Nor can it capture all of the phenomenological features of mental effort in making up or changing one's mind. These subjective properties cannot be visualized on any brain scans. For these and other reasons, the goal of using imaging to establish a causal connection between the brain and the mind remains elusive. Neuroimaging alone will not tell us whether the violent offender and psychopath introduced at the beginning of this section could control and were responsible for their behavior. It will not enable us to distinguish between not having the capacity for reasoning and impulse control and having but failing to exercise this capacity. Images of the brain will not threaten our practice of praising people for positive actions either. Scans of normal brain structure and function will not lead us to believe that we are any less praiseworthy for what we do. They will not threaten our capacity to control how our motivational states issue in our actions or our conviction that we are autonomous agents. In the absence of a causal connection between the brain and behavior, one cannot claim that the brain determines behavior. For this same reason, there is no basis on which to claim that neuroscience implies that our belief in free will is an illusion.

Given its limitations, brain imaging should, at most, supplement, not supplant, existing criteria of responsibility in the moral domain and criteria of liability in the legal domain. Because it is still an imprecise science, it will be some time before diagnostic brain imaging becomes a useful tool for evaluating human behavior. If it does, then it most likely will be used to support mitigating or excusing conditions on grounds of significant brain abnormalities that interfere with the capacity for reasoning and impulse control. Even so, as a society we will still have to decide whether or how information about the brain can or should be used for such things as evidence in criminal law, analogous to the way in which DNA evidence is now used. Brain imaging will probably play a limited role in these decisions. Many factors outside the brain will always influence our judgments about responsibility.

Predictive Neuroimaging

Diagnostic and predictive forms of brain imaging are used for different patient populations. While the purpose of the first is to confirm a suspected condition, the purpose of the second is to estimate whether individuals with certain risk factors for neuropsychiatric diseases will develop them. Although these individuals are considered to be at risk, they are asymptomatic. One of the risk factors is genetics, and predictive imaging might be helpful in identifying individuals at high risk of mental illness on the basis of genetic inheritance. In this respect, predictive imaging can be more useful than diagnostic imaging as one component of endophenotype analysis of genetically complex neuropsychiatric diseases. This is especially relevant to later onset forms of these diseases. Imaging may reveal subtle changes in brain morphology and biochemistry that may be markers of neurodevelopmental disorders such as schizophrenia or neurodegenerative disorders such as Alzheimer's. Early identification of these markers may lead to pharmacological interventions that might prevent or slow the progression of these diseases or alleviate their symptoms.

In schizophrenia, for example, MRI studies have shown that structural brain abnormalities are already present by the time patients are first evaluated. There appear to be ongoing changes in the brains of schizophrenic patients during the initial years after diagnosis despite antipsychotic drug treatment. Structural and functional imaging may enable psychiatrists and neurologists to track the progression of these abnormalities. In particular, periodic imaging can show the progressive reduction in gray matter in the frontal lobe. This feature may indicate brain pathology when compared with the normal trajectory of volume enlargement in the brains of adolescents.[46]

In one study, brain scans of adolescents considered to be at high risk for schizophrenia showed reduction in the volume of gray matter in the frontal and temporal lobes, as well as in the anterior cingulate gyrus and the temporal gyrus.[47] The reduction became more apparent once they had developed psychotic symptoms and a diagnosis of schizophrenia was made. These anatomical abnormalities, together with functional abnormalities associated with excess dopamine, have been linked to the disrupted cognitive processing, poor executive functioning, and blunted emotions that are symptomatic of the disease. Most significant about this study was that the early imaging could predict that the patients would eventually develop full-blown symptoms.

Schizophrenia is perhaps the most debilitating of psychiatric disorders. It is such a devastating disease because it strikes people at an age when they are still developing their mental capacities and life potential. The magnitude of suffering and lost opportunities for people with the disorder is substantial. Even with antipsychotic treatment, the prognosis for schizophrenics is often poor, and many are unable to have normal lives. Imaging may facilitate early detection and intervention that might improve the prognosis. This is especially significant in the early-onset form of the disease because of the rapidly changing neuronal circuitry in adolescents. The dynamic nature of neurons at this early age may make them more responsive to pharmacological agents and thereby increase the probability of a therapeutic effect on the affected brain regions.

It has been estimated that between 60 and 80 percent of dopaminergic neurons may have been lost in patients with Parkinson's disease before the appearance of any symptoms of motor dysfunction. Imaging may be able to detect this loss and lead to early pharmacological intervention that may delay the onset of symptoms and slow the progression of the disease. This would result in better quality of life for affected individuals. Imaging may also detect signs of Alzheimer's disease before the appearance of memory loss, personality change, and dementia. PET scans can display the characteristic amyloid plaques and neurofibrillary tangles of this disease. Imaging might even be perfected to the point where it could show the first signs of loss of cholinergic neurons in the hippocampus, prefrontal cortex, and other brain regions. Some researchers and clinicians believe that this feature precedes the plaques and tangles in the pathogenesis of the disease. Although its predictive power is still relatively weak, further advances in neuroimaging may enable neurologists to estimate at a young age who would develop Alzheimer's. Electroencephalography (EEG) can reveal brain abnormalities that might predict whether people in their sixties and seventies will develop dementia. Yet these indications, at best, appear around 10 years before the onset of symptoms, and imaging may reveal signs of dementia at a much earlier stage of life. Periodic PET scans can reveal subtle changes in the hippocampus, prefrontal cortex, and other regions of the brains of Alzheimer's patients as the disease progresses over time.

In addition, fMRI scans can enable neurologists to monitor the effects of drugs such as donepezil and memantine for treatment of Alzheimer's. The first of these drugs blocks the overproduction of the enzyme cholinesterase and prevents the breakdown of the chemical messenger acetylcholine. The second drug counteracts the overproduction of glutamate, which can kill brain cells. Each of these neurotransmitters plays an important role in the disease. Some studies suggest that the combination of donepezil and memantine may provide some benefit to patients in the early stage of Alzheimer's in terms of cognition and other quality-of-life measures. Structural and functional imaging can provide a clearer picture of the effects of these drugs.

The combination of brain imaging and drug therapy may be particularly beneficial to people with the mutation on the APOe4 allele of the gene for the beta-amyloid precursor protein. These individuals have a very high risk of developing Alzheimer's by the time they are 40. Knowing that there is a strong genetic component to this early-onset form of the disease provides a reason for using brain imaging to detect its earliest signs. A smaller number of cholinergic neurons could be a reliable predictor of Alzheimer's and warrant early pharmacological intervention. If drugs could control levels of acetylcholine and glutamate, then early drug therapy might prevent, or at least delay, the onset of the disease. Similarly, brain scans could be used for adolescents and perhaps also children with a high genetic risk of schizophrenia who already display subtle cognitive symptoms of this disease. Scans showing abnormalities in the frontal and temporal lobes, anterior cingulate gyrus, and basal ganglia might predict schizophrenia and justify early dopamine-blocking pharmacological intervention as well.

It remains unclear which structural or functional brain abnormalities can accurately predict a later onset disease in individuals who are asymptomatic. Although there may be correlations between earlier brain abnormalities and later behavioral abnormalities, these are not equivalent to a causal relation between them. And causation should be the basis for prediction. Brain volume can vary by as much as 10 percent from one person to the next. Having less gray matter in the brain, then, does not necessarily mean that one will develop a psychopathology.

Neither does smaller amygdaloid or frontal lobe volume, or abnormal metabolic activity in either of these brain regions, necessarily mean that a person will commit violent or criminal acts. It is doubtful that neuroimaging could ever predict human behavior. These considerations should give us pause in thinking about early pharmacological intervention on the basis of subtle structural or functional brain abnormalities detected by brain imaging.

This point has especially significant implications for schizophrenia, given the serious side effects of the dopamine-blocking agents used to treat it. Newer generation atypical antipsychotics are not significantly more effective than older generation drugs. The newer drugs are not much better at minimizing side effects either.[48] In fact, all of these antipsychotic agents have been associated with an increased risk of movement disorders such as akathisia and tardive dyskinesia, metabolic and endocrine disorders such as hyperlipidemia and diabetes, and hematological disorders.[49] Administering any of these drugs on predictive rather than definitive diagnostic grounds might mean that an iatrogenic condition would result from treatment for a possible condition that never would have developed. The presumed cure might very well be worse than the predicted disease. This point is important because of the changing neural circuitry in children and adolescents. Administering potent drugs during this period may result in permanent deleterious effects on their brains.

Still, the risk of using these drugs must be weighed against the risk of not using them and possibly allowing full-blown schizophrenia to develop for those who are at high risk of having this disease. This weighing is difficult, because, unlike the APOe4 mutation for Alzheimer's, the genetic mutations collectively implicated in schizophrenia have a lower degree of penetrance. The genetic component in schizophrenia is probably more significant than it is in other psychiatric diseases. Still, any one of the genes associated with schizophrenia has much less than 100 percent penetrance. Whether the mutation expresses itself and is a cause of the disease, and how it affects the severity of the disease, will depend on epigenetic and environmental factors. The results of a recent study comparing the antipsychotic drug olanzapine with a placebo have increased doubts about the benefits of preemptive treatment for schizophrenia. Patients in the study who received the active medication showed only a modest delay in acute psychotic episodes and experienced weight gain and other side effects.[50]

In the case of Alzheimer's, should predictive neuroimaging be offered for a future neurological illness when no cure is available? The crux of the discussion should be whether such imaging offers any benefit to those who undergo it. Currently, there is no clear medical benefit. Predictive neuroimaging would be medically beneficial if it led to a vaccine, cholinesterase inhibitor, or other intervention that delayed the onset of Alzheimer's or controlled its progression. In 2001, the drug company Elan launched a clinical trial in the United States and Europe involving several hundred volunteers to test a vaccine for the disease. But the trial was stopped prematurely when some participants showed signs of brain inflammation after receiving three of the six planned inoculations. Clinical trials of cholinesterase inhibitors such as donepezil have been conducted and have shown some benefits in some patients with early-stage Alzheimer's. In addition, initial studies involving antiinflammatory drugs suggested that they might lessen the risk of developing this disease.

But the results of these studies have not been replicated, and therefore a protective effect of these drugs has not been proven.[51] Although drugs such as donepezil may improve cognitive functioning in early stages of the disease, and although other classes of drugs such as memantine may slow its progression, these drugs cannot reverse the disease. Any beneficial effects of cholinesterase inhibitors and glutamate antagonists have been quite modest.[52] The effects of donepezil in some patients indicate that it may increase the risk of heart disease, which would weaken the reasons for prescribing it. Other studies have suggested that cholesterol-lowering statins and immunizations could be promising treatments for Alzheimer's because of their potential to inhibit the production of beta-amyloid plaques. At this point, however, there is no clear indication that these or any of the other pharmacological interventions mentioned could effectively treat or prevent the disease.[53] Even in the best case scenario, such drugs would likely not be available for another 10 to 20 years. And although drugs that might modestly slow the progression of Alzheimer's could help care-givers, they might do more to prolong patient's suffering if they cannot treat its symptoms.

In the light of these considerations, informing a person that scans of his or her brain show early signs of the dread disease could harm him or her by causing anxiety about the future. Given that this disease involves a gradual erosion of all components of the self, this knowledge could darken one's perception of the future and the remaining years of life. The magnitude of this harm could be greater the earlier in life one had this information. This is analogous in some respects to the potential harm in predictive presymptomatic testing for a late-onset genetic disease like Huntington's. Similar concern applies to brain images suggesting some type of future psychopathology. Adolescents, as well as their parents and other parties, may interpret an abnormality in the orbitofrontal cortex or amygdala as though a mental disorder were somehow written into their neurons. Unless the abnormality is significant, however, there is no solid basis on which to draw such a conclusion. Images showing brain abnormalities may indicate a susceptibility to a neurodegenerative disease or psychopathology. But they do not determine that a person will in fact have these conditions.

On the other hand, knowing that one would likely develop a neurodegenerative disease like Alzheimer's could enable one to plan one's life more prudently. It could mean putting more weight on undertaking and completing projects earlier in life. This knowledge could move one to rationally discount the further future, when one might not have the cognitive capacity to undertake or complete projects or be consciously aware of one's surroundings. In this regard, people could benefit psychologically from predictive information about their brains, even if they could not benefit medically from any intervention.

Similar reasons have been given for predictive genetic testing for Huntington's.[54] But there are significant differences between predictive genetic testing and predictive neuroimaging. The test for Huntington's is highly accurate and can tell a person whether he or she has the genetic mutation that causes the disease. Because the mutation has high penetrance, one can know on the basis of the genetic test whether one will develop Huntington's. Neuroimaging detecting early brain anomalies that may be associated with Alzheimer's cannot accurately predict whether one will develop this disease. For those who already have Alzheimer's, cholinesterase inhibitors might offer a modest delay of memory loss and general cognitive decline. This may be more than what people with Huntington's can hope for, since treatments to control its progression are less effective. Nevertheless, the emotional fallout of information from predictive neuroimaging for conditions without effective treatments can be devastating, regardless of the condition in question. The psychological harm in predicting Alzheimer's may be greater than it is in predicting Huntington's, given the greater degree of uncertainty in brain imaging compared with genetic testing. In the absence of a known causal connection between early brain abnormalities and later neurological and psychiatric disorders, the potential psychological harm to people undergoing predictive neuroimaging recommends that this technique should be conducted with careful regulation and oversight.

Predictive neuroimaging is still in the experimental stage. Its applications are not yet proven. As in other forms of medical research, clinical trials involving MRI, PET, and fMRI scans have been designed where subjects are separated into experimental and control arms. The first group includes people who are considered to have a significant risk of developing one of the neuropsychiatric disorders I have been discussing. For example, the adolescents with early signs of schizophrenia in the study mentioned at the beginning of this section were in the experimental arm of that study. Risk is determined by family history or by the presence of a known genetic cause. Subjects in the control group are not considered to be at risk and serve as a normal standard of comparison for the experimental group.

Suppose that some of the volunteers in the control group in one of these trials are healthy and have none of the typical risk factors, but brain scans show them to have less gray matter in the prefrontal cortex than what is considered normal for the population. As we have seen in schizophrenia, this feature of the brain may be an early sign of psychopathology. This and other anomalies may also be the first signs of neurodegenerative diseases. However, an anomaly in the gray matter or other features of the brain does not necessarily mean that an individual with that anomaly will develop a disease of the brain. Nor can the appearance of brain anomalies early in life predict that those who have them will in fact engage in violent or criminal behavior later in life. Individuals with suspicious brain images might be treated with drugs and exposed to their risks for a psychiatric or neurological disease that would never actually develop. Or a disease indicated by these images might progress so slowly that they would probably die of other causes before the onset of any symptoms.

What should the researcher do with these incidental findings?[55] Should he or she tell these subjects that their brain scans indicate a predisposition to a neuropsychiatric disease? Should the researcher tell this to the parents who consented to participation in the trial on behalf of their children? Given the possibility that a less-than-normal amount of gray matter may be an indication of later mental illness, is the researcher obligated to disclose this information? Or is he or she obligated not to inform them, given the uncertainty about what these findings might predict and the likelihood of causing fear and anxiety in subjects and their parents? If the risk of developing a neurodegenerative disease or a psychopathology is not known, then would there be more harm than benefit from informing controls of the results of these brain scans?

It is crucial that the researcher inform all subjects of the aim of a predictive neuroimaging clinical trial, what brain scans might reveal, and the uncertainty about what these findings might suggest for later onset neurological and psychiatric conditions. Given the ambiguity about the medical significance of brain scans, fully informing patients and subjects requires telling them about the uncertainty in interpreting information derived from these scans. The researcher is obligated to explain and discuss this uncertainty with subjects or their surrogates before the trial begins. This obligation regarding predictive medical information is significantly different from the obligation for physicians to disclose all relevant diagnostic medical information to patients in clinical settings. In these settings, disclosure of medical information is necessary for a patient to give valid informed consent to treatment for a particular condition. Unlike predictive information, diagnostic information is more certain and therefore critical to selecting effective treatment. In predictive neuroimaging trials, it is only when researchers point out the uncertainty about what the information might or might not predict for late-onset psychiatric or neurodegenerative disorders that subjects can give valid informed consent to participate in these trials. This pertains both to subjects assigned to the experimental group of the trial and those assigned to the control group.

Even in the best of circumstances, information obtained from clinical trials can easily be misunderstood. This problem may be more acute in predictive neuroimaging than in other areas of medical research because of people's general difficulty in assessing probability and risk. It is complicated further by the uncertainty surrounding the medical significance of structural and functional brain anomalies. Researchers and clinicians have an obligation to point out to subjects and patients that predictive brain scanning is not an exact science. This can minimize the risk of psychological harm in interpreting the information from the scans. It can help to prevent distress in individuals who might otherwise think that their presumed normal brains were not so "normal" after all.

The uncertainty in these experiments requires that consent to participate in them must consist in more than simply signing a consent form. Instead, consent must be an ongoing process of dialogue between the researcher and the subject. As in any form of medical research, the consent form only documents this process. This includes the researcher's explanation that the purpose of research is to obtain valid scientific information that could benefit future patients. In the hypothetical case at hand, the researcher would be required to explain that the general purpose of the imaging study was to gain a better understanding of the relation between brain anomalies and mental illness. But, again, the fact that our understanding of the brain is limited makes it imperative that researchers and clinicians be especially careful in explaining the design and purpose of these trials to subjects and patients. The same obligation of careful explanation extends from adults to parents of adolescents with early symptoms of schizophrenia, who may be asked to consent to their children's participation in an imaging study. The promise of neuroimaging for predicting a wide range of neuropsychiatric diseases must be weighed against the potential psychosocial harm to individuals who would have to live with what can be ambiguous information about their brains. Because different people may interpret and respond to this information in different ways, weighing the potential benefit against the potential harm of predictive brain imaging should be done on a case-by-case basis.

How a researcher or clinician presents and explains information about the brain to a subject or patient, and how a patient or subject interprets and responds to this information, are not the only ethically significant issues in predictive neuroimaging. In a way that is analogous to the use of genetic information indicating a predisposition to a disease, insurers or employers may use information from brain scans to discriminate against people seeking employment or medical insurance. They may be denied employment or insurance because of the perceived long-term cost and risk of employing or insuring an asymptomatic person with a brain anomaly. With the exception of high-penetrance monogenic diseases, just because one is genetically predisposed to a disease does not mean that one will have that disease. A genetic mutation associated with a disease may or may not express itself in a disease phenotype in every person. Similarly, just because an asymptomatic individual has a structural or functional brain anomaly does not mean that this individual will develop a neurological or psychiatric disease.

Unless there is a known causal connection between a brain scan and a subsequent mental illness with a high risk of violent or otherwise harmful behavior, in most cases, information about the brain should remain confidential. This pertains both to the relationship between researchers and research subjects and to the relationship between clinicians and patients. Because this information is so personal and sensitive, the potential for harm to people in having it disclosed to third parties such as employers or insurers could be substantial.

This does not mean that information about the brain should never be disclosed to third parties. Motor vehicle registries would be justified in requesting information about individuals based on brain scans if they indicated a high probability of psychosis or seizures. Clearly, people at high risk of having these symptoms would pose a significant risk of harm to themselves and others if they drove motor vehicles. Employers might also be justified in requesting this information if it meant that workers had a high probability of developing behavior that posed a risk of harm to themselves or other employees. It may be more difficult to override confidentiality and justify disclosure of information about the brain to health insurance companies. Yet, in these days of managed care and the mandate to control costs by minimizing risk, the standard for confidentiality is becoming increasingly difficult to uphold. It could be challenging to ensure confidentiality of patients' medical information with the move toward electronic medical records, to which third parties could gain access. The Genetic Information Non-Discrimination Act, passed by the U.S. Congress in October 2003, protects confidentiality of genetic information. In October 2005, IBM announced that it would not use genetic information in hiring or in determining eligibility for its health care or benefits plans. Similar legislation and company policies in the future could protect confidentiality of information about people's brains for the purpose of securing and retaining medical insurance.

Predictive neuroimaging may become a useful tool in identifying the first signs of neurological and psychiatric conditions. It may also enable researchers to distinguish between neurodevelopmental and neurodegenerative diseases. It could lead to earlier and more effective pharmacological intervention to prevent or control the progression of these diseases. But it is not known what imaging might predict about future medical conditions, which could lead to considerable abuse, discrimination, and harm. Accordingly, predictive brain scans should be used primarily, if not exclusively, to track nervous system disorders with a known family history or genetic cause indicating a high risk of having them. Subjects in the control arm of a predictive imaging clinical trial should have the right to choose whether or not to have information about incidental brain anomalies disclosed to them. This is in addition to their right to be informed about the design and purpose of the trial. There should also be general agreement within the research and clinical community about the medical rationale for and medical significance of these scans. This should reflect what is currently based on empirical evidence, what might be technically feasible, and what should be done to protect populations at risk. In these respects, individuals undergoing predictive neuroimaging should be covered by the same protections afforded to human subjects in other areas of medical and biotechnological research.[56]

Conclusion

Neuroimaging may help to improve the prediction, diagnosis, and treatment of a wide range of neurological and psychiatric diseases. Brain scans may also shed light on the neurobiological basis of our thought and behavior. They may have implications for free will and moral responsibility, as well as for legal liability. Brain scans could influence judgments about liability, mitigation, and excuse. But images of our brains are not perfect representations of our minds. There is considerable uncertainty surrounding the moral and legal meaning of these images, which should temper claims regarding what they might indicate about our ability to control our behavior. In medicine, uncertainty surrounding the significance of subtle structural and functional brain abnormalities should also temper claims that brain imaging could predict who would develop neuropsychiatric diseases. Neuroimaging should supplement, not supplant, existing diagnostic and predictive criteria in clinical and experimental medicine and diagnostic forensic criteria in the criminal law.

Some may find other emerging forms of neuroimaging to be more disturbing. For example, "neuromarketing" uses fMRI scanning to study consumer behavior.[57] Seeing which brain circuits are activated when people decide to buy items could enable companies to market their goods more effectively. But concerns that using neuroimaging for this purpose is a form of Orwellian thought control seem exaggerated. There is no evidence that marketing agencies could use scanning techniques to implant subliminal messages in the unconscious mind and determine which goods people purchased. Nevertheless, even if imaging could not be used to manipulate people's desires or intentions to buy certain goods, there is a general, if not universal, conviction that consumer preferences should be private and not accessible to other parties under any circumstances. Consistent with the principle of respect for individual autonomy, individuals have the right to privacy of sensitive information about themselves. Information about the brain that must be shared with health care providers should remain confidential in most cases. Because brain imaging cannot read people's minds, there is considerable potential for abuse of information about the brain and its relation to the mind. Polices and laws need to be formulated, implemented, and enforced to prevent such abuse.

All of the issues that I have discussed clearly indicate the extent to which privacy and confidentiality of information about the brain is so medically, legally, and ethically sensitive and significant. For this reason, how imaging studies should be conducted and how information derived from them should be used need to be discussed on a more general level. In the words of LeDoux: "Such studies force us to confront ethical decisions as a society. How far should we go in using brain imaging to read minds, and how should we use the information we discover? It is testimony to the progress being made that these questions need to be asked."[58] More accurately, it is not the presumed ability of brain imaging to read minds, but our tendency to misread minds with imaging, which generates most of the ethical problems in this area.

Pharmacological and Psychological Interventions

The development of new-generation psychotropic drugs over the last 20 years has radically transformed the practice of psychiatry. They have enabled psychiatrists to more safely and effectively treat symptoms of patients with major depressive disorder, attention deficit/hyperactivity disorder, obsessive-compulsive disorder, general anxiety disorder (GAD), and other types of mental illness. In particular, SSRIs have replaced older tricyclics and monoamine oxidase inhibitors as the drugs of choice for treating depression. Drugs that can modulate stress hormones secreted inside and outside the brain and thereby regulate cognition and mood are being developed as a novel class of antidepressants and anxiolytics, which treat anxiety and panic disorders. These include SNRIs and CRF-receptor and beta-adrenergic antagonists.

Although the reasons are unclear, the incidence of mental illness has increased among the general population worldwide. This has resulted in a corresponding increase in the prescription and use of psychotropic drugs. I described some of the adverse effects of neuroleptics in people with schizophrenia in the last chapter. Data indicate that the adverse effects of antidepressants are generally not as serious, though they may include the risk of suicide and are therefore significant. Still, patients taking these drugs are sick, and any risks associated with them must be weighed against their benefits in controlling symptoms and improving patients' quality of life. More controversial is the off-label use of certain drugs to alter normal brain biochemistry and enhance normal cognitive and affective capacities. Those who use psychotropic drugs for this purpose do not have mental illness, yet they may be exposing themselves to some risk.

In this chapter, I consider potential benefits and harms of actual and possible uses of psychopharmacological agents for prevention, therapy, and enhancement. These include using drugs to prevent or erase memories of fear-arousing events. They also include drugs that could alter the neural circuitry of violent offenders. I then explore placebos as a psychological intervention and their effects on the brain and mind, focusing on whether it can be ethical to give placebos to treat symptoms associated with different medical conditions. Finally, I consider possible off-label uses of drugs for enhancing cognition and mood. In addition to questions about potential benefit and harm to individuals, these uses raise the question of whether they would reduce or increase social inequality. These considerations rest on a broader question. Before we pharmacologically tinker with hormones, neurotransmitters, or neurons to improve attention, memory, or mood, we should ask how the relevant brain and bodily systems interact, and whether these interactions serve an adaptive purpose. Whether we intervene in the brain pharmacologically or psychologically should be motivated by whether it is in our short- and long-term best interests to do so.

Therapeutic Psychopharmacology

The SSRIs and SNRIs treat depression by modulating the reuptake of serotonin and norepinephrine in the synaptic cleft between neurons. Other psychotropic agents modulate the dopamine system that can also play a role this disorder. All of these agents can restore the critical neurotransmitters to normal levels. Many patients diagnosed with MDD improve in their cognitive, affective, and volitional capacities as a result of taking antidepressant drugs. Left untreated, the disorder can progress, leading to further deterioration of mental functions. Untreated major depression may also have pathophysiological consequences in systems outside the brain. Figure 5, in chapter 2, illustrates some of these consequences.

Initial studies have indicated that newer classes of antidepressants could stimulate neurogenesis, the development of new neurons to replace those lost through depression. This involves the activation of growth factors in the brain. Studies using PET and MRI have found a correlation between depression and loss of serotonergic neurons in the prefrontal cortex and hippocampus of many patients with this illness. Sustained use of antidepressants may spur the growth of new neurons in these brain regions, especially the hippocampus.[1] With more neuronal receptors for serotonin, SSRIs can bind to these receptors and have a salutary effect on mood by increasing serotonin levels in the brain.

Another reason for using antidepressants to treat MDD is that in many cases cognitive-behavioral therapy and other psychotherapeutic approaches are not sufficient by themselves to restore normal brain and mental functions. As noted in chapter 3, imaging studies indicate that the effect of psychotherapy in the prefrontal cortex diminishes in subcortical regions of the brain. Conversely, psychotropic drugs have a stronger effect on subcortical regions and a weaker effect on the cortex. This is probably because beliefs and other mental states emerge from the cortex and are only indirectly linked to subcortical regions. Because psychological and pharmacological therapies affect different regions of the brain, combining these two modalities may be necessary to effectively treat depression. In this and other mental disorders, not one but many brain regions are implicated.

Although psychiatrists know that psychotropic drugs can modulate subcortical and cortical functions, they do not fully understand the molecular mechanisms of these drugs as they act on the brain. If they do not know precisely how they work, then they cannot know what the long-term effects of these drugs will be on neural circuitry. The fact that some patients taking SSRIs experience serious side effects clearly indicates that these drugs are not always beneficial to those who take them. One goal of long-term use of antidepressants is to reverse depletion of serotonergic neurons and stimulate the production of new neurons. A possible side effect of the chronic use of these drugs might be a proliferation of glial cells. These could develop into glioblastomas, which are malignant and aggressive brain tumors. Admittedly, this is speculative. Nevertheless, it is a possibility worth considering because of the potential harm from overstimulating growth factors in the brain.

Similar problems in weighing benefits against harms beset the use of anxiolytic drugs. These drugs are thought to act primarily by enhancing the effects of the neurotransmitter GABA, which promotes a feeling of calmness. Like other psychotropic drugs, however, the mechanisms of action of anxiolytics are not completely understood. Benzodiazepines are one class of drugs that fall into this group. Among other things, they can reduce anxiety by dampening the anticipation of future events. One possible side effect of these drugs is anterograde amnesia, the inability to form new memories. Benzodiazepines can interfere with the process of memory consolidation. A drug that eliminated anxiety about traveling, for example, might result in an inability to recall some of the events experienced on a particular trip. Benzodiazepines can also be addictive. The potential harm from chronic use of these drugs must be factored into the potential benefit from reducing or eliminating anxiety. In principle, the anxiety should be severe or at least moderately severe to justify accepting the possible adverse side effects of the drugs.

Depression is an increasingly common and serious illness in youth, affecting 3–8 percent of children and adolescents.[2] The incidence of depression increases dramatically as children move into adolescence. An estimated 20 percent of adolescents have had at least one episode of MDD by age 18, and 65 percent of the same group has reported less severe but significant depressive symptoms.[3] The brains of adolescents and especially children are more labile than those of adults, with structures and circuits developing at a much faster rate. One consequence of this is that the response to psychotropic drugs can be quite different in these distinct patient populations. Some findings suggest that children's brains may be more responsive to psychotherapeutic interventions such as CBT. This might lessen, though not obviate, the need for drugs to treat depression. One concern is that children and adolescents with the disorder may have to wait a considerable period of time before receiving CBT, and there are obvious risks with leaving depression untreated for even a short period of time.

The main worry about the use of SSRIs is that there is a risk of suicidal ideation and self-harm in some young patients taking them. This led the Committee on Safety in Medicine in Great Britain to declare in 2003 that paroxetine was contraindicated and "should not be used in children and adolescents under the age of 18 to treat depressive illness."[4] They reasoned that the balance of risks and benefits of the drug was unfavorable when used to treat depression in this age group. The United Kingdom's Healthcare Products Regulatory Agency (HPRA) went even further, banning the prescription of all SSRIs except fluoxetine to people under age 18. To support this position, one could cite the suicide of an 18-year-old American college student from Indiana in 2003 while participating in a trial for an SNRI, duloxetine. Perhaps the most reasonable policy was the one issued by the

U.S. Food and Drug Administration (FDA) in March 2004. The FDA asked the makers of 10 new-generation antidepressants to include a warning on labels about a possible connection between the use of these drugs and suicide in pediatric and adult patient populations.[5] In December 2004, the HPRA issued a letter stating that, in the light of the risk of suicide among young adults taking SSRIs, these patients should be closely monitored.

Prescriptions for antidepressant and antipsychotic medications have increased significantly in the last decade. This is due in part to the reluctance of health insurers to pay for psychotherapy and other time-consuming and labor-intensive nonpharmacological treatments. It is also due in part to aggressive marketing by pharmaceutical companies. Methylphenidate (Ritalin) is another drug whose prescription rate to treat ADHD in children has increased exponentially in recent years. Symptoms of ADHD include an inability to control impulses and filter incoming environmental stimuli, which is necessary to concentrate and attend to specific tasks. The disorder has been associated with abnormal functioning in the prefrontal cortex and basal ganglia. Methylphenidate is a CNS stimulant and dopamine reuptake inhibitor that can help individuals with the disorder to focus their attention by regulating the underlying neural mechanisms in these two brain regions.

Many people believe that ADHD is more overdiagnosed and overtreated than childhood depression. Although many children and adults have this disorder, it is unclear when symptoms are serious enough to justify drug treatment. As with depression, some have questioned the need for and efficacy of drugs for ADHD when compared with psychological interventions. Methylphenidate and other stimulants can increase blood pressure and heart rate, which may increase the risk of stroke and potentially fatal cardiac arrhythmias. There have also been a few cases of psychosis involving hallucinations in children taking stimulants for ADHD. These safety concerns led an advisory panel of the FDA in early 2006 to recommend that stimulant labels include drug-risk warnings.

These concerns notwithstanding, serotonin agonists and dopamine agonists do help many people to control symptoms of mental disorders and enable them to have normal mental function. While SSRIs have been associated with an increased risk of suicide, this risk must be weighed against the risk of suicide from untreated depression. In fact, results from two studies financed by the National Institute of Mental Health (NIMH) published early in 2006 indicate that antidepressants can reduce the risk of suicide among depressed teenagers and adults.[6] The results also indicate that antidepressants can achieve remission of symptoms for a significant number of these people. The risk of suicide from untreated MDD is likely much greater than the risk of suicide from treatment in both adolescents and adults with the disorder. Most studies of antidepressants have found that adolescents with depression are more effectively treated with a combination of CBT and drug therapy than with either treatment alone. Studies involving adults have shown greater general efficacy of combination therapy for this age group as well. Even when psychotropic drugs are medically indicated, effective, and safe in the short term, they raise two main ethical issues.

First, psychotropic drugs can have lasting effects on the brain.[7] They can alter not only the systems targeted to treat a particular disorder but also the neural circuitry of other systems. There is still insufficient data on the long-term effects of psychotropic drugs on developing brains. When intervening pharmacologically in a particular brain system, we need to consider the functions of other brain systems, and whether or how drug therapy might affect them. Brain-altering drugs can have more significant neurological consequences the younger the patient is, especially if they are given before puberty, when the central nervous system is still developing. Altering a neurotransmitter to treat one disorder could unwittingly result in another disorder.

For example, drug therapy for ADHD influences the dopamine system in the brain. Studies using SPECT imaging of children with this disorder have shown malfunctioning dopamine systems. Methylphenidate targets dopamine and activates the brainstem arousal system and the striatal cortex to produce its stimulant effect. This modulates networks controlling impulse control and attention. Schizophrenia and Parkinson's disease also involve dopamine systems, the first caused by too much of this neurotransmitter, the second by too little. Dopamine antagonists treat schizophrenia by inhibiting the activity of dopamine receptors. Dopamine agonists treat Parkinson's by increasing the activity of dopamine receptors. Dysfunction of dopamine in different systems is largely responsible for the problems with cognitive and motor control in these disorders. Like other neurotransmitters, dopamine is distributed through many brain regions. While speculative, it is possible that chronic alteration of dopamine systems in children with ADHD could put them at risk of developing a different neuropsychiatric disorder involving the same neurotransmitter later in life. This possibility should move medical professionals and parents to ensure that a definitive diagnosis of ADHD has been made in every case. Once it has been diagnosed, they should consider not only the potential benefits and risks of pharmacological treatment for ADHD but also the risks of cognitive and behavioral problems from not treating it.

Second, decisions to use psychotropic drugs to treat mental disorders in children are not made by the children but by their parents. Children may be capable enough to understand some aspects of the effects of the drugs and thus can assent to, or participate in, discussions and decisions about treatment. Yet most children lack the cognitive capacity necessary for consent to treatment. They may have to experience the consequences of a decision that was not made by them but for them. Because they are acting on their children's behalf, because the drugs can alter brain circuitry and biochemistry, and because the long-term effects of drug treatment are not known, the parents' proxy consent to treatment presupposes a definitive diagnosis of a severe or moderately severe mental disorder. Mild to moderate mental disorders do not indicate an absolute obligation to intervene pharmacologically. Indeed, in some cases, not treating may be in a child's best interests. While there may be adverse events from chronic use of psychotropic medications over time, in severe and moderately severe mental disorders, the benefits of treating acute symptoms in children outweigh any long-term potential risks. In these cases, there is both a parental and professional obligation to treat the child's condition.

Greater brain plasticity and the inability to consent to treatment require more careful weighing of benefits and risks of psychotropic drugs among youth than any other age group. More studies are needed to clarify the risk of suicidal ideation and emotional lability from antidepressants and other psychotropic drugs in the first days and weeks of use. In addition, longitudinal studies are needed to assess the effects of chronic use of these drugs, not only in children but in adults as well. Before prescribing these drugs, psychiatrists must engage parents in discussing the medical indications for and possible adverse events from using them in children. They must be especially careful in applying and interpreting diagnostic criteria and should consider alternative or complementary treatments, such as CBT.

Novel Psychopharmacological Interventions

In the previous section, I said that depression was associated with abnormalities involving serotonin, norepinephrine, and dopamine. But the pathogenesis of this and related psychiatric disorders is more complex. A disrupted HPA axis has been implicated in some types of depression and anxiety. This suggests that the release of CRF from the hypothalamus, ACTH from the pituitary, and the stress hormones cortisol and adrenaline from the adrenal glands all figure in these disorders. Moreover, the fact that inflammatory cytokines can activate the hypothalamus and influence the secretion of CRF is just one indication that systems outside the brain can have a negative influence on brain biochemistry. For these reasons, depression and certain other psychiatric diseases should be characterized not only as disorders of the brain and mind but also as systemic disorders of the brain, body, and mind. This understanding, combined with data indicating that antidepressants help only about 70 percent of the people who try them, has spurred research into the development of novel treatment modalities for depression, anxiety, and PTSD.[8]

Immunomodulating drugs might be able to control the release of inflammatory cytokines that disrupt the CNS and contribute to the cognitive and affective symptoms of major depression.[9] Alternatively, drugs that could modulate the HPA axis and sympathetic nervous system might control cytokine production and lymphocyte-expressed adrenergic receptors. A different class of drugs that modulate hormones released by the adrenal glands in response to stress might have a similar salutary effect on the brain. These effects would result from targeting mechanisms linking the central nervous, endocrine, and immune systems. Although these mechanisms are not yet fully understood, it is known that the connections between and among these systems form a delicate balance necessary to maintain homeostasis. When intervening pharmacologically in these systems, we need to be vigilant so that drugs that control some disorders do not tip this balance and result in other disorders.[10] The possibility of anterograde amnesia resulting from the use of benzodiazepines for anxiety is just one example of this. It will be instructive to consider examples of more experimental pharmacological interventions targeting systems both inside and outside the brain and to assess their comparative benefits and risks.

The neuropeptide substance P is prevalent in brain regions such as the prefrontal cortex and limbic system and is released in response to stress. There is some evidence that substance P antagonists can stimulate neurogenesis in the hippocampus. Because neuron depletion in the hippocampus has been associated with depression and other neuropsychiatric disorders, this could be an effective treatment for them. Substance P has not yet lived up to the promise it generated when it first appeared in the late 1990s, perhaps because it is still not known whether the loss of hippocampal neurons causes or is caused by depression. More promising are CRF antagonists. The cascade of events resulting in many forms of depression and anxiety appears to be triggered by CRF, and CRF receptors are found throughout the cortex and limbic structures such as the amygdala.[11] It thus has an important function in regulating emotional processing. Potentially, CRF antagonists might treat a broad spectrum of depression and anxiety disorders. Arguably, hypersecretion of cortisol and adrenaline does more to disrupt the HPA axis and results in a broader range of pathologies than hypersecretion of the other hormones we have considered. Accordingly, it will be helpful to focus on two classes of drugs—glucocorticoid antagonists and beta-adrenergic antagonists—that block the action of these hormones and examine their actual and possible effects on the brain and body.

The glucocorticoid cortisol appears to play a causal role in some forms of depression. When secreted in large amounts by the adrenal cortex, cortisol can disrupt the negative feedback mechanisms in the HPA axis, which in turn can disrupt levels of the neurotransmitters involved in the regulation of mood. Chronic release of excess cortisol can also cause neuronal loss in the hippocampus and prefrontal cortex. In theory, cortisol-blocking drugs could prevent the cascade of events that result in these pathologies, preventing these conditions from occurring, or at least alleviating the symptoms associated with them. In fact, one study has shown that the antiglucocorticoid mifepristone (RU-486) can treat symptoms of some patients with psychotic depression.[12] More commonly known as an abortifacient, mifepristone can mitigate the effects of a hyperactive amygdala by blocking the action of cortisol on glucocorticoid receptors in this limbic region. This is one way of resetting the negative feedback mechanisms in the HPA axis, as well as restoring normal functioning of the brainstem and other brain regions implicated in psychotic depression. Granted, these results apply only to a subclass of patients with depression. Nevertheless, they support the view that interacting systems inside and outside the brain may be involved in depression and other mental disorders. The results also suggest that intervening in systems outside the brain may have beneficial neurological and psychological effects for patients.

There is a potential risk in using cortisol-blocking drugs, however. Because cortisol has a modulating effect on the immune system, too little of this hormone could result in a hyperactive immune response and autoimmune diseases such as rheumatoid arthritis. This is partly supported by the finding that many people with rheumatoid arthritis have low levels of cortisol in their bodies. On the other hand, too much cortisol can disrupt critical CNS mechanisms and lead to or exacerbate some forms of depression. It can also suppress the immune system. Treating people with glucocorticoid hormones to control autoimmune conditions such as rheumatoid arthritis might lead to depression. Ideally, any intervention should restore and not disrupt the overall balance between mechanisms and systems in the brain and body. Many drug interventions entail trade-offs between positive effects on some systems and negative effects on others. But when one or more systems in the brain are severely disrupted and refractory to standard pharmacological interventions, the actual benefits of an experimental drug that can control or repair the disruption may outweigh the potential risks and justify its use.

The use of drugs to block the action of catecholamines like adrenaline may be more difficult to assess. As described in chapter 2, adrenaline is released by the adrenal medulla in situations requiring effort to fight against or flee from a perceived or real threat. It is closely related to the other stress hormone, cortisol. One effect of adrenaline is that it can embed emotional memories of fearful or threatening events in the amygdala. Because the emotional memories stored in the amygdala are out of our conscious control, they can be difficult to eradicate and can adversely influence the nature and content of our beliefs, feelings, and other conscious mental states. These memories can cause one to perceive events or environmental cues as stressors or threats. This can trigger a heightened fear response from the amygdala that is out of proportion to the real nature of these events and cues. Such a response puts the brain, mind, and body on a constant state of alert. This describes the pathology of some forms of depression, anxiety, and the emotionally disturbing flashback memories of traumatic events that characterize PTSD.

Some have raised the possibility of using a beta-adrenergic antagonist, such as propranolol, to treat this disorder. This drug blocks the effects of norepinephrine, levels of which rise in the brain in response to adrenaline. The aim of using propranolol for PTSD would be to prevent the embedding of pathological unconscious emotional memories of fearful events in the brain. Or the drug might be used to attenuate the emotional significance of and possibly erase memories that already have formed. Brian Strange and his colleagues have conducted experiments whose results appear to support the preventive hypothesis.[13] At least one other study suggests that fear conditioning is contextual, and that the hippocampus interacts with the amygdala in recording and consolidating fearful and other types of emotional memory.[14] So these two brain regions and the memory systems they regulate are not independent. This is also a plausible hypothesis at the level of the mind, since fearful events we experience often have an episodic, autobiographical quality to them.

The main target of prevention or erasure of pathological emotional memories is the amygdala. Emotional memories stored in this brain region can influence how we perceive events and can affect the quality of our conscious mental states. It is mainly because these memories are unconscious that severe forms of PTSD are refractory to conventional treatments. These treatments usually include some combination of cognitive-behavioral therapy and antidepressant or antianxiety drugs. Virtual reality programs may be more helpful. In these programs, individuals are repeatedly exposed to a simulated version of the event or events they experienced. The aim is to enable those with PTSD to respond appropriately to any stimulus that triggers an emotional memory of the traumatic event. But it is unclear to what extent this treatment could correct mental dysfunction at such a deep unconscious level of the mind regulated by a primitive system in the brain.

In theory, propranolol and other similarly acting drugs could prevent, dampen, or even erase pathological memories. They could serve both a preventive and therapeutic purpose. The goal would be to block the mechanisms through which these memories are recorded and stored. This involves the process of consolidation, whereby an event that one has experienced is first registered by certain neural correlates and is then translated into a permanently stored memory in the brain. Adrenaline appears to play a role in consolidation, acting on the pathway between the hippocampus and amygdala to ensure that an emotional memory is strengthened and stored in the brain. If it takes days or weeks for a memory to be stored in the amygdala, and the storage process depends on a certain level of adrenaline, then conceivably a sufficient dose of propranolol could block the production of adrenaline and prevent storage of emotional memory.

This was the hypothesis of Harvard psychiatrist Roger Pitman, who conducted a study of 40 patients admitted to the emergency room of the Massachusetts General Hospital for various traumatic injuries. Subjects in the study took propranolol or a placebo for 19 days immediately after the traumatic event. The idea was to test whether the drug could prevent the consolidation of negative emotional memories of the event by blocking the action of adrenaline and other stress hormones. Pittman's hypothesis also rested on the fact that memories that already have formed are vulnerable to erasure over time and need to be reconsolidated. Since many of the same molecular mechanisms involved in consolidation are also involved in reconsolidation, it is conceivable that the use of propranolol or other beta-adrenergic antagonists could block the mechanisms of reconsolidation and erase a pathological memory. Many of the patients in Pittman's study had an overactive amygdala and an underactive hippocampus and anterior cingulate cortex. Ordinarily, these brain regions modulate the amygdala and ensure its proper function. Ideally, propranolol would restore normal function in the hippocampus and anterior cingulate and modulate the amygdala to prevent the embedding of emotionally charged pathological memories. After one month, those taking propranolol had fewer PTSD-type symptoms than the control group and over time had more moderate responses to stimuli that resembled the initial traumatic event.

Pittman's experiment demonstrated that these drugs could prevent an excess release of adrenaline and thereby prevent the formation of heightened fear-inducing memories in the amygdala. Or they could at least modulate the emotional response to these memories. Such drugs could be given to soldiers before going into battle, or to paramedics just before responding to a medical disaster. In the light of a recent study showing that about one in six soldiers returning from the war in Iraq have had symptoms of PTSD, anxiety, and major depression, this type of intervention could prevent significant harm to and benefit many people.[15]

One possible consequence of using the drugs for these therapeutic or preventive purposes would be the blunting of the natural fear response. This response is adaptive because it offers us a survival advantage in protecting ourselves from real threats. It becomes maladaptive when it puts our bodies and minds on a constant state of alert and is out of proportion to the actual nature of external events. Losing a normal fear response is equally maladaptive. Could we ensure that a beta-blocker designed to prevent a pathological state of fear did not have the extreme opposite and equally harmful effect? Could we ensure that it would not weaken our natural fear response to the point of making us vulnerable to real threats? Even if these drugs were given in carefully calibrated doses, could we accurately weigh the potential benefit against the potential harm in using them for the preventive or therapeutic purposes that I have described?

Suppose that soldiers in the Iraq war were given propranolol as a form of prevention before combat. The aim would be to ensure that any traumatic experiences would not become embedded in the brain as unconscious emotional memory. This memory could result in a chronic hyperactive fear response when triggered by certain events long after combat. Ideally, the drug would modulate the fear response. Soldiers would respond appropriately to threatening events, but would not form heightened emotional memories of them. Yet, if the drug blunted this response too much, then soldiers could end up being wounded or killed because they would have lost their normal fight-or-flight response. What was intended as a prophylactic intervention to prevent harm could unwittingly result in harm.

Alternatively, suppose that some of these soldiers already had these memories and were diagnosed with PTSD. The drug could be administered shortly after they returned from combat and ideally would weaken or erase it from its storage site in the amygdala. This would be one way of treating the veterans of the war in Iraq who returned home with the disorder. Displaying certain images while the veterans were undergoing fMRI scans could elicit recall of a pathological memory. The blocking agent could be administered at the moment of recall and erase it.

Yet recall of an emotional memory, like reconsolidation of the memory, may involve a sequence of brain events and not just one event occurring at a single instant. Blocking agents could be given repeatedly over time to erase pathological emotional memories. But this would require the highly controlled environment of frequent fMRI scans to detect memory recall and monitor the drugs' effects, which would not be feasible. As with attempts to prevent these memories, attempts to erase them could also cause people to develop inadequate responses to fear-inducing stimuli. They, too, could become vulnerable to threats in everyday life. Furthermore, it is unclear whether a drug aimed at altering emotional memory in the amygdala would have any effect on episodic memory in the hippocampus. These two brain regions are both part of the limbic system that regulates emotional processing and therefore are not independent.

In any case, the action of the drugs would have to be very specific, and it would be difficult to predict that they would not have any adverse effects on other memory systems. This would be a concern even if one dose of a drug at a single instant could erase a pathological memory. The anterograde amnesia from benzodiazepines for anxiety disorders is a case in point. There is no guarantee that targeting emotional memory in the amygdala would not result in collateral damage to episodic or other types of memory in the hippocampus or other areas of the medial temporal lobes. Indeed, the findings of the experiments by Strange and his colleagues seem to confirm this fear. They suggest that the benefits of beta-adrenergic blockade or modulation of emotional memory may entail some cost in inhibiting the encoding of new episodic memories, or the loss of existing episodic memories in retrograde amnesia.

There are important differences between therapeutic drugs targeting memory in mental disorders such as PTSD and a distinct class of therapeutic drugs targeting memory in the neurodegenerative Alzheimer's disease. Drugs used to treat

Alzheimer's aim to prevent additional loss of episodic and semantic memory, especially in the early stages of the disease. Donepezil and memantine are designed to prevent further neuronal loss and atrophy in the hippocampus and prefrontal cortex, which are the principal brain regions implicated in the disease. Propranolol for PTSD aims to erase or prevent pathological emotional memories from forming and being stored in the amygdala.

The long-term effects of propranolol and similarly acting drugs on unconscious emotional memory are not known. In particular, it is not known what dosage of the drugs or what timing of their administration would be optimal for preventing or eliminating pathological fear responses while retaining normal responses to fear-inducing stimuli. The use of beta-adrenergic antagonists might also result in the loss of episodic or other memories that are critical to a person's experience of persisting through time. The potential side effects of preventing pathological memories from forming could be as harmful to individuals as the potential side affects of erasing existing pathological memories. While erasing episodic memories could disrupt the psychological connectedness between one's present awareness and one's awareness of the past, preventing new episodic memories from forming could disrupt the psychological connectedness between one's present awareness and one's anticipation of the future. This could adversely affect one's ability to learn new things and to plan and undertake new projects. So the potential side effects of erasing and preventing unconscious emotional memory are equally metaphysically and morally significant.

Absence of a normal response to fear-inducing stimuli has been noted in subjects with bilateral destruction of the amygdala and inferior temporal cortex.[16] The resulting emotive and behavioral changes are known as Kluver-Bucy syndrome. Even less radical pharmacological blockade of adrenaline in humans could weaken a normal fear response, which could make them susceptible to harm. This emotional symptom would be more significant than the blunted emotional response of psychopaths. It would involve not just the potential to harm others but the potential to expose oneself to harm as well. Beyond a certain point, inhibiting adrenaline could make one much less attentive, less vigilant, and more vulnerable to imminent threats. Among emergency workers such as paramedics, the effort needed to respond to an accident requires the release of a certain amount of adrenaline. Drugs that blocked the release of this hormone could preclude an appropriate response in these situations.

As a beta-blocker, propranolol is used primarily to block or diminish the cardiovascular excitatory response to the stress hormones adrenaline and noradrenaline. It is prescribed as a first-line antihypertensive and antiarrhythmic drug because of the way it acts on beta-adrenergic receptors in the heart. But it is not known how chronic use of this drug might affect other systems of the brain and body involved in the stress response. It is unclear whether the intended blocking or erasing effects of propranolol for treating PTSD would be limited to the amygdala.

Perhaps the main problem with beta-adrenergic blockade of stress hormones is that not all people who experience trauma are susceptible to PTSD and go on to develop this or related psychiatric disorders. The initial response cannot predict who will develop a full-blown disorder. Some people may have sleeping difficulties, nightmares, or obsessive thoughts; but these often disappear not long after a traumatic event. In these cases, individuals might be given a preventive medication they did not need and would be exposed to its potential risks. One of these risks could be the loss of positive emotional memories as well as negative ones. This could occur if these drugs affected multiple memory systems regulated by multiple cortical-limbic pathways. Yet failure to intervene in those who are susceptible might mean losing the opportunity to prevent or effectively treat the disorder. Studies indicate that people with PTSD have smaller hippocampi than those without the disorder. But it is not known whether this is a marker of susceptibility to the disorder or an effect of it. Even if MRI brain scans could identify those who were at risk, it would not be feasible to scan the brain of every patient admitted to the emergency room following an accident.

Still, if propranolol could prevent, erase, or at least attenuate the pathological memories of PTSD, then its use could be justified on the ground that a life of psychic suffering is worse than the loss of some positive emotional or episodic memory. The potential benefits of the drug therapy could outweigh the potential risks, significant though they may be. When a condition is intractable to all other interventions, severely affects one's quality of life, and poses a significant risk of harm to oneself and others, considerations of immediate efficacy can override considerations of long-term safety. Perhaps the safest and most effective intervention would be one that dampened the negative emotional effect of the memory. It would not erase the memory of the event itself but would modulate a person's emotional response to it. Whether or to what extent the emotional content associated with an event could be separated from recalling it remains to be seen. Researchers at McGill University have conducted studies based on this idea and are expected to publish their results later in 2006.

In a recent report, the U.S. President's Council on Bioethics warned against manipulating memories. It expressed concern that therapeutic forgetting could subtly reshape who we are.[17] Unpleasant memories are a necessary imperfection in our human nature. Preventing or eliminating them through psychopharmacology could result in an undesirable alteration of our humanity. But this position fails to adequately appreciate the differences between conscious episodic memories of actions we have performed and unconscious, emotionally charged memories of events that have happened to us. This position fails to draw the critical distinction between memories that are unpleasant or disturbing and memories that are pathological. The second type of memory is at the core of psychiatric disorders like PTSD and severe depression and causes considerable suffering in the people affected. The council did acknowledge that some memories are so traumatic that they can destroy the lives of these who suffer from them. The use of psychopharmacology to blunt emotional memory may be justified or even necessary in certain extreme situations, as in the military example I have discussed. However, the council also warned that the power to blunt memories could adversely affect their truth and meaning for us and might incline us to do things we might not otherwise do. This power might allow us to act without empathy, shame, or remorse.

Yet for people with PTSD and similar disorders, the psychopathology may make them incapable of feeling empathy, shame, remorse, or other states mind. In severe cases, reasons for treating these disorders by altering emotional memory outweigh reasons for retaining it and any associated truth or meaning. Treating these disorders with beta-adrenergic antagonists or other psychopharmacological agents is not meant to alter or enhance a healthy self but to restore a sick self to a normal healthy state. Even if these drugs altered the brain and mind, it obviously would be more preferable to eliminate pathological memories than to retain them.

Some individuals who experience anxiety before public speaking or musical performance might consider using propranolol to block the release of adrenaline and its effects on the brain to reduce or prevent anxiety. But taking such a drug repeatedly might have the general effect of blunting the natural fear response to actual threats. In that case, an intervention used to prevent a putative psychopathology could result in a different, though real, psychopathology. Anxiety should be moderately severe to severe to justify the use of a beta-adrenergic antagonist. Because they may entail significant risks, long-term use of these drugs should be limited to psychopathologies, not simply unpleasant states of mind that may interfere with performing at a certain level. These drugs may have other undesirable effects.

A musician who took propranolol to feel less anxious and perform better told me that it blunted his emotional experience of musical performance. It suppressed the "adrenaline rush" he ordinarily felt when performing without the drug and left him with only a vague memory of some of his performances. These are some of the actual costs of keeping one's cool through pharmacological means. In addition, it is possible that beta-blockers could blunt positive emotions such as joy and empathy mediated by cortical and limbic regions other than the amygdala. If these drugs were taken to enhance one's performance, then one might also question whether one's achievements were due to something other than one's own efforts. Not all people would be disturbed by this thought; but some would be.

Pathological mental phenomena are not an isolated set of mental states but part of a holistic mental network. The type of memory involved in the fear or anxiety response is just one of many different mental capacities. It may be naive to think that we could tinker with this type of memory without also affecting other cognitive and affective capacities. We need to recognize the complex interaction of different mental capacities, and the brain systems that underlie them, before tinkering with unconscious or conscious forms of memory. All of these considerations indicate that more studies like those of Strange and Pittman are needed to accurately assess the safety and efficacy of beta-adrenergic antagonists for prevention or treatment of depression, anxiety, and PTSD.

Other possible therapies for psychiatric and neurological disorders include gene therapy for depression. It may become possible to deliver particular genes into the brain that would block the expression of the short version of the 5-HTT allele. As explained in chapter 3, this allele predisposes some people to depression by influencing how their brains respond to stressors. Because these stressors are features of particular environments, the action of the delivered gene would have to be sensitive to the external natural and social environment as well. Robert Sapolsky has raised the possibility of developing gene vector therapies that would use conditional expression systems.[18] That is, the vector would be designed so that the expression of the new gene would depend on the same environmental stimuli that cause or exacerbate psychiatric symptoms. This would be one promising therapeutic application of pharmacogenomics.

As ingenious as this idea is, it would be difficult to realize in clinical practice. Targeting genes and gene products in the body requires highly specific viral vectors. Even if the vectors could deliver the genes to the intended site, they could trigger an inflammatory immune response or, worse, activate oncogenes that could cause cancers. This was the recent tragic outcome of initially successful gene therapy for two children in France with severe combined immune deficiency. They subsequently developed a form of leukemia. Because of the blood–brain barrier, delivering the desired genes into the critical brain regions would not be an easy task. They could be delivered to the brain through the spinal cord. But the brain and central nervous system are more complex than other systems of the body. With so many interacting pathways, it would be difficult to estimate the effects of viral vectors and new genes on the CNS.

Another potential treatment for fear-related mental disorders would be the removal of the gene regulating the expression of the protein strathmin. This idea is based on results from a study using mice.[19] In addition to the stress hormones discussed earlier, strathmin plays a role in the formation and storage of unconscious emotional memories in the amygdala. Identifying and targeting amygdala-specific genes could lead to amygdala-specific drug therapy that would be more precise and possibly more effective than propranolol. Yet it could also be riskier than propranolol. Tinkering with genes involved in the regulation of unconscious emotional memories has the same potential to blunt normal responses to fear-inducing stimuli as beta-adrenergic antagonists. The mice in the study just mentioned became less timid and more aggressive after the gene regulating the expression of strathmin was removed from them. Removing this gene entails the additional risk of disrupting growth factors and tumor suppressor genes in the brain. It is not clear than deleting a gene regulating the fear response would be any safer than inserting a gene for the same purpose.

A different type of gene therapy has been proposed as a potential therapy for the degenerative motor neuron disease ALS. Using mouse models, researchers injected a viral vector carrying a neurotrophic factor, insulin growth factor 1 (IGF-1), directly into the muscles of mice that had mutations in the superoxide dismutase gene (SOD1).[20] These mutations are believed to cause a subclass of cases of this disease in humans. Disease progression in the mice was delayed, and they survived longer than untreated mice. The researchers were able to inject the vector carrying the gene into the brain through the spinal cord, bypassing the blood–brain barrier. As with gene therapy for psychiatric disorders, though, the unpredictability of the effects of viral vectors on neuronal cell bodies other than those targeted indicates that we are a long way from knowing whether this technique is safe. Although ALS is such a devastating disease that it might justify using treatments entailing considerable risks, it would be difficult to defend using any intervention on humans without an accurate assessment of these risks. Until there is a better understanding of how viral vectors and neurotrophic factors function in animal models, it will be some time before clinical trials on humans could be justified.

Another area of pharmacological intervention worth considering is the use of dopamine and opiate antagonists to treat addiction to cocaine, amphetamines, nicotine, and other substances. Chronic use of these substances causes dysregulation in the mesolimbic dopamine system. More specifically, it causes hypersensitivity in the brain's hedonic reward circuit, a pathway extending from the dopamine-producing neurons of the ventral tegmental area to dopamine-sensitive neurons in the nucleus accumbens. This dysregulation is responsible for the craving and compulsive seeking and taking of certain substances. Pharmacotherapy has targeted the dopaminergic reward system to treat this disorder.[21] The dopamine antagonist bupropion has been effective in treating nicotine addiction by modulating levels of dopamine and noradrenaline. In addition, the opiate antagonist naltrexone acts similarly in treating opiate and alcohol addiction. These agents have had less positive results in treating addiction to amphetamines.

Vaccines are being developed that might prevent the "high" one experiences after taking a drug. An experimental nicotine vaccine has been tested in a clinical trial at the Lausanne University Smoking Cessation Clinic in Switzerland. The goal is for the vaccine to produce antibodies that will bind to nicotinic receptors in the blood stream and disable nicotine before it reaches the brain. Researchers have found that subjects with the strongest antibody response are the most likely to stop smoking. Yet too strong an antibody response might adversely affect other receptors and possibly healthy cells and tissues. This is what occurs in autoimmune disorders, where there is an overly aggressive antibody response to a pathogen. Nicotine antibodies could remain in the blood of vaccinated individuals for months and thus expose them to this and other risks. Pregnant women and their fetuses could be especially vulnerable to any adverse events from the circulating antibodies. A vaccine would have to target only a specific type of receptor and produce only nicotine-specific antibodies so as not to produce an autoimmune response that could destroy healthy tissues in the body and brain.

Even if a vaccine could block pleasurable sensations, it would not eliminate the craving for a drug, which is the main problem in addiction. One desirable drug intervention would be an agent that could modulate hedonic processing in the dopamine system and promote rational decision-making regarding expected rewards. The aim would be to prevent a person from compulsively forgoing long-term rewards for the short-term hedonic reward that leads to addiction. No such drug is currently available. If one were developed, then its action would have to be precise enough that it would not have any untoward effects on neural circuits underlying other types of cognitive and conative processing. Researchers and clinicians should also be circumspect in using dopamine and opiate antagonists on addicts. Like the other psychotropic drugs discussed earlier, the exact mechanisms underlying the action of these drugs are still unclear, as are their long-term effects on the brain.

Nevertheless, given the consequences of untreated addiction, the potential to correct a dysfunctional hedonic reward system would appear to outweigh any potentially adverse effects of treatment. These effects could be minimized if the drug therapy were tailored to the genes regulating biochemical mechanisms in the mesolimbic dopamine system. An estimated 50 percent of people with substance addiction are genetically predisposed to addictive behavior. Targeting the critical genes, proteins, and peptides in these brain systems could break the cycle that goes from craving to satiety to further craving. This is one more example of the promise of pharmacogenomics and proteomics in treating a wide range of psychiatric disorders. Yet psychiatrists and other professionals treating addicts would have to be careful that their patients' dependence on one substance did not lead to dependence on another, which would obviously diminish or cancel the benefits of treatment.

Simply prescribing therapeutic drugs would not necessarily control or cure addictions. These disorders may be just as much a function of environmental and psychosocial factors as neurological and biochemical ones. An ideal intervention for addiction would be one that altered an addict's beliefs about the availability of a substance, which could block the desire for the drug generated by the beliefs. Arguably the most promising agents in this regard are drugs that inhibit the reconsolidation of memories of the contextual cues that lead addicts to desire cocaine.[22] This intervention is similar in some respects to the use of beta-adrenergic antagonists to inhibit the reconsolidation of fearful memories. Disrupting the reconsolidation of these memories in the limbic system of the brain could prevent beliefs connecting context with drug use and thereby block the desire for the addictive substance. Here, too, though, it is not clear that this effect could be achieved without any adverse effects on other memory systems. A safer and possibly equally effective intervention would be psychological techniques that could enable one to reframe one's beliefs about the environmental cues that trigger craving for cocaine.

Of the different pharmacological interventions considered in this section, drugs targeting specific components of the HPA axis may be the most promising for safely and effectively treating psychiatric disorders. Interestingly, treatments that target pathways connected to but located outside the brain may be effective in controlling these disorders. Dopamine and other antagonists might safely and effectively treat addiction as well. The benefits of novel pharmacological treatments for schizophrenia, or for neurological diseases such as Parkinson's, Alzheimer's, and ALS are less clear. New therapies for psychiatric conditions are not without risks. But these risks have to be weighed against the potential deleterious effects of untreated psychiatric conditions on the brain. On balance, studies suggest that the potential benefit of glucocorticoid and beta-adrenergic antagonists for severe psychiatric disorders, and dopamine and opiate antagonists for addiction, outweigh the potential harm and therefore could justify their use. Nevertheless there may be trade-offs between actual short-term benefit and potential long-term harm. More randomized controlled studies and regulatory oversight are needed to accurately assess the comparative benefits and risks of these drugs and to determine whether or when they could or should be used.

Cognitive-behavioral therapy and other forms of psychotherapy aim to reframe a person's beliefs and other mental states in order to alter pathological patterns of thought. The placebo response may be an even better example of how beliefs can have therapeutic effects on the brain and body. Any action that intentionally or unintentionally produces a placebo response is a psychological intervention that can complement pharmacological interventions in treating pain and symptoms of some neuropsychiatric disorders. It will be instructive to discuss the placebo response in some detail.

Placebos

A placebo is any chemically inert pill or substance that can be an agent of physiological change in the brain and body. More accurately, the placebo as such is not the agent, but rather the patient's belief that the pill or substance is biochemically active and can have physiological effects. This has been called both the placebo response and the placebo effect.[23] The *placebo response* is the change that is observed following administration of a placebo. The *placebo effect* is the response to the placebo minus the physiological changes that would have occurred without it. Some of the effects associated with placebos are pain analgesia, relief of symptoms of asthma, and stabilization of mood in depression. The placebo response appears to be more common in medical conditions where physiological and psychological factors are interconnected. Accordingly, it could be characterized as a psychosomatic phenomenon. Because they are sensitive to a patient's beliefs and other mental states, placebos can be described as a psychological intervention that can treat symptoms of psychiatric, neurological, and other diseases.

Although no one knows exactly how placebos work, many studies have shown that they can cause physiological changes in the brain and body. One study conducted by researchers at the Neuropsychiatric Institute of the University of California at Los Angeles (UCLA) showed that depressed subjects given a placebo displayed changes in brain metabolism.[24] Most interesting about the study was the fact that the regions of the brain where placebo-induced changes took place were distinct from the regions of the brain affected by antidepressant medication. Using PET and quantitative electroencephalography (QEEG) imaging to compare changes in brain function during treatment with drugs and placebos in patients with MDD, the researchers found differences in brain metabolism that correlated with the two treatments. Subjects who responded to the placebo showed increased activity in the prefrontal cortex. Those who responded to the standard antidepressant medication showed suppressed activity in that region and increased activity in lower regions of the brain.

These findings are consistent with the findings of the study mentioned in chapter 3 regarding complementary drug treatment and psychotherapy for depression. Antidepressant drugs were found to have a bottom-up effect on the brain, extending from the brainstem through subcortical regions up to the cortex. Psychotherapy had a top-down effect, influencing the prefrontal cortex but diminishing through subcortical regions. This makes good sense, since beliefs emerge from and are regulated by the cortex. Significantly, these findings support the view that combined drug therapy and psychotherapy can be effective in treating depression because of the way these interventions act on complementary brain mechanisms regulating mood. The UCLA researchers claimed that their study confirmed that the placebo was an active treatment. But nothing in the pill itself produced the changes in the subjects' brains. Instead, the response was produced by the patients' belief that the pill was active.

The power of belief to alter brain metabolism may extend into lower regions of the brain. In a study at the University of British Columbia (UBC) in 2001, one group of patients with Parkinson's disease were injected with apomorphine, a drug that mimics dopamine.[25] Another group of Parkinson's patients expected apomorphine but were injected with a biochemically inactive saline solution. The PET imaging showed that the substantia nigra region of the patients who were given the saline produced just as much dopamine as those who were given the active drug. Like other uses of placebos, the effect was short-lived. Dopamine production ceased as soon as the patients were told that they were receiving saline. But the most significant outcome of the study was that the expectation of a biochemical effect could result in a real biochemical effect on regions of the brain below the cortex. More recent clinical trials testing glial-cell-line-derived neurotrophic factor (GDNF) for Parkinson's appear to support this point. Patients in the trial who improved the most had not received the active agent but a placebo.

A causal explanation of the placebo response has been elusive. But a plausible teleological explanation is that the placebo response is the combined action of the brain and mind in helping a diseased or otherwise dysfunctional human organism to regain homeostasis. I explained in chapter 2 that beliefs and other mental states emerge from the brain as a higher order sensory processing system that enables a human organism to distinguish between benign and threatening events. It is also plausible to suppose that beliefs can modulate dysregulated physiological functions due to a hyperactive sympathetic nervous system. This system in particular has been associated with depression, pain, and other conditions that respond to placebos, due possibly to the effect of placebos on the parasympathetic nervous system. The placebo response could be characterized roughly as one form of the body's relaxation response, a counter to the stress response.

Studies conducted by neuroscientist Fabrizio Benedetti and his colleagues have shown that the placebo response results from the release in the brain of endogenous opiates, which are natural painkillers.[26] These substances are produced when the brain anticipates pain relief. Benedetti and his colleagues also found that when subjects were given a substance that counteracted the effects of these opiates, their response to placebos stopped. The anticipation of pain relief is a function of combined conscious expectation and unconscious conditioning based on conscious and unconscious memory of an association between a pill or injection and a psychosomatic effect. Analgesia is not the only form of placebo response, as shown in the Parkinson's study on dopamine release. Although there is no evidence to suggest that the placebo response can cure or control disease over long periods, the available evidence does indicate that it can relieve pain, negative mood, and other symptoms of disease over short periods. The brain's ability to respond to placebos may be an inherited adaptive capacity that confers an evolutionary advantage on humans by enabling them to cope with diseases and to survive for some time in spite of them.[27]

In most uses of placebos, the effect stops as soon as the patient knows that the pill or substance he or she is taking or receiving is not biochemically active. This confirms that it is not the placebo as such but the patient's belief that is the agent responsible for the biochemical changes in the brain or body. Yet this raises the question of whether it can ever be ethical to give a placebo to a patient. When a physician gives a pill or injection to a patient, there is an implicit understanding that the pill or solution is biochemically active. If the substance is inactive and the physician gives it to the patient with the intention of generating a placebo response, then he or she is engaging in beneficent deception and is lying to the patient. But if the physician tells the patient that the pill is inert, then this information would prevent the placebo response. It would prevent the patient from believing in the power of the pill to produce a biochemical effect in his or her brain or body. On the other hand, not telling the truth would violate the principle of respect for patient autonomy and the related principle of informed consent. The physician would not be fully informing the patient about the true nature of the pill. If fully informed consent is necessary for any treatment to be ethical, and giving placebos violates informed consent, then giving a placebo is unethical and can never be justified. The argument that giving placebos is unethical can be defended on grounds of patient autonomy and physicians' obligation of disclosure. Placebos may heal; but the healing is based on a lie.[28]

It seems unfair to take a doctor to task for not fully informing a patient that he or she is giving the patient a placebo. Most psychiatrists do not know exactly how antidepressants and other psychotropic drugs work on the brain, or why a particular drug is effective for one patient but not another. Similarly, no one knows exactly how placebos affect the brain or body, though it is known that they can affect them. One could argue that a doctor would not be fully informing a patient about the nature of an active medication if he or she could not entirely explain its biochemical mechanisms and how they affect serotonergic, dopaminergic, or other neuronal receptors. The only difference between the placebo and the antidepressant is that one is biochemically active and the other is not. Just because an agent is biochemically active does not mean that it will have salutary effects on the brain and relieve disease symptoms. If one simply argues that it is unethical to give a placebo because it is deceptive and fails to respect patient autonomy and informed consent, then one fails to appreciate the nuances of the placebo response. This response involves a complex combination of cognitive, emotional, and social factors. One has to consider all of these factors to convincingly argue that it is unethical for a physician to give a placebo to a patient. One cannot reduce it to the process of a physician presenting information about a pill or injection, and a patient making a purely cognitive decision to accept or refuse the pill or injection on the basis of that information.

The placebo response depends on the patient's belief that the pill or injection is biochemically active and that it will cause biochemical changes in his or her brain or body. But there is more behind the response than belief alone. This cognitive attitude is imbued with conative and affective content. That is, the belief that the pill is active and effective is a function of the desire that it be effective, as well as the hope that it will be. The belief is also a function of the expectation of efficacy, which may be strongly shaped by a patient's previous experience with drugs perceived as similar to the new pill. Conscious expectation of relief is further influenced by unconscious conditioned bodily responses to medications taken as pills or injections. So the placebo response involves conscious and unconscious cognitive, conative, and affective mental states.

An important psychological attitude that emerges from the combination of belief and hope is the patient's trust in the physician as someone who always acts in the patient's best interests. Trust consists of both cognitive and affective features and can be shaped by social expectations of what physicians can or should do for patients. These social expectations may be sensitive to cultural factors that also shape the patient's perception of his or her relationship to the physician. In most cultures, the physician is perceived as a healer who stands in a therapeutic relationship to the patient. The *belief that* the pill will be effective is influenced by the *belief in* the physician as an advocate for the patient, and this second type of belief is influenced by psychosocial content.[29] The psychosocial context influences expectation, and expectation is crucial for a placebo response. It is a function not just of simple beliefs and desires but also of the more general cognitive and emotive associations patients make between physicians and health. A constellation of biopsychosocial factors is necessary to adequately frame the question of whether it is ethical or unethical for a doctor to give a placebo to a patient. If it is unethical, then it is because the physician trades on the patient's beliefs, desires, emotions, and expectations in a way that violates the trusting relationship between them.

In the UCLA and UBC studies, it would be enough for the researcher to tell the subjects that they would receive either an active treatment or a placebo. The researcher would not have to tell them which of the two interventions they would in fact receive. Telling the subjects that they might receive either intervention would be enough to satisfy the requirement of informed consent. The trials were designed in such a way that the researchers could test the placebo response without deceiving the subjects. Some might insist that there are differences between research and clinical care, and that there is a higher ethical standard in the clinical setting for doctors to tell patients exactly what they are taking. But here, too, there are situations in which it is permissible to give a placebo because there is no deception or violation of the patient's trust in the physician.

Suppose that a psychiatrist asks a patient to take two pills a day for his depression. One of these pills is a placebo, the other a proven active medication. The psychiatrist asks the patient to take the pills in the order in which she has arranged them, an arrangement ensuring that the patient will take one active pill and one placebo pill each day. Some days, the active ingredient will be taken first, followed by the placebo. Other days, the order will be reversed. Either way, the patient will not know whether the particular pill he is taking is active or inert. The dose of the active medication will be enough to effectively treat the depression. Although the psychiatrist informs the patient that one of the pills taken each day is a placebo, she does not tell him which pill it is. She does tell him that her intention is to see whether combining the pills in this way will be more effective than giving the active medication alone. The psychiatrist even discusses the phenomenon of the placebo response with the patient.[30] Significantly, any biochemical response in the patient's brain related to the placebo will depend not so much on anything the doctor has said as on the patient's belief or expectation each time he takes a pill. If there is a placebo effect, it will be influenced by the fact that one of the pills is active and by the patient's belief that each pill he takes is or may be active. The patient, not the doctor or the inert pill, is the therapeutic agent. The doctor only facilitates the process that results in the placebo effect.

As this case is described, the psychiatrist is not deceiving the patient in administering the two pills. She has provided the patient with all the necessary information about the pills and has informed him of her intention in asking him to take them in the designated way. Because the patient's response is based on his belief and expectation and not on any deception from the psychiatrist, it would not be ethically objectionable to give a placebo with the aim of testing the placebo response in the patient. The uncertainty that the psychiatrist has built into the treatment plan for her patient does not amount to deception.

In theory, taking the two pills might benefit the patient more than if he took the active medication alone. This claim must be made tentatively, however, since it is questionable whether active drug effects and placebo effects are additive.[31] If the placebo produced a positive biochemical response, it would probably occur in the left prefrontal cortex, which regulates the processing of positive beliefs and emotions. If it occurred, then it would appear to confirm the results of the UCLA study. Placebos and active medications work on complementary neurobiological mechanisms at different levels in the brain. This could be more cost-effective and time-efficient than combined medication and psychotherapy, assuming that the placebo would produce the same response as psychotherapy.

Consider now a different case. A patient has a type of cancer that is in its terminal stage. Her pain management has become challenging for two reasons. The pain is becoming increasingly resistant to the morphine delivered through an intravenous drip. She is also concerned that increasing the dose of morphine will make her incoherent, which would interfere with her ability to interact with her family. Her physician tells her that he will begin alternating the intravenous morphine with a saline solution, the amount of which she can continue to control with a hand-held pump. This feeling of control is one element that can help to diminish her pain because it can influence her perception and experience of pain. In this respect, the therapeutic agent is not the physician or the IV drip but the patient. The physician explains that alternating the two substances may be the best way to relieve her pain and enable her to remain coherent enough to interact with and enjoy the presence of her family.

As noted, placebos can be effective analgesics. This is due primarily to the fact that pain is a multidimensional experience with physiological, behavioral, and psychological dimensions. As Donald Price and Howard Fields describe it, "pain has both a sensory-discriminative and an affective-motivational dimension."[32] The sensation of pain is caused by the action of afferent nerves in the peripheral nervous system. But it is well known that the expectation of pain can increase its intensity and duration, and that the expectation of pain relief can diminish pain. One recent study confirms at least the first aspect of this phenomenon. Volunteers were falsely told by researchers that they would receive a heat stimulus that would be more intense than it was. The intensity of the pain the volunteers experienced correlated with what they were told, not with the actual intensity of the stimulus.

Functional magnetic resonance imaging showed increased activation in the anterior cingulate and other brain regions while the volunteers were expecting pain.[33] More generally, these results confirm that a mental representation of an anticipated sensory event can influence neural processes underlying actual sensory experience. This is one respect in which the mind can have a causal influence on the brain. Some aspects of pain are a learned response and may be treated with behavioral therapies that alter patients' perception of their experience. These therapies can have measurable effects on such brain regions as the somatosensory cortex, which is where much of the processing of pain stimulation takes place.

In the hypothetical case at hand, the patient may believe that alternating the morphine and saline will relieve her pain, even though the saline is biochemically inactive. This effect may be more likely to occur than with a pill because the intravenous drip is a more believable and technically convincing agent. Intravenous medications have a more immediate biochemical effect than oral medications. The literature shows that placebo injections are more effective than placebo pills, and that placebo morphine (saline) is more effective than placebo aspirin.[34]

Because the physician has informed the patient that he is giving her a saline infusion, he is not deceiving her. He need not also tell her that the saline is an intravenous placebo lacking the biochemically active properties of morphine. Any pain relief as a placebo effect will be a function of the patient's expectation based on what the doctor has told her, as well as her memory of past effects of the morphine infusion. On these grounds, there is nothing objectionable about giving the placebo morphine. One might claim that the physician was not fully informing the patient about the intention to produce a placebo response and was in this sense deceiving the patient. Even if some medical information were withheld, however, this objection would have to be weighed against the fact that the placebo analgesia is a form of palliative care. In these instances, relieving pain and improving the patient's quality of life have more ethical weight than strict autonomy and fully informed consent.

Depending on a patient's desires, beliefs, and emotions, placebos can produce beneficial biochemical changes in the brain and body and therefore can be an effective psychotherapeutic intervention. Provided that they are given as supplements rather than substitutes for active medication, placebos have a favorable risk-benefit ratio: they either relieve symptoms or they have no effect. The only risk pertains to possible psychological harm to the patient from being deceived into thinking that he or she is receiving an active medication. Yet if physicians give placebos to patients in the ways I have described, they do not deceive them and do not violate their trust or the ethical principles of patient autonomy and informed consent.

A more recent experiment used a topical ointment to investigate the psychological and neurological mechanisms that underlie placebo analgesia.[35] The aim of this study was to test the hypothesis that the anticipation of pain relief can result in pain reduction. Placebo-induced changes in brain activity were visible on fMRI imaging. Participants in the trial who showed increased activity in the prefrontal cortex in response to a stimulus also showed decreased activity in pain-sensitive brain regions. The results indicated a correlation between the anticipation of pain relief and actual pain relief. They also suggested a top-down mechanism whereby the activity of the prefrontal cortex modulated other brain regions more directly involved in the experience of pain.

This experiment is more ethically controversial than the other examples I have presented because the participants were deliberately deceived about the design and purpose of the trial. Participants were told that they were taking part in a study to test brain responses to a new analgesic cream. In fact, they were given a placebo cream to test the placebo effect. Because they were deceived, the participants did not give informed consent to enter the trial, which would have required full disclosure by the investigators of its true purpose. If the participants did not give informed consent, then presumably the trial was not ethical, since any ethically justifiable clinical trial requires full informed consent from those who participate in it. Yet, given that the aim of the trial was to test the hypothesis of placebo analgesia, informing the subjects of that aim would have prevented the investigators from achieving it. Full disclosure would have altered the beliefs that are critical to the placebo response. Would any clinical trial of this nature be unethical because it failed to meet the ethical requirement of informed consent?

In response to criticism that the trial involved the deliberate deception of the participants, the investigators argued that limited use of deception could be justified in research in which full disclosure changes participants' behavior.[36] They pointed out that Institutional Review Boards (IRBs) at Princeton University and the University of Michigan approved the study. More important, they argued that the benefits of the research outweighed the risk of harm and that deception was necessary for the research to be conducted. On this ground, they concluded that the research did not violate the principle of informed consent, broadly construed. But this seems too weak an interpretation of informed consent to have any ethical force. Besides, it sounds counterintuitive to say that subjects in a study can give an ethically acceptable degree of informed consent while being deceived about the design and purpose of that study. A critic of the experiment proposed that prospective participants be told before the study that its aim and procedures would not be described accurately, and that they be accurately informed following completion of the study.[37] This would make the study ethical, though it would probably preclude an effective test of the placebo hypothesis.

An ethically acceptable alternative might be to test the placebo cream with a different cream or drug that has proven analgesic effects. Participants would be randomized into two groups: one receiving the proven therapy, the other receiving the placebo. All participants would be told before the trial that they would receive either the proven therapy or the placebo. But they would not know to which group they would be assigned. Because many in the placebo group would believe that they were receiving the active treatment and would anticipate an analgesic response, fMRI scanning would show results similar to those of the actual trial just discussed. This would be a more ethically acceptable way of testing the hypothesis. Nevertheless, it likely would not yield the same information about placebo analgesia as a study involving deception. There would be at least some differences in the subjects' beliefs about pain relief, which consequently would affect brain responses to the cream.

As noted, the clinical trial for Parkinson's shows that placebos can have more than just analgesic effects. Subjects who believed that they were receiving a dopamine agonist were able to induce their brain into producing dopamine. Even if there are no problems with deception and consent at the outset of any experiment involving a placebo, there is a question about how long it could be ethical to give a placebo. If a subject's or patient's belief that a pill or solution is effective produces positive physiological effects, then could the placebo be given indefinitely? We can respond to this question in three ways. First, all available evidence indicates that the placebo effect is temporary. There seem to be limits to the positive physiological effects of belief. So even a sustained belief in the efficacy of an inert pill or solution will not likely produce a sustained biochemical or physiological response. Second, if placebos are only effective for shorter periods, then giving a placebo instead of an active medication for a longer period to a patient with a serious psychiatric or neurological condition would entail a significant risk of harm for that patient. The risk of leaving a serious condition untreated for too long would be too great to justify continued use of the placebo. There would not be any risk, though, if the placebo were given as a supplement rather than a substitute for an active medication. Third, even if the placebo response had a sustained physiological effect, a clinician or researcher at some point might have to resort to some form of deception of the patient or subject to sustain the effect. This could violate his or her professional integrity and respect for patient autonomy and hence be unethical.

The pervasiveness of the placebo phenomenon in clinical care and medical research suggests that the standard interpretation of informed consent may be a myth. It is not just a matter of a clinician or researcher explaining a treatment or trial to a patient or subject, who then agrees or refuses to take the treatment or enter the trial on the basis of that explanation. A wide range of biological and psychosocial factors may influence how patients and research subjects respond to information about a proven or experimental treatment. At the very least, the practice of obtaining consent from people needs to be more sensitive to these factors and the ways in which they shape how people actually think, feel, and act.

Forced Behavior Control

All of the pharmacological interventions discussed thus far could be described broadly as different forms of behavior modification. Neuropsychiatric disorders can impair cognition, conation, mood, or movement. The aim of pharmacological intervention for these disorders is to restore brain functioning to a normal level so that mental and physical abilities can be restored to normal levels as well. With novel or experimental drugs, it is presumed that those who take them do so voluntarily, are informed of their potential benefits and risks, and are competent to decide to take or refuse these drugs on the basis of this information. In cases of noncompetent children with psychiatric disorders, it is presumed that parents act in their child's best interests when they consent to drug therapy on the child's behalf. Voluntary behavior modification is one thing; involuntary behavior modification is quite another. Can forcing a person to take psychotropic medication ever be justified, even if the intention is to correct a psychopathology?

In the United Kingdom, the Mental Health Act permits psychiatrists to enforce treatment when the patient's illness has undermined his or her capacity to understand the need for it. In the United States, there are legal precedents for the right of competent patients and prisoners to refuse treatments that alter one's thought processes and interfere with one's ability to communicate. This right rests on First Amendment protections against forced government intrusion into the mind. For example, in the case of *Kaimowitz v. Michigan Department of Health* (1973), a Michigan circuit court found that the involuntary use of psychosurgery under the sexual psychopath law violated an involuntarily detained prisoner's First Amendment right. This ruling was upheld despite the fact that Kaimowitz had signed a form consenting to the intervention. In *Rogers v. Okin* (1979), a Massachusetts district court found that patients had the right to refuse psychotropic drugs if they interfered with their ability to think. The court argued that the Constitution recognizes a liberty interest in avoiding the unwanted administration of antipsychotic drugs.

The issues of decisional capacity and forced pharmacological treatment figured prominently in a case reviewed by the Supreme Court of Canada in 2003 (*Starson v. Swayze*). Scott Starson was an engineer and computer programmer who also had a gift for physics. Diagnosed with bipolar disorder, he was found not criminally responsible for making death threats. He was detained in a psychiatric hospital, where he received various psychotropic medications for his mental condition. Starson argued that the drugs prevented him from thinking at his full capacity and that he had the right to refuse them. But a psychiatrist (Ian Swayze) responsible for his care argued that Starson lacked the mental capacity to know what was in his best interests and to understand the need for the prescribed medications. If true, this would have justified treating him against his will. The Ontario Consent and Capacity Board confirmed Swayze's finding of incapacity. But the Superior Court and Ontario Court of Appeal overturned the board's decision. The Supreme Court of Canada dismissed Swayze's appeal. On the basis of his testimony and behavior, the Supreme Court ruled that Starson was not incapacitated but had the capacity to know what was in his best interests. He was capable of making decisions about psychotropic medication for his condition. Starson was deemed competent enough to know the difference between the consequences of having or forgoing treatment. His capacity to make decisions about treatment and his right to refuse it were upheld. If Starson's behavior entailed a significant risk of harm to himself and others, though, then forced treatment could have been justified on preventive grounds.

A different aspect of the same general issue arose in *Washington v. Harper* (1990). Here the U.S. Supreme Court held that the government could not use psychotropic drugs to silence or punish prisoners without due process. And in *Riggins v. Nevada* (1992), the Court ruled against medicating prisoners solely to make them competent to stand trial.[38] In both *Harper* and *Riggins*, the Court ruled that the Constitution permits the involuntary administration of antipsychotic drugs to make a defendant competent to stand trail. But it ruled that this is permitted only if the treatment is medically appropriate, is unlikely to have side effects that could undermine the fairness of the trial, and is necessary for important trial-related interests. In *United States v. Sell* (2003), the Supreme Court adopted a more conservative stand. Charles Sell was a dentist charged with a series of offenses, including attempted murder. Psychiatrists diagnosed him as a having a delusional disorder. Despite following the lower courts in judging that Charles Sell was not dangerous to himself or others, the Supreme Court approved the forced medication of Sell solely to render him competent to stand trial. The rationale was that the state had a compelling interest in holding the trial. This could mean that psychotropic medication could be given involuntarily to restore competence or to ensure that a person remained competent.

The Court's ruling in *Sell* could be challenged on two counts. First, because the medication would be forcibly administered for reasons other than health, it would not be in his best medical interests. Second, it would violate the defendant's First Amendment and Fifth Amendment rights to be free from governmental control of his thoughts and emotions. The second reason supports the generally accepted position that drugs affecting the mind should be treated differently from drugs that affect only bodily function.[39] Forced medication would not have been in Sell's nonmedical best interests either, since nothing about his condition entailed a risk of harm to himself or to others.

Still, there may be cases where the correlation between a brain abnormality and violent behavior is so strong as to suggest that one may be the cause of the other. Here we could ask whether it would be in a convicted violent offender's overall best interests to forcibly alter his or her neural circuitry with drugs to correct the abnormality. We could ask this even though forced pharmacological intervention would ignore consent and would not obviously be in his or her best medical interests.

Pharmacological intervention might restore normal cognitive and emotional processing in cortical-limbic pathways and enable an offender to gain some control of his or her violent impulses. In addition to structural abnormalities in the prefrontal cortex, many violent offenders have too little serotonin and too much dopamine in their brains. Too much dopamine can result in irritability and impulsivity, while serotonin can have a calming effect on behavior. Studies using PET imaging have shown correlations between impulsive aggression and low levels of serotonin in the orbitofrontal cortex and anterior cingulate. Low serotonin levels can impair one's ability to regulate cognitive and affective functions. Combining a serotonin agonist with a dopamine antagonist could raise levels of serotonin in the OFC and anterior cingulate and modulate a hyperactive amygdala to inhibit aggressive violent behavior. What if this type of intervention could modulate these impulses and thereby prevent the person from committing additional violent acts? Would there be reasons against forcibly using psychotropic drugs for this purpose?

The question is especially contentious in the case of young offenders with significant structural and functional abnormalities in the prefrontal cortex and anterior cingulate. Many individuals with these abnormalities have no capacity for moral sensitivity. Biological factors possibly beyond their control might determine a bleak future of psychopathology and further violent or otherwise harmful behavior. The study mentioned in chapter 2 regarding the strong genetic component in psychopathy appears to support this claim. Unless a person had structural or functional brain damage that was beyond repair, intervening pharmacologically at an early age to correct or reduce brain dysfunction might prevent a lifetime of criminal behavior and incarceration. The personalities of these individuals would be altered as a consequence of using psychotropic drugs, and they would not give voluntary informed consent to the intervention. For these individuals, the drugs would not restore a fractured self to a normal integrated set of psychological properties. They would alter these properties, alter their sense of psychological unity, continuity, and agency, and result in a different self.

But would forced pharmacological intervention be ethically objectionable if their pathological personalities entailed a high risk of harm to themselves and others? Even if one answered this question affirmatively, the prospect of personality change would have to be weighed against the prevention of harm through involuntary intervention. Moreover, although drug treatment would alter their mental states, the altered selves would arguably be more desirable than the former violent selves. The former but not the latter would be the type of self with which any rational, self-interested person would want to identify.

Young offenders would not fit easily into this model, however. On the one hand, the fact that their frontal lobes were not yet fully developed theoretically could make pharmacological intervention an effective form of prevention. It could help to modulate still-developing brain pathways underlying reason and emotion and enable them to restrain violent impulses. On the other hand, the fact that young offenders have immature frontal lobes suggests that their brains would be more susceptible to any adverse effects from psychotropic drugs than the brains of adult offenders. If they lacked decisional capacity and thus lacked the right to consent to or refuse treatment, then presumably the idea of forcing treatment on them would not be so ethically objectionable. Yet because of their labile brains, damage to regions underlying agency and personality could be more significant for them than for older individuals. This would make them an especially vulnerable population. For this and other reasons, pharmacological behavior control could be justified for only the most violent of young offenders, if at all.

In cases where a violent offender had decisional capacity, in principle, he or she should have the choice of whether to have or to forgo behavior modification. This would include the understanding that forgoing it would mean incarceration or other limits on one's liberty. The individual who would receive treatment would decide which of the alternatives was more or less undesirable. This would include the understanding that pharmacological intervention to modulate cortical-limbic pathways might entail a substantial change of personality. For violent offenders who made this choice, psychotropic drug treatment could be ethically permissible because they would choose it and it could prevent the harm associated with additional violent acts, incarceration, or execution. Some would object to this point and argue that giving a person a choice between behavior-modifying drugs and incarceration would be coercive and therefore not truly voluntary, since either option would not be desirable for the offender. It would be equivalent to forced behavior control. Given the circumstances, though, it may be the best choice available to that individual. Philosopher Patricia Smith Churchland suggests that, in some cases, this type of intervention should at least be considered:

> Certainly, some kinds of direct intervention are morally objectionable. So much is easy. But *all* kinds? Even pharmacological? Is it possible that some forms of nervous-system intervention might be more humane than lifelong incarceration or death? I do not wish to propose specific guidelines to allow or disallow any form of direct intervention. Nevertheless, given what we now understand about the role of emotion in reason, perhaps the time has come to give such guidelines a calm and thorough reconsideration.[40]

Cognitive and Affective Enhancement

Many drugs have therapeutic off-label uses for which they were not originally intended. They were not part of FDA approval of the drug and are not included in its labeling. Some of these uses are discovered through serendipity, others through monitoring effects of drugs in phase IV clinical trials. One example is gabapentin, an anticonvulsive drug that has been used to treat chronic pain and anxiety, in addition to epilepsy. Mifepristone for psychotic depression is another. Some drugs designed to treat neuropsychiatric disorders can enhance certain cognitive functions. Methylphenidate can help people with ADHD to focus attention and carry out multiple cognitive tasks. This same drug might also help university students and others who do not have this disorder to increase their concentration and perform better on exams. In addition, the cholinesterase inhibitor donepezil, used primarily to treat Alzheimer's, has been shown to improve the retention of information among middle-age pilots practicing on flight stimualtors.[41]

Perhaps the most intriguing of these drugs is modafinil. It was approved for the treatment of narcolepsy in 1998 and is now prescribed to treat sleep apnea and shift-work sleep disorder as well. All three of these conditions are caused by dysregulated circadian rhythm/sleep-wake cycles in the central nervous system. Modafinil reduces daytime sleepiness among shift workers, reducing the incidence of motor vehicle accidents caused by people who otherwise would fall asleep at the wheel. The benefits of the drug are clear. But modafinil is also being used as an agent to promote alertness in people with regular sleep-wake cycles. In fact, 90 percent of all prescriptions of the drug are for this and other off-label uses. Those taking the drug would have prolonged periods of alertness and would function at a high cognitive level on much less sleep than what is considered normal. Experiments involving B-2 bomber and commercial airline pilots on transcontinental flights have shown that this drug can keep them alert and engaged in mental activities despite prolonged sleep deprivation. In some respects, modafinil would function like methylphenidate and other stimulants that can improve people's cognitive capacity to focus attention on specific tasks.

It is not known exactly how modafinil works. Researchers believe that the drug activates dopamine, which then activates norepinephrine and histamine in a process that blocks the hypothalamus from promoting sleep. They believe that modafinil does not produce the hyperactive and addictive effects of stimulants like amphetamines and cocaine because of its selectivity in targeting the dopamine pathway that controls wakefulness. This selectivity may explain why modafinil does not appear to have any undesirable side effects.

If modafinil were used to extend a person's alertness beyond a normal range, it should be described as a form of cognitive enhancement. It would not be accurately described as therapy if its intention were to promote alertness for 20 or more hours. More accurately, it would be described as a nontherapeutic intervention. The inability to be alert for such a long period of time, or the inability to function cognitively on four hours or less of sleep per night for days, would not be considered an illness on any plausible interpretation of the term. Initial studies suggested that modafinil would not be significantly more effective than caffeine in enhancing attention. But let's assume that it is more effective than caffeine and that it can increase alertness or attention for long periods. Let's also assume that it would not cause hyperactivity of the CNS or other systems in the body. Would there be any medical or ethical reasons for objecting to its use?

One concern arises from the theory that sleep, specifically rapid-eye-movement (REM) sleep, is required for memory consolidation.[42] Sleep deprivation would limit the amount of REM sleep and could adversely affect the capacity to form new memories. But if the action of modafinil were specific enough, then it could act on the hypothalamus and other sleep-regulating areas without affecting the hippocampus and other regions that regulate memory formation and storage. Jerome Siegel has challenged the view that REM sleep is necessary for memory consolidation.[43] He has argued that people with drug-induced blockade of REM sleep would have normal or even improved memory. Deprivation of REM sleep does not appear to interfere with the ability to obtain new information. In fact, short-term sleep deprivation has been proposed as a treatment for major depression. Although the underlying molecular mechanisms of this phenomenon are unclear, it is believed that sleep deprivation mimics the effects of SSRIs. Because sleep deprivation would interfere with the decrease in levels of serotonin during REM sleep, it would result in an overall increase in the amount of this neurotransmitter in the brain. This could benefit depressed people by stabilizing their mood.

But long-term REM sleep deprivation may not be so beneficial. As Siegel argues, constant release of monoamines such as serotonin to sustain prolonged awareness of the environment may desensitize neurotransmitter receptors. Rapid-eye-movement sleep appears to inhibit monoamine release and to allow the receptors to rest and reset themselves to retain sensitivity. Thus, even if long-term sleep deprivation does not interfere with memory formation, it may have deleterious effects on other aspects of cognition, as well as on mood. Two additional hypotheses have been proposed to explain the physiological benefits of sleep.

One hypothesis is that non-rapid-eye-movement (NREM) sleep provides a period of low metabolic demand in the brain, allowing neuronal energy resources to be replenished. This is necessary for the brain to meet high metabolic demand during wakefulness.[44] Drugs that limited NREM sleep could interfere with the brain's ability to perform cognitive tasks. A second hypothesis is that sleep plays an important role in maintaining neural plasticity.[45] Limiting sleep through pharmacological means could impair the brain's ability to adapt to changing environments or to adjust to injury. People who are chronically sleep-deprived (fewer than six hours per night) generally are at greater risk of morbidity and mortality than those who sleep six to eight hours per night. The shorter sleepers have a higher incidence of cardiovascular problems, such as hypertension and stroke, and neurological problems and are more susceptible to infection because of weakened immune systems. Sleep deprivation may also be a risk factor for metabolic and endocrine disorders such as obesity and diabetes. Chronic use of a drug like modafinil to limit sleep might cause or exacerbate these conditions. There is also the possibility that flooding histamine receptors to enhance alertness could set off an inflammatory response in other parts of the body. It would be difficult to ensure that the effects of drugs acting on histamine and other sleep-regulating neurotransmitters would be limited to the hypothalamus alone.

More recent studies support the view that slow-wave sleep is critical for consolidation of newly acquired memories in animals.[46] Constant manipulation of the natural alertness system could have harmful consequences. The main issue regarding modafinil is that the biochemical mechanisms and the long-term effects of this and related alertness-enhancing drugs are unknown.[47] A sufficient number of longitudinal studies are needed to accurately assess these effects and determine whether the benefits of the drugs outweigh the risks.

Another potential form of psychopharmacological enhancement would involve drugs that targeted memory. Unlike the use of beta-adrenergic antagonists to inhibit the formation of pathological emotional memories, these drugs most likely would be designed to increase the encoding and storage of long-term semantic memory and to expedite its retrieval in short-term working memory. The alpha2-adrenergic receptor agonist guanfacine has shown beneficial effects on working memory and attention in monkeys and patients with ADHD. But one study investigating this drug's cognitive-enhancing properties found no improvement in volunteers' working memory or executive functions.[48] More promising are drugs designed to increase memory encoding and storage by acting on the transcription factor cyclic adenosine monophosphate (cAMP) and the protein it modulates, cAMP response element binding protein (CREB). This protein is a transport factor responsible for switching on and off the genes involved in long-term memory formation and storage. Memory-enhancing drugs would activate CREB through a series of molecular interactions. The drugs would stimulate the neurotransmitter glutamate at synapses, which would then activate the NMDA receptor and increase the supply of CREB inside cells and strengthen memory consolidation.[49]

The types of drugs I have been discussing in this section could improve attention and memory. Intelligence consists of a complex set of mental traits that includes but is not limited to attention and memory. Still, these are two important components of intelligence that play a crucial role in reasoning, problem-solving, and other mental tasks. There are social and additional neurobiological aspects of pharmacological interventions to enhance attention and memory that warrant ethical concern. Let's consider each of these aspects in turn.

Intelligence can be both an intrinsic good and a competitive good.[50] It can enable one to appreciate art, history, literature, or music, and in this sense can have value in and of itself. But intelligence is more ethically significant as a competitive good. It can give some people a competitive advantage over others in gaining employment, income, wealth, and a higher level of well-being. This advantage, and the social inequality that results from it, might be perceived as unfair because intelligence is a set of cognitive and other mental capacities that one has or lacks through no merit or fault of one's own. Some have argued that the best way to ameliorate this situation would be to offer cognitive enhancement drugs to all. The goal would be to reduce unfairness, but without eliminating beneficial options.[51] If we could ensure universal access to drugs that could enhance the cognitive capacities that are components of intelligence, then presumably this would reduce social inequality and unfairness. It would give everyone an equal opportunity for access to the type of education and employment that would guarantee a moderate to high level of well-being for everyone. But this would not necessarily follow. Equal access to a competitive good, or to the means that would facilitate such access, would not imply equal outcomes from the use of these means.

Different parental attitudes to related competitive goods such as an elite education and lucrative jobs could mean substantial differences among children in the extent to which enhancement technology was utilized. Some parents would be more selective than others in sending their children to better schools or in arranging for private tutors. In these respects, equality in access to cognitive enhancement would not automatically result in equality of opportunity for academic achievement among children. Moreover, some adolescents and adults would use cognition-enhancing drugs for trivial activities. Instead of using methylphenidate to enhance alertness or other drugs to enhance memory in order to perform better on the SAT or university exams, some people would use these drugs to memorize phone numbers or sports statistics. Or they might use them for pathological pursuits such as gambling. Not everyone would use these drugs in a beneficial way. So there would be inequality of outcomes of cognitive enhancement with respect to the competitive goods at issue. Any beneficial options of enhancement would likely come on top of existing social inequality. It would more likely maintain or increase than reduce inequality in whether and to what extent people gained competitive goods.

Even if everyone used cognition-enhancing drugs in the same beneficial way, it would not guarantee that everyone would gain the desired goods. Because they are competitive, the goods in question are limited and not open to everyone. Competition is fundamentally a zero-sum game.[52] The gain for some in achieving these goods will mean a loss for others in not achieving them. In this respect, giving beneficial options to all in the form of universally available cognition-enhancing drugs would not result in everyone realizing their desired goals.

Universal access to drugs intended to enhance cognition is not a likely scenario. Instead, access to these expensive drugs would be based on the ability to pay for them. Because some people are financially worse off than others through no fault of their own, this would seem unfair to those who could not afford to pay for the drugs. They would not have the same access to the drugs as those who were financially better off. But any claim of unfairness would have to be supported by data on the long-term benefits and risks of the drugs. The relevant data are not currently available. If the benefits and risks of these agents were not known, then there would be no basis on which to claim that unequal access would be unfair for those who could not afford them. The claim about unfair access rests on the questionable assumption that the drugs would have only beneficial outcomes. Yet it is possible that those who used the drugs over time might experience more harmful than beneficial effects. They could end up being worse off in terms of their mental and physical health than those who could not purchase the drugs. Inequality in access to cognition-enhancing agents between the financially better off and worse off would not necessarily be unfair to the latter.

There is another reason for questioning claims about fairness in access to cognition-enhancing drugs. Safety issues aside, it is not clear that these drugs would have the same beneficial effects for everyone who took them. Given differences in people's brains and their varying responses to psychotropic drugs, it is possible that some people would derive only a modest benefit from taking them, or no benefit at all. One cannot assume that just because these drugs may have positive effects on the brains of some people, they would have positive effects on the brains of all people.

Interest in drugs that target memory systems has been driven largely by the desire to retard memory loss in the elderly. But drugs are being developed to enhance normal memory in the younger population. Memory-enhancing drugs would probably target pathways between the hippocampus or other structures in the medial temporal lobes and the prefrontal cortex. The medial temporal lobe system regulates the encoding and storage of episodic and semantic memory. The prefrontal cortex retrieves these memories for cognitive tasks in working memory. Two famous cases of patients with brain injuries support the hypothesis that memory systems operate independently of each other. On the basis of these cases, it is intuitively plausible to suppose that enhancing semantic or working memory would not adversely affect procedural or episodic memory.

In one case, a male patient known as "H.M." had a bilateral resection of the medial temporal lobe to treat epileptic seizures. An unfortunate consequence of the surgery was that H.M. experienced both anterograde and retrograde amnesia. He was unable to remember events that occurred after the operation, as well as events occurring several years before the operation. Yet he retained memory of his childhood. In addition, his semantic and procedural memory were spared. His general intelligence, perceptual functions, linguistic ability, and factual knowledge and skills all remained intact.

In a second case, a male patient known as "K.C." sustained a brain injury in a motorcycle accident. This resulted in damage to multiple brain regions, especially the medial temporal lobes. He had anterograde amnesia of both personal experience and factual information, but his retrograde amnesia was asymmetric. "K.C." could not recall any personal events before the accident; but the semantic knowledge he acquired before it was still intact. His knowledge of mathematics, history, and geography was not significantly different from that of other people at his educational level.[53] Although the regions of his brain regulating his episodic memory were severely affected, the regions regulating his semantic memory were not affected.

These two cases suggest that different memory systems in the brain, and damage to them, can be highly selective. They also suggest that CREB-boosting drugs could enhance the storage and retrieval of semantic memory without affecting conscious episodic memory or unconscious procedural memory.[54] If memory systems operate independently of each other, then we should be able to use "smart drugs" to target the desired system without having to worry about any collateral damage.

But other research suggests that cases like those of "H.M." and "K.C." may be the exception rather than the rule. There are reasons to believe that the functions of different memory systems depend on widely distributed regions of the brain. It is possible that brain damage could adversely affect more than one memory system. Damage could result in diffuse memory impairment regarding facts and events.[55] If different memory systems are connected, could enhancing the formation, storage, or retrieval mechanisms of one type of memory impair the same mechanisms of other types? More specifically, could increasing the storage capacity of semantic memory impair the capacity to retrieve memories of facts and concepts in working memory?

These questions are motivated by an evolutionary interpretation of memory. The limits we have in our capacity to remember only so many facts and so many events may be part of a mechanism that is critical to our survival. Each memory system may have optimal levels of formation, storage, and retrieval. In that case, trying to increase the storage capacity in one system could have deleterious effects on formation or retrieval in that same system. It could also have deleterious effects on formation, storage, or retrieval mechanisms in other memory systems. Even if we could isolate memory systems and increase the storage of semantic or episodic memory without affecting other systems, it is unclear whether this might affect the ability to retrieve these memories. Ideally, we would want to use drugs that both increased memory storage and made memory retrieval more efficient across all memory systems. But enhanced memory storage would not necessary result in enhanced memory retrieval. Excess storage of semantic or episodic memory might impair the retrieval of such memories in working memory. Or it might result in overloaded working memory, which could impair the ability to execute cognitive tasks. It is also possible that quicker memory retrieval might impair the brain's ability to form and store new information.

The idea that there is an optimal level and rate of memory storage and retrieval is based on the hypothesis that there is an optimal balance between two types of CREB in the brain: "activator" CREB and "blocker" CREB. The first type of CREB activates the genes and gene products necessary for the encoding or formation of long-term memory, while the second type of CREB inhibits the formation of additional long-term memory.[56] Or, if memories have been formed already and are in storage, blocker CREB removes them from circulation in the pathway between the hippocampus or other areas of the medial temporal lobes and the prefrontal cortex by interfering with retrieval mechanisms. By doing this, it prevents "noise" that would interfere with our ability to concentrate on immediate cognitive tasks and to anticipate the future. This makes good evolutionary sense. It is advantageous for us to recall facts and events, or to learn new facts, only to the extent that they are important for our survival. Put another way, the organism finds certain information worth pursuing in relation to its present tasks. The organism does this through access to its past provided by certain memory mechanisms. It is not obvious that storing many more memories beyond what is useful could benefit us in this regard, or any other.

Too much blocker CREB could result in forgetfulness and, in severe cases, dementia. Too much activator CREB could result in an overproduction and oversupply of memory, the brain and mind being cluttered with memories of facts and events that served no purpose. Drugs designed to enhance memory would aim to increase the amount of activator CREB. But if there is an optimal balance between the two types of CREB, and between remembering and forgetting, then drugs that increased memory storage could upset this balance. One possible consequence of this would be impaired memory retrieval. Farah expresses a similar concern: "We understand very little about the design constraints that were being satisfied in the process of creating a human brain. Therefore, we do not know which 'limitations' are there for a good reason . . . normal forgetting rates seem to be optimal for information retrieval."[57] She warns of "hidden costs," and that evolutionary considerations should make us wary of the prospect of cognitive enhancement as a "free lunch."

The recent spate of injuries among professional athletes seems an apt analogy here. The use of anabolic steroids has increased the muscle mass of many athletes, enhancing their strength and skills. But this has resulted in an increase in injuries to muscles, ligaments, and bones. One explanation for this phenomenon is that the increased body mass is too much for the body's skeleton and other structural features to support. The increased bulk is not something for which the human body was naturally designed. We can also ask whether the brain could support increased memory without any adverse effects.

Another possible consequence of increased memory would be difficulty in learning new things, which depends on a certain degree of forgetting. The most famous case of this condition was the patient Shereshevkii, as reported by the neuropsychologist Alexander Luria. Shereshevkii's formidable ability to remember facts and events resulted in his inability to process new information. His seeming inability to forget nonessential facts and events made him unable to hold down a career, other than that of a memory performer.[58]

A fictional illustration of this condition is the character Ireneo Funes in Jorge Luis Borges's short story "Funes the Memorious." Following an equestrian accident in which he sustains a brain injury, Funes remembers every detail of everything he experiences. Speaking to the narrator, Funes says, "My memory, sir, is like a garbage disposal."[59] He becomes an invalid, a prisoner of a hyperactive system of memory consolidation and recall, unable to learn new things and anticipate the future because he cannot tolerate any additional experience. The narrator suspects that Funes "was not very capable of thought. To think is to forget a difference, to generalize, to abstract. In the overly replete world of Funes there were nothing but details, almost contiguous details" (36). Funes's overloaded semantic and episodic memory systems severely impair his working memory. He is unable to execute such cognitive tasks as problem-solving and decision-making. Funes is also unable to anticipate and plan for the future, because he cannot forget any of the particular features of his experience. Borges writes that Funes died of "pulmonary congestion," a metaphor for his overloaded memory. The upshot of these considerations is that we should be wary of making the inference that if memory is good, then more memory is better.[60]

The problems of memory overload that I have described could be avoided by separating retrieval of recent memory from retrieval of remote memory. Presumably, researchers could avoid any adverse effects by enhancing the storage and retrieval of recent memory while allowing normal forgetting rates of remote memory.[61] Perhaps drugs targeting the mechanisms of working memory could have this effect. But even recent memory can involve many trivial details that could clutter the mind. It is unclear how specially designed drugs could weed out recent memory of trivial facts from recent memory of useful facts, or whether quicker retrieval would not have any untoward effects on useful memory formation and storage. Again, the idea of an optimal balance within and among memory systems serving an adaptive purpose seems quite plausible. It is doubtful that artificial manipulation of naturally de-signed memory systems that have served us so well could improve these systems. It is equally doubtful that this could be done without entailing any risks.

Unlike replacing or adding silicon chips to upgrade or increase computer mem-ory, memory systems in the brain could not easily be upgraded or expanded by activating neurons with certain drugs. Memory-assist devices, such as Palm Pilots, can function as a form of semantic memory when the brain has lost some of the neuronal connections that sustain this memory system. But these devices are lim-ited in providing us with all the memory we need to perform a full range of cog-nitive functions. Retrieving information from these devices is also different from retrieving them from the brain. Human memories are not encoded in specific neuronal connections but are distributed through multiple neuronal pathways. These pathways mediate not just semantic but other memory systems as well. In addition, entering information into a memory-assist device is very different from taking a psychoactive drug to enhance memory. Unlike the first action, the second action can directly alter neuronal connections, which may have unforeseeable consequences that may be neither beneficial nor benign.

A different worry is that altering regions of the brain that control cognitive functions might disrupt emotional functions. Cognitive and emotional processing are part of an interconnected system in the mind regulated by interconnected cortical-limbic pathways in the brain. Because of these interactions, trying to en-hance cognitive processing could impair emotional processing. A drug that made a person "smarter" might also make that person emotionally flat. Even the thera-peutic use of psychopharmacological agents could have this effect. Anecdotal ev-idence suggests that dextroamphetamine (Adderall), which is in the same class of drugs as methylphenidate, can have adverse effects on mood. One woman taking the drug—to improve attention, memory, and other cognitive abilities that had become impaired due to an earlier series of concussions—noted: "I worked like a demon, but I found myself disconnected. At the computer I was entirely focused, but off duty, certain pleasures, like wandering around aimlessly in my own mind, were no longer available to me."[62] This account raises a concern similar to the one raised earlier about the potential blunting effect of propranolol on positive emo-tions and felt experience. Any benefits of these drugs may come at the cost of becoming disengaged from one's emotions. It is also possible that, given the connection between cognition and emotion, too much of one and too little of the other could impair some forms of reasoning. The constellation of psychological effects of cognitive enhancement might not be so desirable.

No one knows what the long-term cognitive, affective, or conative effects of alertness- or memory-enhancing drugs might be. Admittedly, this concern is not unique to enhancement drugs but applies to therapeutic drugs as well. Still, it is one thing to administer a drug with potential adverse effects for therapeutic treatment of a mental disorder. It is quite another to administer a drug with potential adverse effects to enhance normal mental functions. Until there is a better understanding of the risks of drugs intended for cognitive enhancement, the potential harm from long-term use of these drugs justifies limiting them to short-term use in special circumstances and only when there is a compelling reason to use them.

Cognitive enhancement must be distinguished from mood enhancement. The concept of using SSRIs as "mood enhancers" does not refer to the treatment of major depression, severe anxiety, or even milder mental disorders such as dysthymia. Instead, anecdotal evidence suggests that many people use these drugs to overcome shyness and alienation, or to create a general feeling of well-being. These are people with normal mental functions who take the drugs to feel "better than well."[63] Psychiatrist Peter Kramer cited some of this evidence in his popular 1993 book *Listening to Prozac*.[64] This book includes discussion of patients who are prescribed and take SSRIs such as Prozac to boost self-confidence and self-esteem.

But claims that antidepressants or other psychotropic drugs are prescribed and taken to enhance normal affective capacities are exaggerated. These claims make light of the fact that the majority of people who take these drugs do so because of the debilitating affective, cognitive, and physical symptoms of major depression. The aim of these drugs is not to make people feel better about themselves but to restore people who are sick and who suffer from mental illness to normal levels of mental and physical functioning. Some may take these drugs to enhance mood, but most do not. Certain antidepressants may be used as an alternative to hormone replacement therapy to treat symptoms of menopause. If these symptoms had a significant negative effect on a woman's quality of life, then using an SSRI or SNRI to treat them would hardly qualify as enhancement. For those whose affective symptoms fail to meet clinical diagnostic criteria of major depression, anxiety, and similar disorders, any positive effects of these drugs are probably minimal. As psychiatrist Greg Sullivan explains: "If someone is pleased with the effects of an SSRI, that usually is an indication that the drug has had a significant impact on serious symptoms, including those caused by a chronic low-level depression (dysthymia). . . . But SSRIs are not 'happy pills,' and people without significant mood or physical dysfunction do not generally get much benefit from them, certainly nothing that would make them sustain their use."[65] Similarly, Farah notes: "the small literature on short-term SSRI effects in normal subjects suggests no change in either direction on positive effect, only a selective decrease in negative affect."[66]

There are potentially serious side effects of SSRIs in people whose levels of serotonin, norepinephrine, and dopamine are normal. Because antidepressants increase the availability of these neurotransmitters, they can result in mania in some biologically vulnerable people. Hypomania can be confused with a cheerful character, and taking drugs to enhance mood could unwittingly cause this mental disorder. In addition, these drugs may trigger the serotonin syndrome. This syndrome is usually caused by a combination of two drugs, one of which is an SSRI. It is a consequence of excess serotonin in the central nervous system. Its symptoms can include euphoria, drowsiness, overreaction of reflexes, rapid muscle contraction, high body temperature, confusion, hypomania, and, in severe cases, coma and death. The serotonin syndrome occurs in approximately 14 to 16 percent of persons who overdose on SSRIs.[67] In a well-known case, a combination of meperidine and phenelzine resulted in this syndrome and the death of 18-year-old Libby Zion in March 1984. Given the possibility of this syndrome, when considering using SSRIs for mood enhancement, we would do well to follow the adage, "If it ain't broke, don't fix it!"

Suppose that certain drugs could be designed to safely enhance mood. Suppose further that other drugs could safely enhance attention, reasoning, and problem-solving. People with normal cognitive and affective mental states could take them to become more focused, alert, and feel better about themselves without having to worry about any long-term adverse side effects. Would there be any reason to object to taking these drugs to substantially alter psychological properties and create new, happier, and more intelligent selves? One response would be that the self thereby created would not be an authentic self. Although the person would take the drugs voluntarily, the real agent of the change in cognition or mood would not be any desire, belief, or effort of the person but the pharmacological agent. It seems contrary to the idea of authenticity for one to identify with psychological properties generated by drugs that substantially altered normal brain biochemistry. Authenticity presupposes the capacity for self-conscious reflection on one's desires, beliefs, intentions, and other mental states. The drugs could interfere with this capacity by altering the contents of consciousness.

This hypothetical scenario of mood enhancement is significantly different from the hypothetical case of the artist with dysthymia in chapter 2. There the question was whether the patient should be treated for a mild mental disorder due to a mild brain abnormality. He had to weigh the benefits of restoring brain function to a normal level in treating the disorder against the loss of a mildly depressed state with which he identified and which he believed enriched his life. Similarly, beta-adrenergic antagonists would be used to prevent or eliminate pathological emotional memories in conditions such as PTSD and thus retain or restore normal affective capacities. Here the issue is whether it would be desirable to pharmacologically alter brain and mental functions to raise them above a normal level. If the altered mood were induced through artificial means and was alien to the psychological properties we associated with normal brain function, then one could question whether these would be properties of an authentic self, the sort of self with which one would want to identify in the long term.

Some have described the use of drugs to enhance normal cognition and mood as "cosmetic neurology."[68] Their concern is that these uses of psychotropic drugs will alter the meaning of "illness" and "health." Others, including some members of the President's Council on Bioethics, have expressed existential worries about the possible use of these drugs for such things as the selective erasure of unpleasant memories. They worry that this could radically change our experience of suffering and, more fundamentally, what it means to be a person. But as long as we define mental health in terms of a reasonable threshold capacity for basic mental functions, it is unlikely that cognitive or affective enhancement will threaten our definitions and understanding of "health," "illness," "suffering," and "personhood."

It is also unlikely that drugs or transcranial magnetic stimulation could erase unpleasant episodic memories and leave all pleasant episodic memories intact.[69] This idea suggests that we could neatly separate some memories from others because they are located in particular neurons or sets of neurons. It suggests that we could select specific memories for deletion by identifying specific neurons in a brain scan. Yet erasing certain unpleasant memories would probably result in the erasure of pleasant ones as well, given the connections between different memories and memory systems. There is no memory bank in the brain that might allow us to be so selective in depositing and saving some memories while withdrawing others.

If we define personhood minimally in terms of the capacity for self-conscious awareness, then psychopharmacological enhancement would not necessarily alter our understanding of what a person is. Nor would it alter our general conception of personal identity. But it could alter the identity of a particular person who took such a drug and thus could have both metaphysical and ethical implications. More precisely, it would not alter the *numerical* identity of the person, since we would still be able to physically identify an individual as the same person from earlier to later times. But it could alter the *qualitative* identity of the person by altering the psychological properties in terms of which he or she experiences his or her self as persisting through time.[70]

Psychopharmacological enhancement could also alter qualitative identity by altering the behavior in terms of which others identify an individual as the same person at different times. Qualitative identity grounds our prudential concern about how each of our lives goes and our normative practices of holding others praiseworthy, blameworthy, and responsible. The radical personality change in Phineas Gage, mentioned in chapter 3, is an example of a change in qualitative identity. The change led his family and friends to say that the person following the brain injury was "no longer Gage." Cognitive or affective enhancement would not necessarily disrupt episodic memory, in which case the psychological connections and continuity between one's present conscious awareness and the past would remain intact. But it could change the way one formed intentions, undertook projects, and realized these intentions and projects in the near and further future. In this sense, enhancement could influence the psychological connectedness and continuity between one's present and one's future. Cognitive enhancement could alter agency and thereby alter the subjective experience of persisting through time. But it would not undermine agency if the altered intentions were the known or foreseeable consequence of a free and deliberate act of taking an enhancing drug.

If the psychological properties of the person with enhanced mood or cognition were substantially different from the psychological properties of the person who took an enhancement drug, then it would not be clear *who* benefited from it. To say that a person benefits from a drug intervention implies that that person is made better off than he or she was before the intervention. This requires a comparison between two states of affairs in which the same person exists. Yet if the drug caused a substantial change in the person's psychological properties, then one could question whether such a comparison could be made. For the person who took the drug intuitively would have become a qualitatively different person. The psychological connectedness and continuity necessary for personal identity through time would have been disrupted. If these psychological relations were disrupted and the relevant comparison could not be made, then one could not claim that the person benefited from enhanced cognition or mood. Even without adverse side effects, these considerations give us reasons to question the desirability of using psychotropic drugs for enhancing cognition or mood when no mental disorder exists.

Suppose, again, that enhancement drugs were proven to be safe as well as effective. But they would not be available over the counter. Suppose further that a person wanted a drug that would enhance his or her cognitive skills or mood and asked a doctor to prescribe it for him or her. Assuming that the drug was safe, there would be no risk of harm to the individual, and the doctor would be permitted to prescribe it. But there would be no therapeutic relationship between doctor and patient, given that the individual in such a case would not have a disease or illness in any sense of these terms. Even if we construe "therapy" loosely, it is unclear how an intervention that did not restore a patient to, or maintain a patient at, a normal level of mental or physical functioning could be described as therapeutic. The relationship in the case imagined here would not be therapeutic, since there would be no condition justifying medical intervention for treatment or prevention. Thus the doctor would have no duty of beneficence and no obligation to prescribe the drug simply because the individual wanted it.

Modafinil may be prescribed as an alternative to methylphenidate for the treatment of ADHD. Given that ADHD is a psychiatric disorder, this use of the drug would clearly be therapeutic. There may also be compelling reasons for prescribing modafinil for people who need it to perform specific occupational tasks. Airline pilots on transcontinental flights and night-shift workers would fall into this group. Given the cognitive requirements of these tasks, it is questionable whether using the drug to keep them alert would be accurately described as enhancement. Whether the use of a drug is described as therapy or enhancement depends not on the drug itself but the purpose of its use. Doctors are obligated to treat neurological, psychiatric, and other diseases and thereby alleviate pain and suffering in patients who have these diseases. This often involves prescribing certain medications. In cases like the two just mentioned, doctors may prescribe medications necessary for certain types of work. But they are not obligated to make people more competitive or happy. If a person had access to cognition- or mood-enhancing drugs through some other (legal) means, then that person alone would be responsible for any untoward effects of taking them.

Some have speculated that the possibility of neurocognitive enhancement could fundamentally alter the physician-patient relationship.[71] Whether it does this will depend on physicians' views on what it means to have a therapeutic relationship with patients, whether this is a fiduciary relationship, and what it means to act in patients' best interests. It will depend on how physicians conceive of and exercise their professional autonomy in discharging their duty of care to patients. There may be considerable variation among physicians in how they exercise this autonomy.

Conclusion

I have considered different pharmacological interventions for different neurological and psychiatric disorders. I pointed out the difficulty in assessing the safety and efficacy of chronic use of these drugs for therapy or prevention because their long-term effects are unknown. More studies are needed to accurately assess these effects and to adequately weigh the probable benefit against the probable harm to the people who take them. I also discussed the placebo response and argued that it may be ethically permissible for a doctor to use certain psychological techniques in order to produce such a response in a patient. Turning to the potential use of psychotropic drugs for cognitive or mood enhancement, I pointed out that brain systems are designed in such a way that these drugs might not always have a salutary effect. Given the natural design of brain systems, it is unclear whether such drugs could improve the functions of these systems. Trying to increase the functions of some systems might impair the functions of others. Psychopharmacology for the sake of enhancement could result in some form of harm.

The human nervous system is much more complex and sensitive to stimuli than any other system in the human body. For this reason, and because the brain regulates our thought and behavior, the potential magnitude of harm from intervening in the brain must be taken seriously. The plasticity of the brain and the risks in manipulating it also distinguish cognitive and mood enhancement from other forms of bodily enhancement, such as cosmetic surgery. If chronic use of psychotropic drugs to enhance mental traits entailed only minimal benefit and a significant risk of harm, and they were not medically indicated to treat a disease, then there would be no good medical or ethical reasons for doctors to prescribe them to patients. Indeed, they might be prohibited from doing this on grounds of nonmaleficence. Even if drugs that enhanced cognition and mood were effective and safe, doctors would not be obligated to prescribe them to people for these off-label purposes just because they wanted them. In addition, these drugs would more likely maintain or increase than reduce social inequality. Equal access to these drugs would not ensure equal outcomes. One could also question whether drug-induced enhancement would be contrary to the nature of our true selves.

The therapeutic use of psychotropic drugs cannot control or alleviate the symptoms of all psychiatric and neurological disorders. In some cases, these conditions are intractable to pharmacological intervention. Neurosurgery, neurostimulation, and psychosurgery may be medically indicated. These interventions raise a different set of ethical questions, which I will discuss in chapter 5.

Neurosurgery, Psychosurgery, and Neurostimulation

Some psychiatric and neurological disorders are intractable to all drug therapy, and surgery is the only way to control their progression and relieve their symptoms. Surgical intervention in the brain is much more invasive than psychopharmacology and, as such, carries a unique set of risks. These include infection from incisions, respiratory failure from general anesthesia, and damage to brain tissue and systems resulting in various forms of neurological impairment. Alternatively, electrical or magnetic stimulation of particular regions of the brain may effectively treat the symptoms of some neuropsychiatric disorders and obviate the need for conventional surgery. These techniques are less invasive than surgical resection or ablation and less likely to result in neurological sequelae.

In this chapter, I discuss some of the ethical issues surrounding these techniques. I distinguish neurosurgery for tumors and neurological disorders such as epilepsy from psychosurgery for psychiatric disorders such as severe depression and OCD. The rationale for this distinction is that the second class of disorders has a distinctive psychopathology typically not associated with the first. Although both forms of surgery alter brain structures, each aims to correct a different type of functional abnormality. Moreover, unlike neurosurgery to remove tumors, correct malformations, or implant tissue in the brain, psychosurgery to treat severe depression, obsessive-compulsive disorder, or other psychiatric conditions is considered an intervention of last resort. I discuss the weighing of benefits and risks in determining whether neurosurgery or psychosurgery can be justified. The issue of consent from patients figures more importantly in brain surgery than in any other area of neuroethics. This is because of the invasiveness of the procedure and the risk of significant neurological impairment following surgery. It is also because the competence necessary for consent may be impaired by dysfunction of the organ that is both the intended area of intervention and the basis for competence and consent. In addition, I consider different forms of neurostimulation from electrodes implanted inside the brain, as well as from devices outside the brain. These techniques include deep-brain stimulation for motor-control disorders such as

Parkinson's disease, transcranial magnetic stimulation, and vagus nerve stimulation for depression and anxiety. They also include computer–brain interface technology for other neurodegenerative disorders, such as ALS. In the last section, I explore a possible use of neurostimulation for managing pain. In many cases, all of these interventions can be safe and may be the only means of effectively treating and controlling certain disorders of the brain and mind. But they may be more ethically controversial than psychopharmacology because they can more directly alter the neural basis of a person's thought and behavior.

Neurosurgery: Risks and Benefits

Unlike the risks of psychoactive drugs, the risks of neurosurgery are well known. Surgery to excise a tumor or repair an aneurysm in the brain may remove an immediate threat to a person's life. But it may also result in such adverse effects as personality changes, impairment of memory and language, visual field and motor difficulties, and seizures. Nevertheless, on balance, neurosurgery is preferable to drug therapy for some disorders.

Consider epilepsy, for example. Newer antiepileptic drugs are better tolerated and have fewer side effects than previous classes of these drugs. Yet they are not obviously any more effective in treating epilepsy.[1] Roughly one-third of patients with epilepsy continue to have seizures despite using these drugs. Depending on the severity of the disorder, surgery for intractable epilepsy can range from small resection of the cerebral cortex to removal of the anteromesial region of the temporal lobe to removal of an entire cerebral hemisphere. Surgery can control seizures that would otherwise persist with disturbing frequency. Left untreated, seizures can cause chronic excitation of brain circuits, altering the function and structure of neurons, even destroying them. As neurosurgeon Samuel Wiebe explains, "seizure-producing cortex has long been known to be deleterious to the function of the surrounding normal brain, contributing to cognitive and psychomotor deterioration."[2] He notes that 2–5 percent of patients undergoing cortical resections to treat epilepsy experience a range of cognitive and motor deficits. Still, when weighed against the likely consequences of untreated seizures, the benefits of surgery that can end or control seizures outweigh the surgical risks and therefore justify the procedure. Results of a study by Wiebe and his colleagues indicated that surgery for temporal-lobe epilepsy is superior to prolonged medical therapy.[3]

Recall Sister John in the novel *Lying Awake*, which I discussed in chapter 2. What she fears from the surgical removal of the meningioma pressing on her temporal lobe is not so much the potential loss of any of her cognitive or motor functions. Her greater fear is losing the mystical experiences with which she has come to identify and that give meaning to her life. But her neurologist persuades her that failure to remove the meningioma, the source of her visions, would result in an even greater loss to her. What distinguishes this fictional case from generic cases of epilepsy is that, for Sister John, the comparison is not so much between risks and benefits as between greater and lesser senses of loss. In the next section, I will present an actual case of neurosurgery where weighing greater and lesser senses of loss to a patient is an integral part of the moral calculus of risks and benefits.

More precise MRI-guided stereotactic techniques have greatly improved the safety and efficacy of surgical intervention in the brain. These techniques have lessened the risk of sequelae to patients undergoing neurosurgery. Still, the magnitude of the harm resulting from permanent damage to the cortex or other regions of the brain cannot be ignored or minimized. For this reason, many consider neurosurgery an intervention of last resort for neurological disorders. It is worth repeating, though, that roughly one-third of patients with epilepsy have seizures that are intractable to drug therapy and fall into this class.

In some cases of epilepsy, neurosurgery should be considered as a treatment of first rather than last resort. If the cause of epilepsy is a lesion, a developmental problem, a cyst, or a tumor, then seizures may be less likely to respond to medication. If seizures are confined to one area of the brain that can be removed without affecting other areas, then surgery should be done earlier rather than later. Patients with severe epilepsy typically are referred to a surgeon after many years of disabling seizures, which can cause extensive damage to many different regions and functions of the brain. Waiting too long for surgical intervention may result in neurological damage that is too advanced to repair. In all cases of epilepsy, the short- and long-term risks and benefits of neurosurgery must be weighed against the short- and long-term risks and benefits of forgoing the procedure.

Surgery for benign or malignant tumors raises a different set of ethical concerns. Most often, primary brain tumors are gliomas, which grow from glial cells. Astrocytomas and oligodendrogliomas may be slow-growing tumors that cause seizures, though they can cause other forms of brain dysfunction when they are malignant. The most aggressive and fasting-growing malignant brain tumors are glioblastoma multiforme. The prognosis of people with these tumors is poor. Few people survive more than two years after diagnosis because these tumors are aggressive and can kill quickly by local infiltration and increased intracranial pressure. Surgical removal of malignant tumors that are more common in children, such as medulloblastomas, can result in longer term survival. But it can contribute to significant cognitive and other disabilities as well. The standard course of treatment is to remove as much of the tumor as possible and follow it up with chemotherapy and/or cranial-spinal radiation. Many children who receive these three treatments for brain tumors have significant learning and other cognitive impairments following the treatments. In this particular patient population, we need to consider not only the value of life-saving surgery but also the quality of life for patients who survive such surgery.

As substitute decision-makers, parents are presumed to act in the best interests of their children. Agreeing with physicians on a three-phase surgery-chemotherapy-radiation treatment plan for their children is often consistent with these interests. Yet, if the child can only look forward to many years of cognitive and physical disability and poor quality of life as a result of the surgery, then in some cases a decision by parents and physicians to forgo surgery can be justified. Even when a decision not to intervene will result in the death of the child, a shorter life may be preferable to a longer life with significant neurological impairment. The price of a cure might not be so high as to argue that anything other than palliative care should be prohibited. But it could be high enough to argue that forgoing life-sustaining interventions in the brain would be permissible in some cases.

Although benign brain tumors are not as serious as malignant ones in an acute life-threatening sense, they often involve much more complicated medical and ethical decision-making. If benign tumors are only partly surgically removed or left alone, they, too, can become life-threatening and result in significant neurological damage over time. Yet often it cannot be known whether or to what extent these tumors will develop, which is what makes the decision of whether or not to operate so difficult. Neurosurgeons must weigh the risks and benefits of intervening in the brain earlier against the risks and benefits of intervening later or not at all in the light of this uncertainty. Meningiomas fall into this category. More difficult in neurosurgical risk-benefit assessments are pituitary tumors. Although these tumors are usually benign, they control much of the body's endocrine system. Failure to treat them can lead to the hypersecretion of pituitary hormones and disorders such as Cushing's syndrome and hyperthyroidism. Pituitary dysfunction may also have the opposite effect, destroying hormone-secreting tissues and resulting in insufficient levels of hormones in the body. Because the pituitary gland is located at the base of the skull, the slightest error in even partial surgical removal of these tumors can result in damage to the brainstem or other regions that control essential bodily functions. The size and location of such a tumor may limit or even preclude surgery as a treatment option. Some tumors are inoperable.

A "gamma knife" may be an attractive alternative in these cases. It is not literally a knife but a radiosurgical technique that may be effective in treating brain tumors or malformations that have become entangled in critical nerves in the brain. Multiple beams of gamma radiation are targeted to the tumors or malformations to destroy them. This procedure is attractive because, by avoiding incisions into the skull, it is minimally invasive and does not require general anesthesia. It can also avoid damage to nerves and blood vessels in the brain. So it would involve much less risk of infection, hemorrhage, or paralysis. But even low doses of radiation in the brain can have adverse neurological effects, and these effects may not appear until much later in the patient's life. Exposure to radiation can also put one at risk of developing cancer. Although the gamma knife can attain submillimeter accuracy, this would not entirely eliminate the risk of a surgeon or radiologist directing the beam slightly off target. This could alter normal neural circuits. Nor are the long-term effects of radiation beams that hit their intended target on the affected area of the brain known. There is also the question of just how deeply into the brain these beams can penetrate. They may not be able to reach all subcortical regions and ablate all tumors deep inside these regions. Although it may be a feasible alternative to standard surgery for treatment of such conditions as arteriovenous malformation (AVM) and trigeminal neuralgia, and although it may have a broader range of applications as it is refined, gamma radiation is still limited in safely and effectively treating most brain tumors. The gamma knife is not the only technique in radiosurgery. Other techniques are equally effective and are widely used, though they involve many of the same risks.

In some cases, early surgical intervention in the brain to remove tumors may be more beneficial than later intervention, all things considered. This was noted earlier with respect to tumor-related epilepsy. Left untreated, a tumor can grow and damage regions other than those in which it was originally located. If this occurs, then it may be difficult to remove the tumor without damaging these other regions. The risk entailed by the surgery must be weighed against the risk of allowing the tumor to progress. But, again, at the earlier time it may be impossible to know whether or not the tumor will progress. Monitoring the tumor with CT, MRI, or other types of imaging may be the best course of action.

Consider the case history of Lucia Eufemia, a patient treated at the Montreal Neurological Institute.[4] In 1995, at age seven, she was diagnosed as having a pilocytic astrocytoma, a benign and slow-growing tumor in the brain. It was located around the cerebellum and brainstem. Although benign brain tumors do not infiltrate brain tissue in the same way that malignant tumors do, they can push away and damage healthy brain tissue. Because of its location, only slightly more than half of the tumor was removed. The tumor resumed growing a few millimeters every few months. In early 2003, at age 15, Lucia developed paralysis in her right arm, and was experiencing fatigue, nausea, and blurred vision, all the result of the tumor. Chemotherapy and radiation failed to slow its progression, so a second surgery was the only option. Because the tumor was now more extensive, the risk of damage to regions of the brain controlling critical bodily functions was considerable. The slightest error in excising the tumor could result in further morbidity or even death. Yet the long-term risks of not operating would be just as great, given the equally significant risk of allowing the tumor to grow larger. On balance, in early 2003, the risk of operating seemed less than the risk of operating later or not at all, thus justifying the procedure.

To minimize brain damage, the patient remained awake during the surgery. In this way, she would be able to report any unusual or lost sensations correlating with brain damage. Nerves around the patient's skull were frozen, but even without the freezing, Lucia would have felt no pain, because the brain has no afferent nerves to conduct pain sensation. This time around, the surgeons were able to excise 80 percent of the tumor. They hoped that what remained would not grow back or, if it did, would grow very slowly. That could take years, a hope that justified not trying to remove the entire tumor and risking damage that could result in coma and death. The tumor remains in Lucia's brain and is monitored by periodic nueroimaging and other clinical and behavioral measures.

In this type of case, the ethical issue is not simply how to weigh potential benefits against potential risks to the patient. More specifically, the issue is estimating greater and lesser potential risks of operating earlier against operating later, which turns on weighing greater and lesser potential harm to the patient. Is the potential for harm to the patient greater if neurosurgery is performed at an earlier or later time? What complicates this medical and moral calculus is that often only a portion of a benign tumor can be removed if surgery is to remain within the threshold of acceptable medical risk. As a matter of nonmaleficence, surgeons have a duty to not expose their patients to undue risk. But patients, or parents and others who are substitute decision-makers for children, have a prima facie right to decide whether to undergo or allow a procedure that entails some risk of harm to them.

They must give informed consent to the surgery. This is a process consisting of three components. First, the surgeon must disclose to the patient the nature of his or her condition and the risks and benefits of a proposed surgical procedure, as well as any other treatment options. Second, the patient must be competent to understand the information that the physician presents to him or her. Third, the patient freely decides to have or forgo the procedure on the basis of the information presented to him or her.[5] Provided that the patient's neurological condition did not impair his or her competence, or that a surrogate decision-maker chose the course of action that a noncompetent patient would have wanted, neurosurgery in the case at hand would be justified. An important factor in a competent patient's decision may be his or her appraisal of the quality of life he or she would have with or without neurosurgery. There may be instances in which a person believes that the consequences of neurosurgery would leave one with an unacceptable quality of life that would be worse than death. The patient may believe that the effects of curing a brain disease would be worse than letting the disease run its course.

The Iranian Twins

When patients do not have a life-threatening condition, there may be cases where even a high risk of morbidity and mortality may not be enough to prohibit neurosurgery on ethical grounds. Although a surgeon's duty of nonmaleficence to not harm patients has considerable weight, it is not an absolute duty. In living organ donation and transplantation, for example, surgeons expose donors of liver and lung lobes or kidneys to some risk of morbidity and even mortality in procuring these organs. Yet, provided that the donor meets strict psychosocial criteria in the assessment prior to donating and is not exposed to more than a medically acceptable degree of risk, living donation is medically and ethically permissible. Still, there are limits to how much risk is acceptable. Some might argue that, when the risk of mortality from a surgical procedure is considered to be greater than 50 percent, the procedure should not be performed.

This is not a reasonable rule for all cases, though. It would be unreasonable to refuse surgery with a 30 percent chance of success if otherwise the patient would likely die within a few weeks. Surgical statistics alone may not be very helpful. What is needed is a case-by-case balancing of potential benefit and harm to decide whether a particular surgical procedure should or should not be performed on a particular patient. The reasonableness of this position is exemplified in the following case.

Ladan and Laleh Bijani were 29-year-old Iranian twins born joined at the head. When they were two years old, their parents consulted with German doctors about possible separation surgery for their daughters. The doctors told them that at least one of the twins would die in surgery. Ayatollah Ruhollah Khomeini proclaimed that that operation would not be permissible under Islamic law because doctors knew in advance that one twin would die. Twenty-seven years later, Ladan and Laleh decided that they wanted to undergo a long and risky operation to separate them at the head. They made this decision knowing that there was a significant probability that both would die from the procedure. The surgery was the only way for them to have separate and independent lives, free of the extreme physical constrains of a rare congenital malformation. It was performed at Raffles Hospital in Singapore in July 2003.

The most difficult obstacle in separation neurosurgery for conjoined twins is the sagittal sinus, a large vein at the back of the skull that the twins shared. This vein is an essential part of the drainage system that moves blood from the brain back to the heart. If the drainage were to become blocked, the brain could swell or bleed excessively, killing one or both twins. The surgery is riskier for adults than children because the vein and surrounding structures are larger and more interconnected. Children have a better chance of recovering from any neurological insults resulting from brain surgery because their developing brains are better at compensating for this damage. A gradual, multistaged procedure, instead of a single marathon procedure, can further reduce the risk of separation surgery for children. A gradual procedure was used to successfully separate Carl and Clarence Aguirre, two-year-old Filipina twins joined at the top of their heads, at Children's Hospital and Montefiore Medical Center in New York in August 2004. The Iranian conjoined twins underwent one procedure. After 50 hours of surgery, Ladan and Laleh died within 90 minutes of each other from a massive cerebral hemorrhage secondary to a ruptured sagittal sinus.[6]

There are three possible outcomes of separation surgery, which can be ranked in order of desirability. The most desirable is that both twins are successfully separated and survive the surgery, with perhaps some but not significant neurological impairment. The next desirable outcome is that one twin survives and the other dies. This has been the outcome of some separation surgeries involving very young children, though the surviving twin often has some degree of neurological disability. The least desirable surgical outcome is that both twins die, which unfortunately is what occurred for the Bijanis. These three outcomes can be compared with a fourth scenario in which there is no separation surgery and the twins remain joined at the head.

Doctors are not obligated to provide a particular drug treatment or perform a surgical procedure just because a patient requests it. Indeed, even when requested by a competent patient, a procedure that would involve the physician knowingly harming the patient would be prohibited both medically and ethically. Some physicians and ethicists argued that the risk of death from surgery for Ladan and Laleh was greater than 50 percent, and therefore the surgery should not have been performed. But even such a high risk of mortality does not necessarily mean than surgeons would intentionally or knowingly be harming the twins by doing the separation surgery. Medical risk is not the only criterion in assessing benefit and harm to patients. There were both medical and nonmedical dimensions of benefit and harm in this case, and the nonmedical dimension played a critical role in determining whether the surgery was ethically justified.

It is not obvious that the death of both twins would be a worse state of affairs for them than continuing to be joined at the head. Comparing shorter and longer lives of the same two people, one could argue that, given the continued suffering they would endure in their conjoined state, a longer life for them would be worse than a shorter life. What mattered for each of the twins was not simply continued biological life but also, and more important, the quality of that life. Quality of life consists roughly in the capacity to undertake and find meaning in projects connected with one's interests. It presupposes a basic level of physical and mental capacity, which can vary from one person to the next. There is no universal or absolute measure of quality of life, which is largely subjective and a matter of degree.

If the twins considered that their quality of life was very low, then it would not be unreasonable for them to take the risk of death for the chance of a good surgical outcome that would greatly improve their quality of life. Death would be the lesser evil, and continued life would be the greater evil. When compared with continued life joined at the head, death for the twins would not be the greater loss. This reasoning very likely was behind their mutual decision to undergo the surgery despite the risk. It also suggests that the intuitive rule of not performing a surgery entailing greater than a 50 percent risk of death would have been unreasonable in this case.

Would this reasoning make it permissible for surgeons to perform a procedure that entailed less than a relatively small chance of even one twin surviving? Nonmaleficence is not an absolute duty for surgeons. Yet, as moral agents, they have a duty to protect patients from significant risk of harm or death, which the odds in this case would indicate. Presumably, they would be prohibited from performing such high-risk surgery. Some might appeal to the doctrine of double effect (DDE) to support this argument. Thomas Aquinas first formulated this doctrine in his analysis of justifiable homicide in self-defense. It refers to actions that can have both good and bad, beneficial and harmful, effects. The DDE says that it is permissible to perform an action that has an unintended but foreseeable bad effect if the act is intended and has a good effect, the bad effect is not a means to the good effect, and the good effect outweighs, or at least compensates for, the bad effect. Defenders of DDE might claim that the separation surgery in this case was impermissible because it failed to meet the third condition. The survival of one twin might compensate for the death of the other. But the relatively high risk of both twins dying from the surgery suggested that there probably would not be any good outcome that could compensate for the bad outcome. Because of this, and because being joined at the head is not a life-threatening or terminal condition, defenders of DDE might conclude that the separation surgery on these adults should not have been performed. Continued life joined at the head arguably would be better than two deaths.

By focusing only on survival versus death, however, DDE fails to consider the quality of life for the twins. This factor was critical to their decision to undergo the surgery. Benefit and harm in such a case must be more broadly construed to include not just quantitative medical factors but qualitative nonmedical factors as well. If separation surgery prevented the greater harm of continued life as conjoined twins, and death for both twins was the lesser harm, then it seems that separation surgery was reasonable and hence justifiable in this case. Surgeons would be justified in trying to prevent the greater harm by operating. Put another way, one could argue that continued life for the twins would have a net disvalue and that death would be value-neutral. Given that the quality of their continued lives joined at the head would be very poor, they would not be deprived of any compensating goods by dying sooner. An outcome of neutral value is preferable to an outcome of negative value. This reasoning would also justify the operation. Provided that the twins were competent and freely consented to the surgery, and that the surgeons were acting in the twins' all-things-considered best interests, the separation surgery was ethically permissible.

Similar reasoning would justify consent of competent and informed parents for their children to undergo separation surgery. Given the moral calculus of potential benefit and harm with and without the surgery, there is no significant moral difference between direct consent by adults and proxy consent by parents for their children. Parental consent was acceptable in the August 2004 case of the conjoined Filipina twins in New York, as well as the October 2005 case in Delhi of 10-year-old Indian twins Farah and Saba Ahmad conjoined at the head. Unlike the situation of the Filipina twins, Farah Ahmad had two kidneys, while her sister Saba had none. She would need a kidney transplant if she survived the operation. Assuming that the transplant had to be done shortly after the brain surgery, this would complicate Saba's recovery and reduce her chance of long-term survival. Given Saba's poor prognosis, it would be permissible to treat the twins unequally in the separation surgery. It would be permissible to maximize the probability of survival and a good neurological prognosis for Farah, even if it minimized the probability of survival for her sister. An outcome in which one survived with good neurological function would be better than an outcome in which both died. Arguably, such an outcome would also be better than one in which both twins survived with poor neurological function. Whether one agrees with this claim depends on how much moral weight one gives to survival and how much to well-being over the remainder of the twins' lives. Giving more weight to well-being would still involve some uncertainty. It would depend on the quality of each twin's own future life experience, which would have a subjective component that could not be predicted or measured at the time of the surgery.

Neural Transplantation

The prospect of fetal tissue and fetal, adult, and embryonic stem-cell transplantation in the brain is different from separation surgery in at least two respects. First, this type of transplantation is part of regenerative medicine, which aims to regenerate cells, tissues, and organs that have failed or are failing due to trauma or degenerative diseases. Second, transplantation of cells and tissues into the brain is still experimental. Some clinical trials have been conducted to test the efficacy of fetal-tissue and neural stem-cell transplantation. But these trials have failed to produce the desired results, and this type of transplantation is years away from standard clinical application. The goal of fetal or embryonic stem-cell transplantation in patients with Parkinson's disease, for example, would be to replace dopamine-producing neurons that have been lost. In Alzheimer's, the goal of such a procedure would be to replace neurons in the hippocampus and cortex regulating memory and other cognitive functions. Fetal tissue and stem-cell transplantation might also regenerate neurons that have been damaged or destroyed from strokes or spinal cord injuries. Like separation surgery, though, this type of surgery raises the ethical question of how much risk is permissible.

Transplantation of tissue grafts from aborted fetuses into the substantia nigra region of the basal ganglia in the brains of Parkinson's patients began to be performed on an experimental basis in the 1980s. In 1999, the National Institutes of Health (NIH) sponsored a double-blind, placebo-controlled clinical trial to determine whether this surgery was effective.[7] Patients in the intervention group received general anesthesia. Burr holes were drilled in their skulls, and the fetal tissue was implanted in the designated region. Patients in the control group received general anesthesia, though the burr holes did not penetrate the cortex. Both groups received a low dose of the immunosuppressive drug cyclosporine for six months postoperatively and continued to receive drug therapy for their disease. To ensure that the trial was blinded, the surgical and evaluation sites were in separate locations. The surgeon was the only member of the research team aware of each subject's group assignment.

Let's assume that the standard levodopa drug therapy for many Parkinson's patients is only marginally effective.[8] Can any benefits from learning whether fetal-nigral tissue transplantation can regenerate dopamine–producing neurons justify exposing research subjects to its risks? If the transplant procedure proves to be effective, then many patients who are or will be suffering from Parkinson's could benefit from these trials. If the procedure proves to be ineffective, then many patients will be spared the medical risks and financial burdens of an unproven operation. But the risks to the subjects in these trials are significant. General anesthesia can lead to respiratory failure. Although general anesthesia is now safer than before, it still entails respiratory risks to patients who undergo it. Moreover, subjects might become infected from the burr holes and have their immune systems weakened by the cyclosporine. Patients who receive the implants are exposed to greater risk because of the needle penetration to the brain. There is also some risk of damage from the surgery to other regions of the brain controlling memory and other cognitive functions, as well as personality. Some subjects in a recent trial testing fetal-nigral transplantation developed dyskinesias.[9] It would appear that the risks to both groups are significant enough to outweigh any potential benefits to them or to future patients.

Obtaining informed consent from the research subjects in these trials is necessary but not sufficient for the trial to be ethically justified. In addition, the research must not expose the subjects to undue risk. Researchers and clinicians are permitted to expose research subjects and patients to some degree of risk, but not to undue risk. Some might argue that the risk in this or other surgical trials is high enough to prohibit them. In addition, some might argue that the "sham" surgery for patients in the placebo arm of the trial is doubly unethical because the surgeon is deliberately deceiving the patients into thinking that they are receiving the fetal tissue implants. Nevertheless, only such a trial can determine whether fetal tissue surgery is more effective than standard drug therapy in treating Parkinson's. Among other things, a clinical trial can test for false positive results from the surgery when it is practiced on a purely innovative or experimental basis.[10] These trials might yield results that could lead to better treatments for this disease and benefit future patients.

In severe cases of Parkinson's, where drug therapy has been ineffective in controlling symptoms, the participation of subjects in fetal tissue transplant surgical trials is not obviously unethical. When comparing life with uncontrollable bodily movements and cognitive and affective deterioration against the risk of postsurgical morbidity or mortality, some patients may rationally believe that the potential benefits of the surgery are worth the risks. Patients in both experimental and control arms of the trials may have the same belief, since positive results for those receiving the implants would mean that those receiving the sham surgery would subsequently receive the implants and experience the same therapeutic effect. Moreover, they might believe that the risk of morbidity or even mortality from the surgery is the lesser harm and that continuing to suffer from the disease is the greater harm. This would make it reasonable for them to enter the trial. They might conclude that undergoing actual or sham surgery on balance would be in their best interests. In severe cases of Parkinson's, it might be permissible to perform fetal-nigral tissue transplantation on competent, consenting patients, despite what at first blush might seem to be a medically and ethically unacceptable degree of risk.

Whether one agrees or disagrees with this claim may depend on whether one gives more ethical weight to patient autonomy or to physician nonmaleficence. But these two principles need not, indeed should not, be seen as mutually exclusive. On the contrary, the surgeon's belief about his or her duty to benefit and not harm a patient should be influenced, to some degree at least, by what constitutes benefit and harm for the patient. An individual with Parkinson's may decide that participating in a surgical clinical trial or undergoing an experimental surgical procedure overall would be more beneficial than harmful to him or her and therefore in his or her best interests. These will include both medical and nonmedical interests.

Fetal, adult, and embryonic stem cells may be more promising for neural transplantation, given their potential for self-renewal and to differentiate into many different cell and tissue types in the body. Neural stem cells could regenerate neural tissue damaged from neurological disease and thus could be an important part of regenerative medicine. Hematopoietic stem cells are perhaps the most familiar adult stem cells. They are found in bone marrow and are the source of many kinds of blood cells. These particular stem cells are multipotent, meaning that they can generate a variety of cell types, possibly including two types of brain cell: neurons, which relay neural signals; and astrocytes, a class of glial cells that provide a supportive environment for neurons to function properly. Fetal stem cells found in umbilical cord blood resemble hematopoietic stem cells and could have the same neural regenerative potential. Embryonic stem (ES) cells would have the greatest potential for neural regeneration. This is because they are pluripotent, or capable of differentiating into virtually any cell type. The fact that they are much more versatile than other stem cells suggests that it might be easier to coax them into neural cells. Embryonic stem cells hold considerable promise for treating a wide range of neurodegenerative diseases. But implanting these cells into the brain would not necessarily mean that they would produce the desired results.

With a few exceptions to date, clinical trials for neural stem-cell transplantation have shown that the therapeutic promise is far from being realized. For most neurodegenerative disorders, the procedure is not yet medically feasible.[11] This is because researchers still do not know how to tweak and prompt stem cells so that they would differentiate into specific neural cells. Experiments involving mouse models have suggested the possibility of using ES-cell-derived astrocytes as vectors for the delivery of gene therapy to treat gliomas and other CNS tumors.[12] But it is far from clear whether the genes would integrate into the targeted brain regions in humans and function as intended. As noted in chapter 4, vectors in gene therapy experiments have been associated with the subsequent development of some cancers. It is possible that stem cells could overly stimulate growth factors in the central or peripheral nervous system, leading to uncontrolled proliferation of cells and benign or malignant tumors. This occurred in a case presented at the Children's Hospital of British Columbia in September 2004.

A 10-year-old girl had developed severe cognitive, behavioral, and motor handicaps as a result of herpes simplex encephalitis during infancy. Unwilling to accept the prognosis of permanent cognitive and physical disability, her desperate parents contacted a doctor in Russia. The doctor claimed to have regenerated neural tissue and restored neurological function in patients by transplanting fetal stem-cell tissue into the cerebral-spinal fluid (CSF). The parents traveled to Russia, and their daughter had fetal tissue injections into her spine in the lumbar region in a procedure known as intrathecal stem-cell infusion. Unfortunately, her neurological function did not improve. Even worse, the transplanted tissue began to proliferate unexpectedly in her spine. Although it did not develop into a malignant tumor, the proliferating tissue did impair her ability to walk, causing paraplegia. It was discovered that the abnormal growth came from the foreign tissue, because it contained male chromosomes and a male genetic karyotype. At this point, the parents returned to Vancouver and brought her to the pediatric neurological clinic at the British Columbia Children's Hospital. High-dose steroids helped. But the growth could not be surgically removed, and there was a high likelihood that the tissue would continue to grow and cause further and more severe disability.

This case illustrates that it is still not known how transplanted stem cells can be controlled. In particular, the case illustrates the need for more studies and substantial empirical data to understand how stem cells can affect growth factors in the spinal cord and brain. When used as unproven therapy, fetal stem-cell tissue transplants can harm a patient more than the neurological disorder the procedure is intended to treat. It is especially difficult to justify exposing a patient to such a potentially life-threatening risk of harm caused by uncontrolled growth of implanted embryonic or fetal stem-cell tissue when the patient's condition is not terminal. This raises the following question. Could an experimental surgical procedure be given for a debilitating neurological condition with no proven treatment, even when the condition is stable and not terminal?

In a nonterminal case, any experimental and thus unproven treatment should not pose more than a minimal risk of harm to the patient and should have some expected benefit. In a terminal case of a relentlessly progressive disorder where death is imminent, the acceptable ratio of probable harm to benefit should shift. In the second case, the promise of a potentially significant benefit can offset the potential for further harm to the patient. Surgical intervention would be justified, and a neurosurgeon would be justifiably exercising his or her moral agency, because the surgery would be intended to prevent the perceived greater harm of death. What complicates the ethical assessment in the nonterminal case is that the patient's quality of life may be a critical factor in weighing potential benefit against potential harm to him or her. This can be difficult to assess if the patient is unable to effectively communicate what his or her quality of life is and surrogates such as parents make this judgment for him or her. Desperation or frustration with the patient's condition and limited treatment options can distort these substitute judgments. As a result, they may not accurately reflect the experience or wishes of the patient and may not be in the patient's best interests. Indeed, these judgments could result in procedures that cause more harm to the patient, as occurred in the case of the 10-year-old patient I have been discussing.

But there is a general presumption of parental autonomy in deciding which treatments to give children. Quality-of-life considerations can legitimately fall under this autonomy, provided that they are made in consultation with the physician or medical team providing the treatment. Parents, in principle, should have the autonomy to decide on a treatment for their child, even if it entails some risk. They can consent to the treatment if it could be therapeutic despite the risk. They can also consent to it if they believe that the quality of their child's life without the treatment would be so low as not to be worth living. This is controversial, however, because there is no clear objective measure of quality of life that applies equally to all persons. It can be especially controversial in children and incompetent adults, who may not be able to give a clear indication of their subjective experience to others. Yet in many cases, a general sense of a person's experience with medical conditions can be gleaned from his or her behavior.

When the risk of neurological impairment from a procedure is significant, the patient lacks the competence to consent to the procedure, and the patient's condition is severe but not terminal, surrogates such as parents and physicians involved in the patient's care must together assess the patient's quality of life. On the basis of the patient's behavior, they can decide whether his or her quality of life is low enough to justify a risky procedure. A good example of a risky procedure requested by some parents on quality-of-life grounds is placing a child with cerebral palsy in a hyperbaric oxygen chamber. While the intent of this procedure is to increase oxygen to the brain and control the symptoms of the condition, it entails a risk of further morbidity and mortality for children who undergo it.

In cases where stem cells are implanted in the brain, they might integrate improperly into neural circuits. Stem cells intended for the hippocampus might migrate to the temporal lobes and cause epileptic seizures. If the cells were from allografts transplanted into the brain from a different person or embryo with a different genotype, they could trigger a harmful immune response. Embryonic stem cells carry the same surface antigens that the immune system recognizes as pathogens and might result in the same immune rejection that occurs with transplanted organs. Closer immune or human leukocyte antigen (HLA) matches could reduce the likelihood of this occurring.

The potential problem of an adverse immune response could be avoided by creating stem cells from one's own somatic cells. They could be created through therapeutic cloning of an embryo from somatic-cell nuclear transfer. In this procedure, the nucleus of a somatic cell is transferred to an enucleated egg, which genetically reprograms the nucleus. As a form of autologous transplantation, injecting one's own stem cells into the brain would greatly diminish the potential for an adverse immune response, since the cells would be genetically identical to the donor. Nevertheless, it is possible that mutations could result from the genetic reprogramming, not unlike the mutations that have resulted from the reproductive cloning of animals such as the sheep "Dolly." Although the risk of immune rejection would be lower in the transplantation of ES cells from one's own somatic cells, these cells could still be immunogenic. Proteins encoded by mitochondrial genes could stimulate the immune system and cause it to reject the new neural cells.

All of these considerations underscore the need for carefully designed and regulated clinical trials for neural transplantation. Although it has not yet been realized, the promise of these techniques for controlling the progression of or even reversing neurodegenerative diseases is considerable. But the risks are considerable as well, as illustrated by the case of the girl with the neurological disorder who had the fetal stem-cell tissue injected into her CSF. This indicates that we have a dual responsibility to people suffering from neurodegenerative diseases.

We have a responsibility to expand research on adult, fetal, and embryonic stem cells that might lead to treatments that could control the progression of these diseases. This includes the use of stem-cell lines derived from in vitro fertilization (IVF) embryos discarded from fertility clinics or harvested from embryos created through somatic-cell nuclear transfer, or therapeutic cloning. Although more stem-cell lines could be derived from the second procedure, religious and politically motivated objections have blocked public funding for this research in the United States. Privately funded embryonic stem-cell research is legal. To date, only the United Kingdom and Denmark allow publicly funded embryonic stem-cell research. There is also the practical question of whether therapeutic cloning would be feasible, given the large number of eggs that would be necessary to perform it. Equally significant is the ethical question of whether there would be any coercion or exploitation of the women who would contribute these eggs.

We also have a responsibility to ensure that neural stem-cell transplantation is safe and effective so that people could benefit from it and not be harmed. This is especially important for the protection of vulnerable individuals such as children, who may not understand the risks of procedures designed to treat chronic neurological disabilities. People other than those with the neurological condition may be making decisions about whether to perform a risky procedure. In cases of severe neurodegenerative disease with no other treatment options, neural stem-cell transplantation may be justified as an experimental procedure. But only closely monitored research involving randomized controlled clinical trials can establish whether this and similar procedures can be safe and effective forms of therapy.

Psychosurgery

The Portuguese neurologist Egas Moniz coined the term "psychosurgery" to describe the procedure of making lesions in dysfunctional circuits of the limbic system, which he believed generated emotions, memory, and personality. His aim was to modify abnormal thoughts and feelings by forcing their neural correlates into different brain pathways. His preferred procedure was the prefrontal leucotomy, or frontal lobotomy. Moniz believed that surgically destroying the frontal lobes of humans could improve severe psychiatric illnesses. The procedure consisted in first injecting alcohol into the white matter of patients' frontal lobes. Moniz and the neurosurgeon Almeida Lima then used a leukotome, an instrument with which they made lesions in each frontal lobe, to sever areas of white matter about one centimeter in diameter. Many applauded the anecdotal success stories of the operation, and Moniz received the Nobel Prize for medicine in 1949 for the "therapeutic" value of leucotomy.[13]

The most enthusiastic proponent and practitioner of psychosurgery was the American neurologist Walter Freeman, who performed some 3,500 frontal lobotomies in the United States in the 1940s and 1950s. Freeman's method consisted in inserting an instrument (an "ice pick") through the skull just above the eyes and swinging it back and forth to disconnect white matter in the frontal lobes and their connections to the thalamus. Although lobotomies relieved some symptoms of severe psychiatric illness, they often had severe neurological and psychological consequences. These included significant personality changes, seizures, apathy, loss of impulse control, and, in some cases, death. Lobotomies ceased being a standard treatment for mental diseases with the advent of antipsychotic and antidepressant drugs.

Given its notorious history, many people are disturbed by the very thought of psychosurgery. In spite of this, it continues to be practiced as a medical treatment of last resort for obsessive-compulsive disorder, severe depression, and anxiety disorders that are refractory to all other treatments. Psychosurgery is relatively rare and involves a much smaller number of patients than other forms of brain surgery. It is still experimental in that the indications and exact procedures are contentious and constantly undergoing revision and review. Although some repudiate these procedures, they usually undergo close scrutiny by panels of psychiatrists, clinical psychologists, neurologists, and neurosurgeons. More selective MRI-guided stereotactic techniques have improved the safety and efficacy of psychosurgery Nevertheless, the risk of permanent damage to brain circuits and of neurological and psychological disability is significant.

Psychosurgery consists in the surgical ablation or disconnection of brain tissue with the intent of correcting abnormal cognitive and affective mental states caused by psychiatric disorders. It alters dysfunctional brain circuits and pathways that underlie different types of psychopathology. The procedure has been refined considerably since the days of Moniz and Freeman and is now more precise and comparatively safer and more effective. In some respects, psychosurgery is analogous to cardiac ablation. For some people, particular cells in heart muscle can cause abnormal electrical impulses in either the ventricle or atrium, resulting in arrhythmias that may be annoying but benign, or life-threatening. Once the source of the rhythm abnormality has been identified, the problematic cells can be obliterated by high-frequency radio waves produced through a catheter that reaches the heart after being inserted into an artery in the groin or neck. This procedure can correct many cardiac arrhythmias. Similarly, psychosurgery aims to correct psychiatric disorders by ablating brain circuits identified as causes of these disorders.

Of all conditions treated with psychosurgery, OCD has perhaps the best risk–benefit profile. Cingulotomy has been the surgical procedure of choice to treat severe OCD that has not responded to any pharmacological agents or cognitive-behavioral therapy. Symptoms of this disorder have been linked to damage to the basal ganglia. But a dysfunctional anterior cingulate gyrus has been implicated as probably the main cause of patients' obsessions with contamination and compulsion to wash their hands. In a cingulotomy, bilateral burr holes are drilled in the skull, and two small holes are made bilaterally in the cingulate. The patient is conscious but cannot feel the metal probe as it slides through brain tissue to the cingulate. The tip of the probe is heated to 70 degrees Celsius for 60 seconds, burning two rectangular lesions, each 2.5 centimeters by 1 centimeter, in the targeted tissue. The purpose of making these lesions is to alter a dysfunctional circuit in the main pathway between the limbic system and prefrontal cortex causing the abnormal cognitive and emotional processing that is responsible for the obsessions and compulsions. The same procedure has also been performed on depressed patients who have not responded to antidepressant medication.[14] Subcaudate tractotomy, limbic leucotomy, and anterior capsulotomy are similar procedures targeting different regions of the brain that also regulate affective and cognitive processing. These types of psychosurgery have been performed primarily to treat severe mood and anxiety disorders.

Data from cingulotomies for OCD performed over the last 30 years at the Massachusetts General Hospital indicate that 30 percent of patients who underwent the procedure experienced significant improvement of their symptoms, while 60 percent experienced mild to moderate improvement.[15] But a significant number of the same patients experienced such serious postsurgery symptoms as personality changes ("frontal lobe syndrome"), apathy, aggressive behavior, amnesia, and difficulty controlling impulses. Some patients attempted suicide. Studies from the United Kingdom and the Karolinska Institute in Stockholm in the 1990s yielded similar results.[16] Other studies have had more positive results, especially regarding alleged negative personality changes resulting from psychosurgery.[17]

The main question here is how much risk is acceptable for a patient to take, given the severity of the condition and the potential benefits of psychosurgery in treating psychopathological symptoms. A related question is to what degree of risk is a surgeon permitted to expose a patient who has been deemed an appropriate candidate for psychosurgery. Risk is more difficult to assess in psychosurgery for psychiatric disorders than in neurosurgery for neurological disorders. For while it is known that psychosurgery can be effective for some patients, it is not known exactly how it works. If the mechanisms through which psychosurgery affects the brain are not well known, then this would seem to increase the probability of unforeseeable adverse events from the procedure. This uncertainty intuitively would recommend a lower threshold of acceptable risk for psychosurgery than for other forms of intracranial surgery.

How much risk the patient is willing to take will depend on how the patient judges his or her quality of life given the symptoms caused by the psychiatric disorder. If the symptoms of OCD, MDD, or GAD make life intolerable for the patient, then it can be quite reasonable for him or her to choose psychosurgery to relieve these symptoms.

How a patient factors quality of life into his or her decision should also influence the surgeon's perspective on the permissibility of the procedure. Surgeons are not obligated to perform surgical procedures just because patients request them. But surgeons do have an obligation to act in patients' best interests. Thus, if a patient's quality of life with a psychiatric illness is bad enough to justify the procedure for him or her, then it seems prima facie permissible for the surgeon to perform it. The surgery can be in the patient's best interests, which the surgeon has a general obligation to respect when acting not only as a medical but also as a moral agent. A surgeon who performs such a procedure is discharging his or her duties of nonmaleficence and beneficence to the patient when the condition is refractory to all other treatments, the patient can no longer cope with the symptoms, and there is no relief in sight. When these conditions are met, psychosurgery is permissible, despite the possible postoperative effects that I have mentioned. On balance, the benefits of the surgery medically and ethically outweigh the risks. Yet because of the magnitude of the harm that patients undergoing it could experience, psychosurgery should only be considered when all other treatment alternatives have been exhausted and therefore as a treatment of last resort.

Risk–benefit assessments in psychosurgery are closely related to the ethical issues involved in obtaining informed consent from patients undergoing the procedure. Some patients may undergo psychosurgery out of a desperate desire for relief from their symptoms. This desperation may impair their ability to rationally weigh the potential benefits against the potential risks and make a rational decision to have or forgo the surgery. To be sure, there are other medical conditions in which patients may desperately desire relief from their symptoms through pharmacological means. What is distinctive about psychosurgery for psychiatric disorders is that these disorders can impair one's ability to understand the potential benefits and risks of the procedure. And yet the source of this impairment is the very target of the procedure. Because of this, and because of the magnitude of the potential neurological and psychological harm from psychosurgery, the threshold of decisional capacity to consent to psychosurgery should be higher than it is for other medical interventions.

More than 20 years ago, James Drane proposed a sliding-scale model for patient consent to treatment.[18] The stringency of consent was a matter of degree, depending on the severity of the medical condition, the alternatives for treatment, and the degree of risk associated with the proposed procedure or therapy. On this model, the least stringent level pertains to life-saving situations, where the patient is acutely ill, there are few or no treatment alternatives, and the available treatment is safe and effective. The most stringent level pertains to chronic, non-life-saving situations, where the risks of the proposed treatment are significant, the benefits are questionable, and there are alternative treatments.

We can adopt Drane's model to guide us in assessing consent to psychosurgery. My analysis suggests that consent to psychosurgery lies at the higher, more stringent, end of the consent scale. One qualifying factor is that the psychiatric conditions for which the procedure is indicated are often not strictly speaking life-threatening, though there is a risk of suicide. Yet the magnitude of the potential harm from psychosurgery to the patient is considerable. Any adverse events from the surgery could alter memory, personality, and other psychological states the integrity and continuity of which allow for a decent quality of life. Another important factor is that psychiatric disorders often involve impairment or loss of the capacity to give informed consent. They can directly affect the mental capacity to reason and make decisions about treatment.

Accordingly, a careful neurological and psychological evaluation of the patient must be made before he or she can be considered as a candidate for psychosurgery. Obsessive-compulsive disorder may not involve the same degree of cognitive and affective impairment and thus not the same degree of impairment in decisional capacity as mood disorders. Nevertheless, people with this disorder often have difficulty with reasoning and decision-making. This is mainly because the anterior cingulate, which is dysfunctional in OCD, plays an important role in regulating the cognitive and affective processing necessary for one to make rational choices. A family member or other person who knows the patient should participate in discussing the benefits and risks of the surgery with the medical team. But unless the patient's basic competence to reason and make decisions is in question, he or she alone can consent to psychosurgery. Consent to psychosurgery can be problematic in cases of severe depression, however, when the patient's mood disorder may leave him or her with impaired or no decisional capacity. Provided that it is clear to all relevant parties that they are acting in the patient's best interests, an appropriately designated surrogate can consent to the surgery on the patient's behalf. This can be justified when the condition poses a significant risk of harm to oneself or others.

Proxy consent to psychosurgery may also be justified in cases where the psychiatric condition does not pose a significant risk of harm to oneself or others. This situation would occur when the condition is intractable to all other treatments, and the patient's quality of life is so bad that the potential benefits of the surgery outweigh the risks. This last judgment would be based on the patient's behavior over time. If the patient lacks the degree of decisional capacity necessary for consent but retains a certain degree of general cognitive function, then he or she should participate in the deliberations and assent to the decision. By assenting, the patient implicitly agrees with or objects to the decision, even though assent does not have the same ethical or legal force as consent. Similar justification can be given for proxy consent to neurosurgery on behalf of patients with brain tumors causing significant cognitive or affective impairment. In all of these cases, the potential neurological and psychological side effects of brain surgery require that consent be a deliberative process of dialogue between the neurosurgeon and supporting medical team on the one hand and the patient and/or surrogate on the other.

Proxy consent to psychosurgery is arguably weightier and should be held to a higher ethical standard than proxy consent to all other surgical procedures, including neurosurgery. This is because psychosurgery may alter the neural basis of personality and behavior more directly and deeply than other interventions in the brain. Psychosurgery for OCD, anxiety, or depression aims to correct the neural circuits directly responsible for the cognitive, affective, and conative capacities that

constitute personhood and the self. Neurosurgery generally aims to correct structural or functional abnormalities that less directly affect the neural basis of who we
are. This difference is what makes the magnitude of the potential harm of adverse
effects of psychosurgery more ethically significant. In the light of the risk of serious
adverse events resulting from psychosurgery, a group of neurosurgeons in Scotland
has recently formulated and defended "a policy of not offering ablative neurosurgery for mental disorders to anyone who is incapable of providing sustained,
informed consent."[19] As I have argued, though, there is no reason to absolutely
prohibit surrogate decision-makers from consenting to ablative psychosurgery on
behalf of noncompetent patients. If the patient's condition is severe, it does not
respond to any other therapy, and the potential benefits of the procedure outweigh
the risks, then proxy consent can be justified.

In addition to the psychiatric disorders mentioned here, cingulotomy may be
used experimentally for intractable pain. It is believed that the anterior cingulate
plays a role in modulating pain sensation and pain affect. This may be due to its
projections to and from the primary somatosensory cortex. An overactive pathway
in the anterior cingulate may cause or contribute to severe pain. Ablating a portion
of this region may eliminate the overactive pathway and result in better pain
control. Although pain may increase one's feeling of desperation and may impair
one's decisional capacity to some degree, it does not necessarily undermine this
capacity. So there would be no need for proxy consent for this treatment. Like the
other uses of psychosurgery that I have described, cingulotomy for pain relief is
experimental. There are no clinical data on outcomes, which means that it may be
unpredictable with respect to potentially severe alterations in personality and behavior. These factors can complicate the process of obtaining informed consent
from patients considering cingulotomy for pain control. Because the lack of data
implies greater uncertainty with the procedure, researchers have a stronger obligation to explain this uncertainty to patients when presenting psychosurgery as a
possible treatment. This uncertainty also means that the threshold of decisional
capacity for these patients should be very high.

All of the claims and arguments in this section need to be framed by the fact
that ablative neurosurgery remains controversial. Until recently, no prospective
randomized, double-blind, placebo-controlled trials had been conducted to test
the safety and efficacy of these procedures. A trial to test gamma knife capsulotomy
is currently underway at the Karolinska Institute. As the study of fetal-nigral
transplantation for Parkinson's disease showed, it is challenging to do a study of any
neurosurgical procedure with placebo controls in an ethically acceptable way. Yet
clinical trials are necessary to determine just how safe and effective a procedure is.
Moreover, like other surgical and pharmacological treatment for mental disorders,
ablative surgery is not curative but an intervention that aims to control the symptoms of these disorders. Although psychosurgery can relieve symptoms in some
patients, the harm from any adverse events resulting from this procedure would
probably be greater than the harm from any adverse events resulting from pharmacological interventions. Any structural damage to the brain would likely be
permanent. Indeed, the irreversibility of this damage is the most important ethical
issue for both standard neurosurgery and psychosurgery. It is for this reason that

ablative psychosurgery should always be an intervention of last resort for psychiatric disorders. But when the provisos that I have cited are in place, psychosurgery can be an ethically acceptable treatment for severe forms of these disorders.

Forced Behavior Control

Consider now a more contentious question. Would it ever be ethically permissible to use psychosurgery to prevent or treat violent behavior? More specifically, would it ever be ethically permissible to ablate circuits projecting from a hyperactive amygdala to the prefrontal cortex as a form of forced behavior control of violent offenders? In theory, psychosurgery could prevent children and adolescents with neurobiological markers for psychopathology from committing violent criminal acts. It could also prevent adult offenders from committing additional criminal acts. Recall my discussion of Churchland's comments on this and related questions in chapter 4. She implicitly distinguished forced pharmacological intervention from forced surgical intervention as possible forms of behavior control. She suggested only that the first type should at least receive careful consideration as to whether it would be preferable to a life in prison. Beyond this, surgically altering a violent offender's brain against his or her will would strike most of us as inhumane and morally repugnant. Most people would consider such "Clockwork Orange" scenarios to be worse for the offender than long-term incarceration. This conviction would be reinforced by the notorious history of frontal lobotomies. For even the most violent offenders, such radical obliteration of the neurobiological basis of the mind intuitively would violate something that many consider inviolable.

What if a competent violent offender is not forced to undergo psychosurgery but voluntarily asks for it? This individual believes that psychosurgery is his or her only chance of controlling violent impulses and of giving him or her freedom of will and the possibility of parole as an alternative to life imprisonment. Would the procedure be ethically objectionable in this case?

Some might argue that we should not distinguish between elective psychosurgery for the offender and elective psychosurgery for patients with intractable depression or OCD. For, in all of these cases, the procedure could, in principle, benefit those who undergo it. Nevertheless, psychosurgery for a violent offender might involve much more extensive alteration of neural pathways and consequently a more radical change in thought and behavior than psychosurgery for depression or OCD. More important, as is not the case with the latter two conditions, the goal of the procedure for the offender would be preventive rather than therapeutic. The principal aim of psychosurgery would be to eradicate uncontrollable impulses that otherwise would result in violent acts. It would not be given primarily to restore a normal balance of cortical-limbic and cognitive-affective processing for the benefit of the offender. In these respects, psychosurgery even for competent and consenting violent offenders would probably be too radical a form of behavior control to gain social acceptance. Others might argue that, given that psychosurgery and life imprisonment are both undesirable, an offender would not have a real choice and could not voluntary consent to the first option. In that case, psychosurgery would effectively be forced behavior control. For these reasons, many would find this use of psychosurgery to be ethically objectionable.

It would also be extremely difficult to argue that, as moral agents, neurosurgeons would be permitted to perform the procedure as a form of harm reduction. It is questionable whether any potential benefit to an individual from surgically altering the neurobiological basis of his or her personality could offset the potential harm to that individual. Nor is it clear that any potential benefit from the prevention of additional harm to others through psychosurgery could offset the potential harm to the offender. If altering the brain for preventive or therapeutic behavior control ever became ethically acceptable, we very likely would draw the line at pharmacological intervention and absolutely rule out psychosurgery.

Neurostimulation and Brain–Computer Interfaces

There are exciting and promising alternatives to standard and ablative neurosurgery for the treatment of many neuropsychiatric disorders. In some of these disorders, stimulation of neural circuits may relieve symptoms and dramatically improve patients' quality of life. There are two general types of neurostimulation. In the first type, activating electrodes implanted in certain regions of the brain stimulates neurons and neural pathways in these regions. In the second type, the brain is activated not by implanted electrodes but by electrical or magnetic pulses directed to the relevant neural circuits from an external source. The second type of neurostimulation is less invasive and, as such, does not involve the same degree of risk associated with infection from surgical incisions in the skull, as occurs in psychosurgery and the first type of neurostimulation. This would appear to make it a medically and ethically preferable alternative to more invasive brain lesioning. But these forms of brain neurostimulation are still in early stages and continue to be experimental.

The first type of neurostimulation has also been described as deep-brain stimulation (DBS). Electrodes implanted in a region of the brain are connected to batteries in a pacemaker implanted near the collarbone. Patients hold a device that they can switch on and off and thereby control the amount of electrical stimulation to the brain. The pulsing electrodes can normalize neuronal signaling. This technique can help patients to regain some physical functions that have been impaired or lost as a result of neurodegenerative disorders. The technique has been especially helpful in restoring coordinated movement for patients afflicted with the motor control problems in advanced Parkinson's disease. Electrical stimulation can modulate two structures in the basal ganglia, the globus pallidus interna and the subthalamic nucleus, and keep them from being hyperactive or hypoactive. It can compensate to some degree for the effects from the loss of dopamine neurons that play a critical role in regulating motor functions.[20] The delivery of electrical pulses can reduce both the rigidity and tremors that are symptomatic of Parkinson's. DBS may enable patients who are physically "frozen" to walk and otherwise move freely. It may also enable patients with involuntary bodily movements to have more control of these movements.

In addition, DBS might help people with Tourette's syndrome, a motor disorder characterized by repetitive muscle movements and, in some cases, involuntary swearing and cursing. Stimulation of electrodes implanted in the anterior cingulate gyrus, caudate nucleus, and basal ganglia enables some people with this syndrome to regain control of their movement and speech. This technique can enable people with these disorders to regain their capacity for agency and consequently a critical component of their selves.

For people with these conditions, DBS has turned situations of despair and unbearable suffering into situations where they can resume a normal or near-normal life. It can mean the difference between having no control and having a considerable degree of control of one's body and life. The same technology could also be used to prevent or treat epilepsy. A device implanted in the temporal lobe could automatically release a very low dose of an antiepilepsy drug or deliver an electrical signal that could block seizures. This technique has other possible therapeutic uses. In 2002, an ethics commission in France approved clinical trials using neurostimulation for OCD.[21] In contrast to the brain lesioning in psychosurgery, neurostimulation has the advantage of being reversible and therefore less potentially destructive. The electrodes can be removed, and patients can control the function of the electrodes by switching them on or off. This also makes it easier to justify conducting blind, placebo-controlled clinical trials and to obtain informed consent from participants in research in an ethically acceptable way.

Still, DBS may have unforeseen adverse consequences. Implanting or stimulating electrodes just 1 millimeter off target could cause seizures. Such mistakes could also cause patients to become cognitively impaired, emotionally flat, and, in some instances, suicidal. Even when the targeted area is stimulated as intended, activating the basal ganglia in isolation from other brain circuits that also play a role in motor coordination, such as the cerebellum, may give the patient only a limited degree of control of motor function. Neurologists have reported that one patient treated with DBS for Parkinson's developed mania and other abnormal behavior. Adjustment of the stimulation relieved these symptoms, but at the cost of a return of his debilitating motor symptoms.[22] Moreover, isolated stimulation of one region involved in motor control could interfere with the functions of other regions regulating this same capacity. This could defeat the purpose for which the technique was designed. Another concern with DBS is that infection and edema may develop at the sites of stimulation, as has been reported in some cases. For these reasons, the commission overseeing the OCD study in France set strict experimental conditions for using DBS. These included careful selection of subjects (only those whose OCD was refractory to all other treatments), obtaining informed consent, and careful evaluation of results. Belgian neurosurgeon Bart Nuttin and colleagues drafted ethical guidelines for the use of DBS to treat a range of neuropsychiatric illnesses and published them in August 2002.[23]

It is worth emphasizing that DBS can mean the difference between having some or no control of one's body. How a person assesses the risk of entering an experimental trial or of being treated with neurostimulation will be influenced by that person's subjectively experienced quality of life with Parkinson's or OCD. If the disorder is severe and the person's quality of life is very low, then he or she may reasonably conclude that the potential benefits of the technique are worth the risks. It may be in his or her best interests to enter an experimental trial testing the technique or to be treated with it in a clinical setting. Nevertheless, researchers conducting the trial must inform individuals of the potential risks before they can consent to participate in the trial. This would include informing them that there may be unknown risks in stimulating the brain.

More patients with advanced Parkinson's may choose neurostimulation since Amgen, the maker of glial-cell-line-derived neurotrophic factor took this drug off the market in late 2004 because of safety issues. This was arguably the most promising drug for Parkinson's because it contained neurogenerative factors that might have spurred the growth of new dopamine-producing neurons. Some drugs that continue to be prescribed for Parkinson's can have disturbing side effects. For example, a number of patients taking the dopamine agonists pramipexole and ropinirole became compulsive gamblers. The drug, which mimics dopamine and compensates for depleted levels of this neurotransmitter, caused a disproportionate stimulation of one type of dopamine receptor in some patients who were taking it. This caused dysregulation of their hedonic reward circuit in the limbic system, which then led to the pathological gambling.[24]

Virtual reality therapies are being developed as a nonpharmacological alternative treatment for Parkinson's and stroke-related motor disorders. Electrodes are attached to a patient's arms and shoulders to record electrical activity of muscles in an arm or other affected areas. Patients watch a three-dimensional monitor where colored balls appear to fly toward them. They are instructed to use a weakened arm as if to catch the ball. The aim is to rewire the brain and thereby restore some of the lost motor function. It will be some time before these programs are available for therapy in a clinical setting.

When pharmacological treatment is no longer an option, patients with advanced Parkinson's may rationally believe that neurostimulation is in their best interests and request it. This, in turn, should influence how researchers or clinicians discharge their duties of nonmaleficence and beneficence in deciding whether to offer neurostimulation to patients. Generally, the fewer the treatment options and the more severe the symptoms, more weight should be given to the potential benefit and less weight to the potential risk of this particular treatment.

Neurostimulation could also be used to treat severe depression and anxiety disorders. In patients who fail to respond to antidepressant medication, stimulating the prefrontal cortex may correct an imbalance between an overactive amygdala and an underactive cortex and thereby restore normal cognitive and emotional processing. Stimulation could excite neuronal activity in the cortex and inhibit neuronal activity in the amygdala. One recent study has shown that DBS modulated elevated activity in the subgenual cingulate region and produced clinical benefit in six patients with refractory depression.[25] These results are particularly promising because they suggest that DBS can influence functions of all the brain regions implicated in depression. This would make it a superior treatment to pharmacotherapy and CBT, each of which affects only a subset of the brain regions underlying the disorder. The results of this study suggest that, in addition to its therapeutic potential, DBS may lead to a better understanding of what occurs in the brains of individuals with depression. More generally, electrodes implanted and stimulated in the brain can modulate overactive or underactive circuits and relieve symptoms of both motor and mood disorders. As in the case of the Parkinson's patient treated with DBS, it is possible that this technique could result in mania or other abnormal states of mind and behavior when used to treat patients with depression. This risk would be a function of the fact that DBS must be repeated in order to have positive effects on mood. It can also amplify the effects of antidepressants. Questions remain about the significance of the DBS study for depression because the experiment did not control for the placebo effect.

The behavioral symptoms of mood and anxiety disorders are subtler than those of Parkinson's or OCD. This complicates drawing a direct link between brain stimulation and behavior or symptom control. Furthermore, locating the organic cause or causes of mood and anxiety disorders is more difficult. The etiology of these disorders may include psychological factors such as beliefs and emotions that have a more widely distributed neurobiological underpinning involving more than just motor areas. In addition, the nature and content of these mental states are influenced by stimuli in the natural and social environment. Neurostimulation cannot regulate or cancel the effects of all these factors. Its efficacy as a treatment for a broad range of neuropsychiatric disorders may be limited.

Electroconvulsive therapy (ECT), transcranial magnetic stimulation (TMS), vagus nerve stimulation (VNS), and echo-planar magnetic resonance spectroscopic imaging (EP-MRSI) seem attractive treatment alternatives to DBS, especially for depression. For they avoid surgical intervention in the brain altogether. Among these techniques, only VNS involves surgical implantation of a device in the chest and neck. None of these techniques involves implanting electrodes in the brain. So there is no risk of infection in the brain or of electrodes moving into and exciting unintended neural circuits, which could cause seizures or strokes. Each of these procedures can stimulate different brain regions in ways that can benefit patients.

In ECT, electrodes are applied to the head, and a series of electrical shocks are delivered to the brain to induce seizures. This procedure appears to restore the proper balance of neurotransmitters in the pathway between the prefrontal cortex and the limbic system. Repeated sessions of ECT have significantly improved symptoms in some patients whose depression did not respond to antidepressant medication.[26] Also aiming to restore cortical-limbic balance is TMS, which consists in delivering a localized magnetic pulse to the brain through the scalp by application of handheld coils. This technique is preferable to ECT because it requires no direct electrical connection to the brain. It can excite neurons in the prefrontal cortex of a patient with depression, or one who has had a stroke, and thereby improve mood and cognitive function.[27] This technique could also be used to modulate overactive circuits in the temporal lobes that have been implicated in epilepsy. This could result in fewer seizures.

In VNS, while the target of stimulation is the brain, stimulation of the vagus nerve occurs outside the brain. For this reason, VNS is distinctive among these techniques. This technique has been used experimentally to treat epilepsy, bipolar depression, and chronic pain. The FDA recently approved VNS for treatment-resistant depression. A VNS device functions very much like a pacemaker for the brain. It stimulates the left vagus nerve in the neck with a series of electrical pulses. These pulses travel through surgically implanted wires attached to a pulse generator in the chest. The technique stimulates the connection the vagus nerve has to limbic structures, the thalamus, and the somatosensory system in the brain, all of which regulate a range of perceptual and affective states. It thus modulates widespread patterns of brain activity. Although VNS has been effective in controlling epileptic seizures in children, overall it has had mixed results as a treatment for neurological and psychiatric conditions in clinical trials on humans.[28] Some researchers have postulated that activation of the vagus nerve with certain antiinflammatory drugs may slow the progression of certain tumors in the brain. It would do this by suppressing inflammatory cytokines associated with tumor development.[29] This suggests that the therapeutic possibilities of VNS could go well beyond those of other forms of neurostimulation and underscores the distinctive nature of this technique.

The fundamental problem with neurostimulation, as with many other techniques I have discussed, is that medical researchers still do not know precisely how they work. Despite being less invasive than ablative neurosurgery, ECT, TMS, and VNS may prove to be no more medically or ethically acceptable as treatments for chronic neuropsychiatric diseases. In particular, ECT has been known to result in significant memory loss in some patients. Moreover, like internal and external forms of electrical neurostimulation, external magnetic stimulation of the brain may adversely affect circuits other than those targeted by the procedure. Some of these techniques may have limited efficacy because they can penetrate only so far into the brain. In TMS, because the device can excite only the cortex, the strength of the magnetic field falls off sharply beyond a distance of only a few centimeters. In addition, TMS may have only short-term effects on the targeted areas of the brain. Subcortical as well as cortical regions of the brain have been implicated in many, if not most, neuropsychiatric disorders. Clinical trials aiming to increase the depth and duration of TMS to treat depression are underway in the United States. It remains to be seen whether these trials will achieve their desired effects.[30] Earlier, I noted that TMS could result in fewer seizures for patients with epilepsy. Yet the main risk of this technique is that could have the opposite effect and cause seizures in patients with a range of neuropsychiatric disorders. The risk of this occurring would be greater in repeated TMS (rTMS), which may be necessary for positive results because the effects of this technique are transient. The challenge for this type of neuromodulation is to stimulate the critical brain circuits and restore or maintain the right balance between excitatory and inhibitory neurons.

The electrical fields generated by EP-MRSI can go much deeper into the brain, making this technique a potentially more effective form of therapy. This is a scanning procedure used to monitor the metabolism of medications in the brain. In an imaging study of patients with bipolar depression at McLean Hospital in Belmont, Massachusetts, researchers discovered by serendipity that the magnetic fields generated by these scans stimulated regions of the patients' brains that modulate positive emotions. The stimulation had such a salutary effect that many patients came out of the study in a cheerful mood.[31] While these results are promising, studies involving more than just imaging are needed to form an accurate safety profile and determine whether EP-MRSI would be an effective treatment for depression.

In all of these techniques, the main ethical concern is that there is considerable uncertainly about their long-term effects. Many studies suggest that different forms of noninvasive electrical and magnetic neurostimulation are effective; but the risks are not well known. Neural stimulation can either excite or inhibit neurons. Some of these techniques involve both excitation of some neurons and inhibition of others. This can make it difficult to balance and control the effects of stimulation. The effects would also depend on what frequency is used and which areas of the brain are stimulated. Accordingly, more long-term randomized placebo-controlled trials involving a significant number of individuals are needed to accurately assess the benefits and risks of these procedures. Such trials are also needed to determine whether they are safer and more effective treatments than drug therapy or psychosurgery for a broad spectrum of neuropsychiatric disorders.

This will be a challenge, given that people's brains are wired differently. The location of the neural source or sources of a mental disorder may not be the same for two different people with the same disorder. Nor will two patients with the same disorder and similar symptoms necessarily respond to neurostimulation in the same way. Generally, though, the same strict experimental conditions should be applied to studies involving all of these techniques, regardless of the degree of invasiveness. In addition, informed consent must be obtained from patients and research subjects, or from appropriate surrogates. This requires that the researcher or clinician explain the potential benefits and risks of these techniques and point out the uncertainty in making such an assessment. The medical uncertainty about the long-term effects of what are still experimental techniques indicates that any clinical applications of neurostimulation would be ethically justifiable only when the conditions they were designed to treat were refractory to proven treatments.

Brain–computer interfaces (BCIs), also described as neural prosthetics, may be the most fascinating of the new neurotechnologies. These systems do not deliver electrical currents or magnetic impulses to the brain. Instead, they enable people to control patterns of neural activity through their thoughts to indirectly perform movements when paralysis prevents them from moving directly on their own. One form of BCI uses electroencephalography to discern brain waves through sensors attached to the scalp. A newer form uses neural implants that are connected to a computer through cables attached to the head. This is superior to the EEG version, because electrodes located under the skull are more sensitive to neural signals than sensors placed outside it. The electrodes are implanted in the motor cortex and can discern patterns of neuronal activity indicating an intention to initiate a particular physical movement. People with neural implants in this region of the brain can translate their thoughts into actions by manipulating a cursor with these thoughts. They can perform such actions as moving a robot arm by mentally sending signals to the computer and thereby performing the point-and-click action ordinarily done with the hand. In animal studies testing this technology, monkeys were able to control robot arms with their own brain signals, which were detected by implanted electrodes connected to a computer.[32]

Neural prosthetics using implanted brain chips hold considerable promise for people who are partially or completely paralyzed from spinal cord injuries or motor neuron diseases like ALS. This technique may enable them to translate thoughts into words and actions and thus regain some degree of control over speech and bodily movements. They could cause prostheses to move by processing their intention and decision to move through the computer. Or they could speak and communicate through computer voice devices. BCIs could dramatically improve the quality of life of many people who otherwise could not speak or who had little motor function.

Experiments using this technology have been conducted over the last 20 years. Recently, the FDA approved what may be the most advanced BCI clinical trial, using implants in the brains of five paralyzed people.[33] The goal of the trial was to enable patients to operate a computer and perform computer-based activities by thought alone. The first person to receive such an implant has been able to use his thoughts to control a computer cursor and move a robotic arm, open and close a prosthetic hand, and change the channel and volume of a television set. This type of neural remote control is distinctive from the other types of neurostimulation I have described and discussed because only BCIs are thought-controlled devices. This is precisely what makes them both exciting and controversial.

Leaving aside the hypothetical scenario of some people manipulating BCIs to control other people's thought and behavior, there are ethical issues with these devices even when they are within the control of one person. These issues revolve around the question of just how much control a person can have of his or her own brain signals. This in turn raises the question of how much control one can have over the functions of the implanted brain chips, computer, and prosthesis or other devices that constitute the interface system. Those with chips implanted in their brains can think about executing a bodily movement, and that thought alone can elicit patterns of neuronal activity in the motor cortex that can cause the movement. At the mental level, this would involve forming an intention to move and executing that intention in a decision to move. Intentions can be described as plans consisting of a complex set of desires, beliefs, and reasons.[34] But forming an intention or plan and executing it are two separate mental acts. Both mental acts depend on normal functions of the orbitofrontal and ventromedial frontal cortex, but not necessarily the same set or sets of neurons. One can form an intention to act but not execute that intention in a decision and action by changing one's mind at the last moment. One may decide to act on a different intention instead, or decide not to act at all. It is not clear exactly how or to what extent these distinct mental acts are regulated or coordinated by different regions of the cortex. Even the most basic bodily movement involves thousands of motor neurons.

This is pertinent to the question of neural control and free will because a sufficient sense of control of one's desires, intentions, and decisions requires the ability to change one's mind. It is unclear how BCIs would enable one to prevent the system that is mediating thought and movement from causing the movement of a limb or prosthesis if, at the last millisecond, the patient decided not to execute an intention to move. If the BCI system could not distinguish between intending to perform an action and executing that intention and deciding to act, or between the regions of the brain that mediated these distinct mental acts, then it is possible that the system could make people perform some movements involuntarily. The basic problem is that it is not yet known how well humans can control brain signals, or the bodily movements these signals regulate. It is not known precisely how a mental act such as forming an intention or making a decision can cause a computer to trigger an event in the motor cortex that issues in a bodily movement.

To complicate matters further, people with long-standing paralysis may use different mental and neural processes in operating BCIs. Ordinarily, a voluntary arm or leg movement is preceded by an unconscious belief that one can move the limb. Over time, paralysis may result in the loss of this belief. Instead, paralyzed individuals using a BCI would be consciously imagining or simulating bodily movements that they would have performed directly if they were physically able to do so. Imagination and simulation probably involve brain regions in addition to the motor cortex and prefrontal cortex. Because more neurons in more brain regions would be involved in producing a bodily movement, it might be more difficult for one to exercise cognitive control over the process that extends from the intention to the action. Recent developments in neural prosthetic studies on monkeys suggest that neural signals could be monitored in such a way as to separate planning from executing movements.[35] But it will be some time before this very precise type of cognitive control of mental states could be realized in humans.

There are more practical concerns with the chip version of this technology. The implanted chips could cause infection in the brain. They could also cause scarring or move from the site of implantation. In either case, the consequence could be the loss of the neuronal signal. It is also possible that chips that had moved within the motor cortex would initiate neural firing that would cause unintended movements or seizures. Or they might move outside the motor cortex into other brain regions and interfere with cognitive or other neurological and physical functions. Much more work is needed to ensure greater neurological and mental control and thus minimize the risk of these adverse events for people using BCIs.

If the technology were perfected to the point where the risks were greatly minimized, at least one ethical question would remain. These devices could enable people with severe disabilities to communicate and move with some degree of freedom. To be sure, this technology would be expensive, though arguably less expensive than 24-hour assisted care. We can assume that BCIs would be more cost-effective for these patients in the long term. Medicaid or other programs could make them available to all people with disabilities who qualified for them. But suppose that some of these individuals refused to use the technology. They might fear that the implanted brain chips would not function as intended and that the chips would make them perform some actions involuntarily. These individuals might feel that they would have more control of their bodies and surroundings by continuing to rely on more labor-intensive and costly forms of assisted living. Could we compel them to use the technology? Or would we be obligated to accommodate them and respect their decision to opt out and reject the use of BCIs?

We would have at least a prima facie obligation to respect patient autonomy in these cases. We should accommodate the wishes of those who are severely disabled and, in this regard, worse off than the majority of people in society. As a matter of fairness, we should give priority to the needs and interests of those who are worse off. The severely disabled are worse off than others because they have greater physical needs. But they have a right to decide how these needs are met in a way that is consistent with their medical and nonmedical best interests. They may rationally reject BCIs because it would not be in their all-things-considered best interests to use them. They may believe that, because the efficacy of this technology would depend on many factors other than their minds and brains, it would give them less rather than more control of their bodies. On these grounds, one could argue that the severely disabled could not be compelled to use BCIs, despite the potential cost savings and other forms of efficiency this technology might entail for their care.

Let's return to neurostimulation and consider a more controversial hypothetical use of this technology. Recall the discussion of out-of-body experiences in chapter 2 and the experiments that produced these experiences. Olaf Blanke did this by electrically stimulating the juncture of the temporal and parietal lobes and their connection to the right angular gyrus. This type of brain manipulation can produce these experiences by altering somatosensory and vestibular information, which can alter a person's subjective experience of and orientation in time and space. It can also create the experience of dissociation of the self from the body. These and other experiments have contributed to the field of "spiritual neurology," the study of the neurological basis of spiritual and religious experience. Recent experiments attempting to replicate the effects reported by Blanke and earlier by Michael Persinger have failed. This has raised questions about the ability to bring about these phenomenological modifications in research subjects undergoing procedures involving stimulation of the temporal lobes.[36]

Mario Beauregard, a brain imager at the University of Montreal, has conducted experiments not involving any brain manipulation that show an equally intriguing result. The experiments involve Carmelite nuns and use PET and fMRI scans to show a correlation between activation of the parietal lobe and a heightened meditative state in these nuns.[37] The meditating nuns in Beauregard's study have reported sensing a greater interconnectedness with their social and natural environment. They have said that when they are in a heightened meditative state, the self seems to dissolve into a larger entity, which they have described as "God."[38] This is less controversial than the OBE experiments because there is no manipulation of the brain.

Suppose that a neurologist could manipulate the temporal-parietal lobe juncture and the right angular gyrus through electrical or magnetic stimulation. The aim would not be to produce OBEs but to alter one's perception of space and time and generate an experience similar to that of the nuns in Beauregard's study. Could this technique be used to treat chronic intractable pain? Would it be ethically objectionable to do so for this therapeutic purpose?

As noted in the discussion of placebos in chapter 4, the anticipation of pain can increase both the intensity and duration of pain for the person who feels it. Anticipation of pain can also increase suffering by causing fear and dread about what one will experience in the immediate or near future. Altering a patient's perception of time by shifting awareness away from the future to the present may reduce fear and thus reduce suffering. This can be accomplished by behavioral and psychological interventions, which can have measurable effects on the regions of the brain that regulate pain. Hypnosis is one such intervention that can be especially effective in reframing one's cognitive and affective states about time and achieving the goal of reducing the perception of pain.

Eric Cassell describes the case of a woman with stomach cancer that illustrates the salutary effect of hypnosis in altering a patient's temporal awareness. After completing a course of chemotherapy, she fearfully anticipated the next treatment. Hypnosis was able to reduce her anticipation of the pain associated with the chemotherapy. In Cassell's words, "they [the treatments] are not there until they suddenly 'arrive' and then they quickly disappear. Although weakness, some nausea, and poor appetite lasted for a brief period post-chemotherapy, the problem had greatly lessened, as had the anticipation of the next treatment."[39]

Antonio Damasio and colleagues have reported a similar effect of hypnosis. In experiments designed to manage chronic intractable pain, hypnotic suggestions were given to a group of patients. The suggestions reduced both their sensation of pain and their emotional reaction to pain. PET scans showed that the hypnosis altered the patients' perceptions of pain by causing changes in the primary somatosensory cortex and the cingulate cortex. These changes reduced pain sensation and pain affect.[40]

Electrical or magnetic stimulation of the temporal-parietal juncture and angular gyrus could have a similar effect. If it could alter a patient's sense of time and shift the patient's awareness away from the future to the immediacy of the present, then this action might alleviate the patient's pain and suffering. This type of neurostimulation would be more likely to achieve the desired effect if it could incorporate the influence of cultural and religious symbols on patients' beliefs, which can influence a range of neuronal connections. If a patient had pain that was intractable to opioid analgesics, then intuitively it would seem permissible to stimulate the relevant regions of the brain to relieve the patient's pain and suffering. In many respects, the aim of this intervention would be the same as the aim of hypnosis or meditation to alter a patient's experience of temporal progression. It would also be similar to virtual reality programs used to shift perceptual awareness in patients with severe burns and thereby diminish their experience of pain during constant dressing changes.[41]

All of these interventions can alter a patient's perception of time and reduce pain perception and pain affect. If hypnosis, meditation, and virtual reality techniques are ethically permissible ways of treating intractable pain, then there is no obvious reason why electrical or magnetic stimulation of the relevant brain regions for this purpose would not also be ethically permissible. Some forms of electrical neurostimulation are invasive and in this respect are unlike meditation, hypnosis, or virtual reality. Yet the intended effect of altering brain and mental states would be the same as in these other interventions. It would not be fundamentally different from using morphine or other opioids to relieve pain. Provided that patients consented to the procedure and that it did not expose them to an undue risk of harm, there would be no reasonable ethical objection to it.

This argument might be more persuasive if temporal-parietal lobe/angular gyrus neurostimulation were used exclusively in palliative care, where patients were too sick to undergo hypnosis or engage in meditation. Because the patient's remaining life span would be relatively short, any risks of adverse neurological side effects would not be of any great consequence. In addition to relieving pain, electrical or magnetic manipulation of the parietal-temporal juncture could alleviate suffering. It could do this by generating the feeling of being interconnected with something larger than the self. Like the nuns in Beauregard's experiment, patients undergoing this type of neurostimulation might be able to transcend their pain and suffering by relating it to, or framing it within, a larger spiritual or humanitarian framework. This would be one way of making pain and suffering meaningful for them.[42] It might enable patients to cope with painful terminal conditions, gaining a measure of control of their situation by generating a feeling of hope through a feeling of connectedness with others.

One objection to this use of neurostimulation would be that it would amount to a radical alteration of the self as an integrated psychological unity persisting through space and time. The alteration would result from a source alien to the self. Yet, if a competent patient chooses it, the patient's condition is terminal with death imminent, and the patient is experiencing severe pain and suffering that is intractable to all other treatments, then the practice could be ethically justifiable. The dissolution of the spatial and temporal representation of the self will come at death in any case. Manipulating the brain along the lines I have described would only slightly move up the moment when one experiences the dissolution of the self at death. This experience is brain-based, regardless of whether it occurs sooner through neurostimulation or later as a natural neurological phenomenon when all brain functions permanently cease.

The ability to produce religious or spiritual experiences by neurostimulation is controversial. Nevertheless, the possibility of stimulating certain regions of the brain as a form of palliation is consistent with accounts of religion or spirituality as an experience that has evolved in humans to enable them to cope with the unpleasant contingencies of life.[43] Certain functions of the temporal and parietal lobes of the brain mediate this experience. It is not implausible to say the Christian idea that the "Kingdom of God is within you," expressed in the Gospel of Luke (17:21) and emphasized more in the Gospel of Thomas, suggests that religion or spirituality, in part at least, is a neurologically mediated experience. Additional support for the view that religious and spiritual experiences are at least partly brain-based can be found in a passage from the Buddhist text *Bardo Thodol* (Tibetan Book of the Dead): "These realms are not come from somewhere outside thyself. They come from within . . . they exist from eternity within the faculties of thine own intellect . . . issuing from thine own brain . . . reflections of thine own thought-forms."[44] It is doubtful that religious experience is entirely a neurological phenomenon. Yet if this experience is at least partly brain-based and can help consenting patients to cope with intractable pain and suffering in terminal illness, then it would not be unethical to generate it by electrically or magnetically stimulating the brain.

Conclusion

In this chapter, I have discussed ethical issues in the weighing of risks and benefits of neurosurgery, psychosurgery, and invasive and noninvasive forms of neurostimulation. With the exception of the use of psychosurgery to forcibly alter violent behavior, most of these interventions in the brain can be ethically justified when certain provisos are in place. Provided that patients are competent, they give informed consent, and the probable benefit to them outweighs the probable harm, these interventions in the brain can be medically and ethically justified. In contrast to neurosurgery and neurostimulation, psychosurgery should be a treatment of last resort. This is because it has a higher probability of resulting in irreversible neurological and psychological disability, and because it is not always effective in controlling or alleviating psychopathological symptoms. For these reasons, the threshold of competency for consent should be higher for psychosurgery than for other interventions in the brain.

In some cases, surrogate decision-makers may consent to psychosurgery on behalf of patients who are not competent, if they are acting in the patient's best interests. There are instances where the patient would, on balance, be worse off without the surgery. I argued that a neurosurgeon's or neurologist's obligation of nonmaleficence to patients is not absolute and can be influenced by competent patients' own assessment of the benefits and risks to them with or without neurosurgery, psychosurgery, or neurostimulation. One problem with these assessments, however, is that we still do not know the long-term risks of these interventions. More longitudinal randomized clinical trials are needed before we have a clear picture of their safety and efficacy.

Some of the neurodegenerative and psychiatric disorders I have described will lead to the demise of the patients who have them. For these patients, death will be defined in neurological terms. But what does it mean to say that a person has died and has ceased to exist? In terms of which brain functions do we define death? Is death exclusively a neurological phenomenon? In what respects does the definition of death depend on our metaphysical definition of persons or human beings? Is there a point beyond which a human being cannot be harmed? I will address these questions and explore some of the ethical implications of brain death in the last chapter.

Brain Death

I have defined persons as individuals with the capacity for consciousness and other forms of mentality. This capacity necessarily depends on the normal functioning of the cerebral cortex and supporting subcortical brain structures. The nature and content of our mental states may also be influenced by certain functions of the immune and endocrine systems, depending on how these systems interact with the central nervous system. In addition, our mental states depend on how we interact with the natural and social environment. Our minds are a reflection of a tripartite model consisting of brain, body, and environment. Although the cerebral cortex is not sufficient for a complete explanation of human mentality, it is necessary to generate and sustain our conscious and unconscious mental life. When the cortex permanently ceases to function, we permanently lose our capacity for mentality and cease to exist as persons. Other brain and bodily structures may continue to function. But these are only features of the organisms we leave behind when we die.

Many neurologists and legal theorists have argued that the irreversible loss of higher brain function alone is not sufficient for a determination of death. They hold that all brain functions, including those of the brainstem, must cease for death to occur. On this view, a human being with only minimal brainstem function continues to exist. In fact, one neurologist has rejected these two positions, arguing that neurological criteria are too limited for defining death. Rather, death should be defined in broader biological terms, since integrated somatic functions may continue, and a human being may continue to exist, even after all brain functions have permanently ceased.

The plausibility of these competing conceptions of what death is and when it occurs depends on what one believes about the sort of beings we essentially are. Are we essentially persons whose existence necessarily depends on the continued functioning of the cortex? Or are we essentially human organisms who exist provided that certain integrated biological functions, which may or may not be mediated by the brain, are intact? The metaphysical argument about what sort of beings we essentially are influences which neurological or biological definition of death we adopt. This definition, in turn, influences ethical judgments about how we can benefit from or be harmed by actions done to us at the margin between life and death.

In this chapter, I defend a narrow neurological criterion of death. This says that the permanent cessation of higher brain, or cortical, function is sufficient for the death of a person. I distinguish between persons and human organisms and argue that we are essentially persons rather than organisms. I elaborate this distinction by considering different conceptions of the soul, as well as different perspectives on when the soul leaves the body. Discussion of some prominent legal cases will illustrate differences in people's beliefs about these issues. I argue that only persons, and not human organisms, can have interests. The capacity for consciousness is necessary to have interests, and this capacity is an essential property of persons but not of human organisms. Insofar as benefit and harm are defined in terms of the satisfaction or defeat of interests, only persons can benefit or be harmed. This argument is critical for exploring the ethical implications of brain death. It is particularly critical for analyzing ethical questions about the permissibility or impermissibility of such actions as withdrawing life-support and procuring organs for transplantation.

Defining Death

It is important to distinguish between the *concept* of death and a *criterion* of death. The concept of death simply says what death is: the end of the existence of some individual. A criterion of death specifies the conditions in terms of which an individual's death can be determined. We need a criterion of death to establish *when* an individual dies. But there are several distinct and conflicting criteria of death and considerable disagreement on which of these is the correct or most plausible way of determining when death occurs. When an individual dies depends on the properties that are essential to the existence of that individual and his or her persistence through time. First I will examine different biological criteria of death. Then I will discuss the ontological distinction between persons and organisms. These discussions will be necessary for analysis of the relevant ethical issues later in this chapter.

Before the 1960s, death was a relatively straightforward phenomenon. Death was defined as the irreversible cessation of cardiopulmonary function. Persons were declared dead when heartbeat and breathing stopped, which resulted in the permanent loss of all brain function. This changed with advances in mechanical ventilation. Patients' breathing and circulation could be sustained and they could be kept alive for some time by artificial means. This made it unclear when death occurred and on what clinical basis death could be declared. It was especially problematic for organ transplantation. Transplant surgeons had to address the question of how organs could be taken from a patient's body when it was not clear whether the patient was dead. In particular, they had to address the question of how a heart that could be restarted could be taken from a patient for transplantation without killing the patient.

To resolve these and related problems, an ad hoc committee at Harvard Medical School was formed in 1968 and formulated a whole-brain criterion of death. This said that death occurs when there is permanent loss of integrated functioning of the entire brain, including the brainstem.[1] In 1981, the President's Commission for the Study of Ethical Problems in Medicine and Biomedical and Behavioral Research adopted a similar position. It defined death as the irreversible cessation of cardiopulmonary (breathing and circulation) function, or the irreversible cessation of all functions of the brain, including the brainstem.[2] This definition was formalized in the U.S. Uniform Determination of Death Act (UDDA) of 1981. On this definition, the whole-brain criterion complements, rather than competes with or replaces, the cardiopulmonary criterion. The UDDA specifies that death can be determined by the irreversible cessation of all brain function *or* by the irreversible cessation of cardiopulmonary function. In the United Kingdom, permanent cessation of brainstem function determines death. In the United States and Canada, the whole-brain criterion has become the legal and clinical standard definition of death and is the most socially accepted criterion for determining when a person dies.

The whole-brain criterion of death can be met in any one of three ways: absence of electrical activity in the brain, as determined by an EEG; absence of blood flow to the brain, as determined by blood-flow studies; or absence of function of all parts of the brain, as determined by clinical assessment. This includes no movement, no response to stimulation, no breathing, and no reflexes.[3] The whole-brain criterion has been challenged on several counts. Physicians typically use absence of brainstem reflexes as the most reliable indication of brain death. Yet these reflexes may continue for some time even after respiration and other functions supported by the brainstem have ceased. Brainstem functions may cease gradually rather than all at once. Moreover, there has been evidence of antidiuretic hormone and pituitary blood flow from patients with no brainstem activity, suggesting continued activity in the hypothalamic-pituitary pathway even after the whole-brain criterion of death appears to have been met.[4] Because of its focus on the brainstem, the whole-brain criterion may not always provide a clear and conclusive determination of when death occurs.

A second challenge is from pediatric neurologist Alan Shewmon. He goes beyond the problem of persistent brain-stem reflexes and persistent hypothalamic-pituitary activity and insists that the determination of death should not be based on brain function at all. Shewmon argues that the brain does not mediate most somatically integrated functions of the body. These functions include, but are not limited to, emanation, detoxification and recycling of cellular wastes through the body, and energy balance involving interactions among the liver, the endocrine system, muscle, and fat. These functions also include wound healing, and fighting of infections through interaction among the immune system, lymphatics, bone marrow, and microvasculature. What Shewmon calls the "somatic integrative unity" of a human organism is not located in the brain.[5] Instead, it is a holistic fact involving mutual interactions between and among different systems of the organism. These systems can function for some time without a functional brainstem.

Shewmon's position challenges the strongest defense of the whole-brain criterion of death. Proposing a revised version of this criterion, neurologist James Bernat argues that "death is defined as the permanent cessation of the critical functions of the organism as a whole."[6] These functions are regulated by what he calls the "critical system" of the organism, which consists in certain integrated activity in the brain. Bernat says that not every brain neuron is necessary to maintain the critical system of the organism. What *is* essential to this system are neurons in the brainstem encompassing the ascending reticular formation and its projections to the thalamus and cerebral hemispheres.[7] These structures are essential to generating wakefulness. Death is the cessation of critical *integrated* brain activity, not cessation of all isolated brain activity. Yet if Shewmon is correct, then a human organism can remain alive in the absence of a functioning critical system in the brain. If a mechanical ventilator can perform the same functions as the brainstem in sustaining breathing and circulation, then it is unclear why any parts of the brain need to remain functionally intact for a human organism to continue living. Indeed, a ventilator could be construed as an artificial brainstem, in which case, theoretically, not even this region of the brain would be necessary to sustain the existence of a human organism.[8]

Shewmon's example of a four-year-old boy diagnosed as brain dead from intracranial edema caused by meningitis appears to support this point.[9] After being transferred from the hospital to home, many of the boy's bodily functions continued with only mechanical ventilation, tube feeding, and basic nursing care. Following a neurological examination, Shewmon reported: "Evoked potential showed no cortical or brain-stem responses, a magnetic resonance angiogram showed no intracranial blood flow, and an MRI scan revealed that the entire brain, including the stem, had been replaced by ghost-like tissues and disorganized proteinaceous fluids."[10] Yet Shewmon also noted that, "while brain-dead," the boy's body "has grown, overcome infections, and healed wounds."[11]

Examples like this, where the psychological properties that we ordinarily identify with a person and their neurological basis in the brain are absent, have led many to reject both the whole-brain criterion and the somatic integrative unity criterion of death. In Shewmon's case, it appears that, in all relevant respects, the boy had ceased to exist, even though his body continued to function at some basic biological level. The whole-brain criterion has been the target of similar objections, some of which were generated by the well-known case of Karen Anne Quinlan.

In April 1975, the 21-year-old Quinlan arrived comatose at a New Jersey hospital after ingesting barbiturates, diazepam, and alcohol. She was put on a ventilator to assist her breathing, but she gradually fell into a persistent vegetative state (PVS).[12] Individuals in such a state are awake but not consciously aware of their surroundings. They have intact brainstem functions but little or no higher brain function. Karen's parents wanted the breathing tube removed, but her doctors refused. The New Jersey Supreme Court ruled in March 1976 that, given her irreversible condition, mechanical life-support could be discontinued, even if it resulted in her death. The court ruled that this action was permissible on the grounds of a presumed privacy right guaranteed by the U.S. Constitution, and that Karen's parents were the appropriate surrogates to exercise that right for her. Karen was slowly weaned from the ventilator and unexpectedly began to breathe spontaneously. She lived in a PVS until June 1985, when all of her bodily functions permanently ceased and she was declared dead.[13]

The declaration of death in the Quinlan case was based on the whole-brain criterion. But for many, this had the unpalatable implication that people could continue to exist in a PVS with only minimal brain function sustaining only some bodily processes and no mental capacity. Cases like those of Quinlan and Shewmon's four-year-old patient have moved many philosophers to propose and defend a higher brain criterion of death. On this criterion, the death of a person occurs when there is permanent cessation of the functions of the cerebral cortex.[14] Regions of the lower brain, such as the ascending reticular formation, are also necessary to support consciousness. This structure regulates levels of arousal and mental activity while a person is awake. But because cortical function is necessary for the capacity for consciousness essential to personhood, permanent loss of cortical function is sufficient for the death of a person. A functioning reticular formation without a functioning cortex may enable a person to remain wakeful, but not to have any conscious awareness of his or her self or surroundings. During the 10 years that Karen Ann Quinlan survived without ventilatory support, she met the criterion of higher brain death. If we identify personhood with higher brain function, then Karen the person ceased to exist in 1975. Her body or organism continued to exist until 1985. Like the whole-brain and brainstem criteria, the higher brain criterion of death is made on neurological grounds. But these three criteria are distinct, because they focus on distinct neurological capacities and processes.

The higher brain criterion of death is a capacity-theoretic criterion. It requires the permanent loss of the capacity for cortical function and the capacity for mentality for a person to be considered dead. This implies that a person can remain alive and persist as the same person for a period of time even when cortical or subcortical capacities are not actualized. The necessary neurological capacity includes not only the cerebral cortex, but also its connections to other parts of the central nervous system and to other systems in the body. For example, patients in a "locked-in" neurological state appear comatose but remain conscious inwardly. These patients have sustained extensive damage to the pons, a portion of the brainstem that assists in autonomic functions and relays sensory information between the cerebrum and cerebellum. A locked-in state may result from a primary brainstem stroke, trauma to the brainstem, or Guillain-Barre syndrome (acute ascending polyneuritis), which affects the cranial and spinal nerves and prevents information from entering or leaving the central nervous system.[15] Patients with Guillain-Barre syndrome may not be able to breathe on their own for a period and require ventilatory support to remain alive. In most cases, though, they can fully recover all brain and bodily functions. They do not lose the capacity for integrated brain function while they are affected by this condition.

In most locked-in cases, some brainstem function is intact and is necessary to sustain higher-brain activity. Yet in what has been described as "super locked-in syndrome," cortical activity can temporarily be retained despite totally absent brainstem function.[16] In effect, this condition temporarily severs the connection between the higher brain and the rest of the brain and body. From the outside, locked-in syndrome mimics but does not actually result in brain death, since an EEG and a PET scan will show intact cortical functioning in these patients. Provided that the critical brain and bodily functions underlying the capacity for consciousness remained intact, a patient could survive in such a state for weeks or longer. Some patients with extensive brainstem lesions have survived for years in a locked-in state. But it is questionable whether one could survive indefinitely in such a state despite continued mechanical ventilation. It is likely that a severely damaged brainstem would eventually lead to general neurological deterioration and cessation of all brain and bodily functions beyond a certain point.

Locked-in syndromes may lead some to question the brainstem criterion of death. Some patients remain alive with higher-brain functions intact without a functioning brainstem. Yet this does not undermine the brainstem criterion if it specifies that death occurs when this part of the brain permanently ceases to function. This is consistent with most locked-in syndromes, where many patients affected by them lose brainstem function for a time but eventually recover it. The only sense in which the brainstem criterion may be inadequate as a criterion of death for human organisms is that mechanical ventilation can perform the same functions in sustaining breathing and circulation. As noted, though, it is unlikely that a ventilator could sustain these processes indefinitely.

In a different situation, some patients may regain consciousness by awakening during surgery when the sedative effects of general anesthesia unexpectedly wear off. They can feel pain but cannot move or speak. This is because the muscle relaxant given with the general anesthesia removes the most reliable indicator of conscious awareness: patient movement. This is another example of patients appearing to be locked into their body, and where the body can give others a false perception of the mental state of a patient. The use of electroencephalography in the technique of bispectral index (BIS) monitoring can prevent this problem. It can provide a constant accurate reading of the depth of conscious and unconscious mental states of patients under anesthesia or sedation. For the patient, the combination of the anesthetic and muscle relaxant can alter the perceived connection between mind and body. But this is only an illusion generated by the effects of the drugs, an illusion that dissolves once these effects wear off completely.

Patients undergoing neurosurgery for cerebral aneurysms may have their body temperature significantly lowered. Induced hypothermia reduces or cuts off blood flow to the brain and thereby reduces the risk of damage to brain tissue from intracranial hemorrhage resulting from surgery. Body temperature may be lowered to as much as 60 degrees Fahrenheit, and patients can be "frozen" for several hours. When patients' bodies are cooled to such a degree, their blood tends to coagulate, which poses the risk of tissue damage from ischemia. Researchers have designed a drug, Hextend (high-molecular-weight hydroxyethyl starch), which consists of a chemical and starch combination that prevents coagulation. Although this procedure puts patients in a state of suspended animation, they are not clinically dead and are not literally brought back to life. This is because blood flow to the cortex and other critical areas of the brain is interrupted for only a limited period of time. When done properly, the procedure ensures that the capacity for consciousness is only temporarily suspended, not permanently lost. In some cases of brain trauma or cerebral hemorrhage, neurosurgeons may use anesthesia to induce deep coma in their patients and relieve intracranial pressure. This experimental procedure may minimize brain damage and promote recovery to consciousness.

Brain function cannot be sustained indefinitely without a blood supply to the brain. Beyond a critical threshold of interrupted blood flow, significant brain damage will occur. This can result in loss of some or all functions of cortical or subcortical regions, or both. In some cases of prolonged hypothermia, anesthesia, or coma, enough higher brain function can be restored following these temporary biological states for conscious capacity and personhood to remain intact. But some cortical structures and functions may have been damaged, which could result in impaired mental capacity. Damage to the hippocampus or other parts of the medial temporal lobes could result in retrograde or anterograde amnesia. Damage to the frontal lobe could result in a radical change in personality or severely impair executive cognitive capacities such as planning and decision-making. Personal identity through time is based on the connectedness and continuity of psychological properties such as desires, beliefs, intentions, and the realization of these intentions in actions. If the nature and content of the patient's psychological properties following the procedure were substantially different from the nature and content of his or her psychological properties before the procedure, then the connectedness and continuity of these properties would have been substantially disrupted. If so, then arguably the person who temporarily lost consciousness would not be the same person who regained it. Intuitively, the original person would not have survived the surgery or the coma. The patient would still be *a* person, but might not be the *same* person if his or her psychological properties were so different before and after the surgery or coma.

Still, the main concern here is with the more basic concept of *personhood* and what it means for a person to remain alive or die, not the more complex concept of *personal identity* through time. Both personhood and personal identity consist essentially in the capacity for a range of psychological properties. In contrast, human organisms consist essentially of biological properties, the properties necessary for the integrated functioning of bodily systems. If a person dies when he or she irreversibly loses the capacity for psychological properties, and if an organism dies when it irreversibly loses its essential biological properties, then it seems that there should be two definitions of death. The first definition pertains to persons and is formulated in psychological terms. The second definition pertains to human organisms and is formulated in biological terms.

Bernat rejects this claim. He insists that "the concept of death is applicable only to an organism because death fundamentally is a biological phenomenon."[17] There is only one definition of death, the death of a human organism, which occurs when all critical biological functions sustaining the organism permanently cease. Bernat rejects the idea, defended by Jeff McMahan in his earlier work, that there could be one conception of death for persons and a distinct conception of death for human organisms.[18] Bernat claims that "personhood is a psychosocial or spiritual concept," and that personhood cannot die except metaphorically.[19] But if one accepts the view that there are clear and distinct ontological criteria for persons based on the capacity for mentality, and that these criteria are fundamentally different from the ontological criteria for human organisms, then personhood is a legitimate ontological category. It is not simply a metaphor or psychosocial construct. Persons literally begin to exist and cease to exist, and their existence overlaps to some extent but is not coextensive with the existence of human organisms.

One could agree with Bernat's claim that death is a biological (neurological) phenomenon but disagree with his related claim that death applies only to a human organism. Despite the ontological distinction between persons and human organisms, the death of a person is, in a crucial respect, also a biological phenomenon. The phenomenological quality and content of one's psychological properties is influenced to some degree by events in the social and natural environment. In this regard, one's mental life cannot be reduced to, or explained entirely in terms of, the biological properties of the brain and body. But one's psychological properties necessarily depend on the biological functioning of the cerebral cortex, and the permanent cessation of cortical functioning results in the end of one's mental life. If persons are defined in terms of the capacity for consciousness, and this capacity necessarily depends on the functioning of the cerebral cortex, then persons die when the cerebral cortex permanently ceases to function. Thus the death of a person *is* a biological phenomenon. But it is not defined in terms of whole-brain, brainstem, or somatic criteria.

Accordingly, there should be three biological definitions of death. The first definition pertains to persons and occurs when all higher brain functions end. The second and third definitions pertain to human organisms, and death occurs when all integrated bodily processes end. These processes do not necessarily include higher or even whole-brain functioning. Bernat's concept of a human organism pertains to one with a functioning integrated critical system based in and projecting from the brainstem. Death occurs when this critical system ceases to function. Shewmon's concept of a human organism pertains to integrated somatic processes of the body not necessarily mediated by any brain functions. Death occurs when these somatic processes end. As noted, unlike the higher brain, whole-brain, and brainstem criteria of death, the criterion Shewmon proposes and defends is not a neurological criterion.

One should not multiply entities or definitions beyond necessity. Yet if persons are ontologically distinct from human organisms, then the claim that death applies only to human organisms leaves it unclear what happens to persons when all higher-brain functions permanently cease. If one accepts this distinction, then one may hold that the question of whether an individual survives a brain injury does not have a single answer. How one responds to this question will depend on whether one takes oneself to be a person or human organism, and which region or regions of the brain are necessary to generate and sustain one's essential properties.

For many, the higher brain criterion of death has the counterintuitive implication that a person can be understood as dead when respiration and heartbeat are still present and the body is still alive. It is also morally disturbing to say that it does no harm to a breathing patient to withdraw life-support or take organs from his or her body. These have been the main objections to the higher brain criterion, and they largely explain why the whole-brain criterion of death remains so widely accepted. As Stuart Youngner and Robert Arnold have pointed out, the whole-brain criterion of declaring death remains the medical, legal, and ethical standard.

Among other things, it allows doctors to turn off ventilators without fear of legal consequences, specifically charges of homicide for killing patients.[20] It also allows cadaveric organ procurement for transplantation without violating the "dead donor rule" (DDR).[21] This rule says that organs can only be taken from bodies of patients who have been declared dead. The DDR requires that donors not be killed in order to take their organs. Youngner and Arnold further note that "no one has seriously considered repealing the laws recognizing [whole] brain death; nor has any national professional organization or religious group called for their abandonment or even modification."[22]

The moral reasons for rejecting the higher brain criterion of death and accepting the whole-brain criterion are not very philosophically persuasive, however. Medical, legal, and social objections notwithstanding, only the higher brain criterion can provide a satisfactory explanation of what it means to have interests and why and when persons can be harmed. Only the higher brain criterion can account for the moral implications of what is done to our bodies at the margin between life and death. This is because the cerebral cortex is necessary for the mental capacity that enables us to have the interests or rights that give us the moral status in terms of which we can benefit or be harmed. Benefit consists in the satisfaction or realization of interests, and harm consists in the defeat or thwarting of interests. One consequence of the higher brain criterion is that the DDR could be violated without harming individuals with no cortical function from whom organs were procured for transplantation. These individuals would be human organisms and, as such, would be beyond harm.

Moral claims about what can benefit or harm us rest on the metaphysical claim regarding the sort of entities we are. If we are beings with an interest in what is done to our bodies and how our lives end, if having interests requires higher brain functioning, and if this functioning is an essential property of persons but not of human organisms, then it seems to follow that we are essentially persons and not human organisms. Still, more is needed to motivate and defend this basic argument. As in my account of mind in chapter 2, what I present here is a plausibility argument for the claim that we are essentially persons rather than human organisms. This claim and argument rest on the assumption that persons are defined in terms of the capacity for consciousness. My approach is consistent with the view that there is no objectively true answer to the metaphysical question of what sort of beings we fundamentally are. This question arises from certain convictions we have about ourselves. My use of "essentially" should be taken as a reflection of these convictions rather than a presumed fact of the matter. Nevertheless, I believe that the case for the view that personhood consists in the capacity for consciousness, and that we are essentially persons, is more intuitive and persuasive than any alternatives.

Persons and Organisms

In order to clarify the ontological distinction between persons and human organisms, it is necessary to introduce some technical metaphysical terms. Sortal concepts are used to establish criteria of identity and persistence at particular times and through time. These criteria specify what counts as being a thing of a certain sort, as well as what counts as continuing to exist as that thing. Substance sortals are distinguished from phase sortals.[23] A phase sortal designates a kind or sort to which an individual belongs through only a phase or stage of its history. "Child," for example, is a phase sortal. Although I was not a child when I began to exist, I later became a child and then ceased to be one, all the while remaining the same individual throughout the various transformations of human development. In contrast, a substance sortal designates the kind or sort of thing an entity is at all times. A substance sortal designates a thing's essential properties, the properties it cannot lose without ceasing to exist as that thing. So when we ask what kind of entity we essentially are, we are asking about a substance sortal rather than a phase sortal. Our substantial nature specifies the conditions under which we exist and when we cease to exist. The fundamental question is whether the substance sortal at issue is "person" or "human organism."[24]

A human organism is a biological entity that can be defined in terms of integrated functioning of its constituent parts. At the beginning of a human life, the integration necessary for an entity to be and persist as a human organism is present, at the earliest, around 14 days after fertilization and the formation of a zygote. This is after the possibility of monozygotic twinning has passed. When such twinning occurs, a zygote divides into two qualitatively similar but numerically distinct zygotes, at which point the original zygote ceases to exist. A human organism cannot begin to exist before this time, because it lacks the property or properties necessary to identify it as a distinct entity. It would be logically incoherent to say that one zygote could divide into two numerically and spatially distinct zygotes and still persist as the same zygote. This is the ontological reason for claiming that a human organism cannot exist until 14 days after fertilization.[25]

The biological reason for this claim is that certain structures in an embryo must be present for any integrated functions to take place. At only a few days after fertilization, a zygote can be described as nothing more than a nonintegrated clump of cells. At the other end of life, a human organism ceases to exist after all integrated functions of the body permanently cease. These functions may be mediated by what Bernat refers to as the critical system based in and projecting from the brainstem. Or they may be mediated by somatic mechanisms outside the brain altogether, as Shewmon maintains. In the first case, a human organism can remain alive without any cortical function. In the second case, a human organism can remain alive even after all brain functions have ceased.

As defined in chapter 2 and earlier in this chapter, a person is a being with the capacity for consciousness, the capacity to be aware of its existence and its surroundings. Some would insist that a person is also a being with the capacity to reason and participate in meaningful relationships. Personal identity consists in the awareness of oneself persisting through time. A person persists through time as one and the same individual in virtue of the connectedness and continuity of certain psychological properties. The psychological properties necessary for personhood and personal identity are generated and sustained by the brain and body. This is consistent with Parfit's definition of personhood: "The existence of a person, during any period, just consists in the existence of his brain and body, and the thinking of his thoughts, and the doing of his deeds, and the occurrence of many other physical and mental events."[26] To borrow McMahan's more concise term, persons are "embodied minds."[27]

Although the main biological basis of the mind is the cerebral cortex, the embodiment of the mind also includes subcortical brain structures, as well as systems of the body that interact with the brain. All of these structures and systems influence the qualitative nature and content of one's psychological properties. These may include cytokines from the immune system and hormones from the endocrine system, both of which can affect the central nervous system and the mental states it generates and sustains. This supports my earlier point that the biological basis of the mind is not entirely neurobiological. The psychological properties that constitute the mind emerge when the brain and body reach a certain level of complexity. Once these properties emerge, they do not become independent from the brain and body but instead interact with them in a nested hierarchy of feed-forward and feedback mechanisms designed to maintain systemic balance in the brain and body.

Persons begin to exist when they develop the capacity for consciousness, and they cease to exist when they lose this capacity. Having or lacking this capacity can be a matter of degree. Many believe that it begins to develop just after birth in infancy. But there is disagreement about when it is lost. Perhaps the most controversial test case for the second issue is Alzheimer's disease. In patients with this most common type of dementia, the capacity for mental life may gradually erode over many years until there is no longer any evidence of mentality and underlying cortical function. Beyond this point, one could say that an individual with Alzheimer's ceases to exist as a person. The capacity for mental life falls along a spectrum. There is a gray area near the degenerative end of the spectrum where it can be difficult to determine whether there is any capacity for mental life in patients with Alzheimer's or multi-infarct dementia.[28] Some have argued that it is mistaken to think that there is a precise point at which death occurs in any human, even one who dies "instantaneously" in a traumatic accident. Death is not an event but a biological process in which all bodily systems gradually cease over shorter or longer periods.[29] This does not mean that there is some intermediate state between being alive and being dead. Beyond a certain point all brain and bodily functions that keep one alive clearly cease, and death can be declared.

Patients with brain injuries resulting in severe alteration or loss of consciousness, but who do not meet diagnostic criteria for coma, can be separated into three categories. In a *persistent vegetative state*, patients are awake but have no conscious awareness of their surroundings. When this condition continues for three months after anoxic injury or twelve months after brain trauma, the patient is considered to have entered a *permanent vegetative state* with no chance of recovering any conscious capacity. Between a persistent and a permanent vegetative state, some patients may progress to a *minimally conscious state*, in which they have some awareness of self and environment.[30] Not all of these patients automatically progress to the permanent vegetative state. The key factor in distinguishing these states is not levels of resting brain activity but differences in the integration of brain functions.

For example, Arkansas resident Terry Wallis was misdiagnosed as being in a permanent vegetative state in 1984 following a brain injury resulting from a motor vehicle accident. It became clear that this diagnosis was incorrect when he began speaking in July 2003.[31] He had remained in a minimally conscious state for 19 years. This example illustrates that, in some cases of patients in prolonged but reversible coma, a minimally conscious state may be mistaken for the permanent loss of critical brain functions. It may be mistaken for a permanent vegetative state. Patients in a minimally conscious state appear vegetative but actually have residual neural resources, which consist in small groups of neurons firing in isolated regions of the brain. The brain activity of patients in this condition falls somewhere between a state where there is some capacity for conscious awareness and a state where there is no such capacity.

Citing a case like that of Terry Wallis, some might argue that it is difficult, if not impossible, to clearly distinguish a patient who is vegetative from one who has some, albeit little, neuronal activity. They might argue that the decision that a patient is vegetative and unlikely to regain consciousness is not based exclusively on clinical criteria. Such a decision could also be influenced to some degree by value judgments of neurologists or other physicians involved in the case. Furthermore, since the brain structures supporting the capacity for consciousness are distributed throughout the cortex and subcortical regions, it is unlikely that we could locate a center for mentality. It can therefore be difficult to specify which brain regions supporting the capacity for mentality cease to function without completely undermining this capacity. This is one reason why, unlike the way a mechanical ventilator might function as an artificial brainstem, it would be virtually impossible to construct an artificial cerebral cortex that could support consciousness on its own.

In most cases, however, brain imaging can be combined with EEG and other techniques to establish a definitive neurological diagnosis. These techniques might include the full outline of unconsciousness (FOUR) scale, which assesses eye, motor, brainstem, and respiratory function to enable more detailed diagnosis of patients with reduced responsiveness. This scale can distinguish between a deep unconscious state, where there is still some brain activity, and whole-brain death.[32] High-resolution imaging could accurately measure cortical function and establish whether the capacity for mentality was present or absent.

Recent studies indicate that fMRI PET, and diffusion tensor imaging (DTI) scans can quantify the most subtle differences in brain activity and provide clear and distinct diagnostic criteria for locked-in syndrome, persistent vegetative state, minimally conscious state, and permanent cessation of brainstem function.[33] These scans can determine whether patients have lost all awareness of their environment, or are minimally aware. They can clarify what might be uncertain using objective diagnostic criteria based on awareness, arousal, movement, and other behavioral features. Individuals in a permanent vegetative state may respond to touch and sound because some of their sensory cortex may still be active. But the frontal cortex that is critical for consciousness and personhood is no longer active. Brain scans could confirm that one region was active while the other was not. Changes in neural activity can be monitored by periodic use of PET, fMRI, or DTI scans over weeks or months. By comparing earlier and later images of brain function, neurological deterioration to a permanent vegetative state can be confirmed. The combination of these techniques and other neurological criteria can determine whether a person continues to exist or has ceased to exist.

This determination is significant for the ontological distinction between persons and human organisms. Specifically, it implies that persons begin to exist later than human organisms and can cease to exist before organisms do. After all cortical function permanently ceases and the person ceases to exist, a breathing and heart-beating body is just the physical organism the person leaves behind. To insist that we are essentially organisms would be to insist that as persons we are only phase sortals who exist as such through only one phase of our lives, since we have the capacity for conscious awareness only during this phase. Several examples can support the claim and argument that we are essentially persons and not human organisms.

Suppose that a three-year-old child has a traumatic brain injury and loses all cortical function, falling into a permanent vegetative state and remaining in this state for fifty years. He is kept alive by artificial nutrition and hydration. These forms of life-support are eventually withdrawn, and he is declared clinically dead after all brain and bodily functions cease. Because he lost all cortical function at the time of his injury, he ceased to be a person after three years and existed as a human organism for fifty years. It seems counterintuitive to say that we are essentially the sorts of individuals who could spend almost all of our lives in a vegetative state. Yet this view is consistent with the idea that we are essentially human organisms. This is even more counterintuitive than the idea that one could be declared dead while one's body was still breathing and alive.

Consider another example. Anencephalic infants are born without a cerebral cortex. But they usually have enough of a brainstem to support bodily functions for a short period of time. These cases are increasingly rare, due largely to such preventive measures as dietary intake of folate during pregnancy. They do occur, though the life span of anencephalic infants is usually only several days. It seems technically possible that life-support could sustain basic integrated bodily functions of these individuals for many years. If it were possible to do this, and these functions were integrated enough to qualify these individuals as organisms, then they could survive as organisms for a considerable period of time. But they never would develop the capacity for consciousness, because they never would develop the higher brain structures necessary for this capacity. They would not even have the potential to develop this capacity. If so, then a human organism need not ever have the potential to develop the capacity for consciousness, or indeed any form of mental life.

Because a functioning brain of a human organism need not have the necessary structures for mental life to emerge, a human organism need not ever become an embodied mind. This suggests that those who never have the capacity for mentality, or those who lack it for the balance of their lives, are not essentially different from others who develop and retain this capacity. They differ from individuals with higher brain function only in that they lack this nonessential property that others possess through only one phase of human existence. But this is radically at odds with the intuitively plausible conception we have of ourselves as embodied minds, as individuals with the capacity for consciousness and an interest in what we do, whether we can interact with others, and how our lives go.

Most of us would consider the two examples I have given to be tragic. Why? They are tragic because the individuals in them either lost or never possessed the essential property of personhood, the capacity for consciousness, over the course of their biological lives. If we are fundamentally human organisms, however, then this attitude is groundless. It should not matter whether one has the capacity for consciousness for a longer or shorter period of one's biological life, because this capacity is only a nonessential property of that life. The asymmetry in our value judgments about these cases suggests that most of us believe that we are essentially persons rather than human organisms. It may be that this ontological question cannot be decided on purely objective grounds. But our beliefs on this matter have to be taken seriously, since to a great extent the ethical significance of many decisions made at the end of human life rests on these beliefs.

McMahan's discussion of the phenomenon of dicephalus includes a third example and argument supporting the view that we are essentially persons and not organisms.[34] In these rare but actual cases, a human zygote divides incompletely and results in twins conjoined below the neck. There are two people inhabiting one body, or organism, between them. In a case presented in *Life* magazine some years ago, dicephalic sisters Abigail and Brittany Hensel had one body but distinct personalities. McMahan says that

> although Abigail and Brittany are two different persons, there seems to be only one organism between them. If so, then neither girl is identical with that organism. . . . But if dicephalic twins are not human organisms, this strongly suggests that none of us is an organism. For, despite their anomalous physical condition, there is no reason to suppose that dicephalic twins are fundamentally different types of being from the rest of us.[35]

McMahan's argument and example are persuasive because dicephalic twins are not a mere logical possibility but an empirical fact.

What makes these twins different persons? Despite sharing one body, they have distinct brains that sustain distinct psychological properties. This does not mean that the biological basis of the psychological properties that make Abigail and Brittany distinct persons is located entirely in the brain. Rather, the endocrine, immune, and other systems in the single body they share interact with the two brains in ways that result in the distinctive quality and content of their mental states. The brain of each twin responds differently to these other bodily systems, as well as to the events they experience in the social and natural environment.

So, even if brain transplants became empirically possible and medically feasible, it would not follow that a person whose brain was transplanted into another body would retain the same psychological properties and would remain the same person. Switching brains between Abigail and Brittany from one head to the other and leaving the one body they share intact below the neck would not mean that the identities of these sisters would remain the same. Such a procedure would likely disrupt the continuity of the unique interactions between each of the two brains and other bodily systems, as well as the continuity of the unique interactions between these systems and the external world. This discontinuity would likely result in a substantially different set of psychological properties following the procedure. It would result in two persons who would be substantially different from the two persons who underwent the procedure.

More important, this explanation does not support but instead casts doubt on the view that we are essentially human organisms. The psychological properties that define personhood and personal identity depend on the functions of the brain and body. But the nature and content of these properties cannot be explained entirely in terms of biological functions. This is consistent with the emergent account of mind, where the psychological properties that constitute the mind emerge when the brain and body reach a certain level of complexity. Psychological properties such as intentionality are needed to represent events in the external world to the brain and make them meaningful to us. The brain and body cannot do this on the basis of their biological properties alone. One could argue that Abigail and Brittany are identical with their organism if we identify their organism with the cerebral cortex and supporting brainstem. Still, although the cortex and brainstem are necessary for Abigail and Brittany to have the capacity for consciousness, they are not sufficient to completely account for the psychological properties of their conscious states. The biological functions of their brains and of the one body they share are necessary but not sufficient to account for the existence of Abigail and Brittany as separate persons. This further supports the view that they, and we, are essentially persons rather than human organisms.

Religious and spiritually inclined people would say that death occurs when the soul leaves the body. But there is considerable disagreement about what the soul is and whether it inheres in the body, the brainstem, an embodied mind, or a disembodied mind. We need to examine different conceptions of the soul, analyzing how these conceptions map onto and clarify the distinction between persons and organisms. We also need to assess which of these conceptions is most in line with our intuitions about the sort of beings we essentially are. This will further set the stage for discussion of the ethical issues surrounding brain death.

When Does the Soul Leave the Body? Terri Schiavo and Nancy Cruzan

Belief in the existence of a soul has both metaphysical and moral implications. A rough definition of the soul is a substance or set of properties that identifies each of us as a unique person or human being. It is in virtue of having a soul that a person or human being has moral status. This moral status gives that individual interests and rights, entailing obligations for others to treat him or her in ways that respect these interest and rights. Let's consider four different conceptions of the soul. There are other conceptions; but the four I present here are probably the most representative of philosophical and religious perspectives.

The first conception describes the soul as an immaterial substance that can exist in a disembodied state. This dualist view is often attributed to Plato, who in the *Phaedo* argues that the soul retains the same range of conscious activity after the nonessential embodied part of the person is no longer alive. Plato identifies the disembodied soul, or mind (*psyche*), with the person.[36] In the later *Phaedrus*, *Republic*, and *Timaeus*, Plato divides the soul into rational, appetitive, and spirited parts. He argues that a person does not cease to exist when all of his or her bodily functions cease, since what essentially counts as that person, the rational soul, is immortal and survives.

Descartes's substance dualism is similar in some respects to Plato's dualism, since Descartes also argues that the soul (mind) and body are distinct immaterial and material substances.[37] He argues that the soul is only contingently and not necessarily related to the brain and body and thus can exist independently of them. Unlike Plato, though, Descartes does not divide the soul into parts. In addition, Descartes holds that mind and body can causally interact through the activity of the pineal gland in the brain. He does not satisfactorily explain how the pineal gland effects or mediates this interaction. Not is it clear how the mind or soul can exist and function without the structures and functions of the brain and body that seem necessary to generate and sustain it. There is no obvious difficulty in identifying the mind with the soul. But the idea of a disembodied substance is too mysterious and leaves too much to be explained to be a plausible conception of the soul.

Alternatively, many accept hylomorphism, which takes a human being to be an essential unity of body and soul. Hylomorphism derives from Aristotle's metaphysics of matter (*hyle*) and form (*morphe*).[38] The soul is the form of the material body, in the sense that it is the main organizing or informing principle of the body. For Aristotle, the relation of the soul to the body is analogous to the relation of the shape of a bronze statue to the bronze that makes up the statue. It is reasonable to say that Aristotle would identify the soul with the design and control of structural and functional bodily processes. He would probably argue that all critical bodily functions cease when the soul leaves the body. Aristotle's account of the soul is consistent with Bernat's account of the body's critical functional center consisting of the brainstem and its projections to other parts of the brain and body.

Some commentators claim that hylomorphism grounds the acceptance of the whole-brain criterion of death in Judaism, Christianity, and Islam.[39] For these religions, the soul leaves the body and the person dies when all brain functions permanently cease. Many within these monotheistic religions believe that following death, the soul can be reunited with the body in an afterlife. According to Aristotle's hylomorphism, however, there can be no disembodied soul or reunification of body and soul. When the soul departs from the body at death, when all brain functions cease, the body that belonged to the person during his or her conscious life decomposes and is not reconstituted as the same body.

A third conception of the soul involves distinct Hindu and Buddhistic interpretations. Vedantic Hinduism generally holds the dualistic view that individual souls pass through a sequence of bodies in the process of transmigration or reincarnation. Each soul contains certain dispositional properties that survive the extinction of consciousness in death and later become embodied in a new psychophysical organism. This imperishable essence of a person is the *atman*, or underlying metaphysical self. It is sometimes also referred to as *jiva* (individual soul), or *jiva-atman*.[40] Although there are some similarities between Hindu and Platonic dualism, Hinduism does not subscribe to the idea of a tripartite soul. Nor does Hinduism subscribe to the notion of causal interaction between mind and body associated with Cartesian dualism. Buddhism denies the existence of a soul as a spiritual substance. It subscribes to the principle of *anatta* (no soul). For Buddhists, what many refer to as "the soul" is not an unchanging entity that survives the destruction of the body. There is no uniquely identifiable eternal self or soul, only a succession of moments of consciousness. We are repeatedly reborn or re-incarnated, not in the sense that a particular conscious self lives again, but in the sense that a continuing karmic pattern of mental and physical acts forms a suc-cession of empirical selves.[41] Each rebirth or reincarnation involves an exchange of one contingent instantiation of consciousness for another.

Despite differences regarding claims about the soul, both Hinduism and Buddhism hold that successive human lives are successive incarnations of the same universal structure. This suggests that there is no clear line of separation between life and death, because there is no uniquely identifiable substance that begins to exist and ceases to exist at specific times. Transmigration or reincarnation is not an event but a process or sequence of events. The soul or essence of a person is not identified with a particular body or brain and, as such, does not cease to exist when biological death has been declared. Yet the idea of transmigration leaves it am-biguous when the soul or essence has moved from one body to another. It is unclear how many dispositional properties or moments of consciousness in the transitional state are sufficient for a human body to retain moral status. It is also unclear when the body might lose this status.

A fourth conception identifies the soul with a unified set of psychological properties associated with the capacity for consciousness. It necessarily depends on the functional capacity of the higher brain and emerges from the brain when it reaches a certain level of complexity. This account of the soul is consistent with the "embodied mind" account of persons. On this account, the soul leaves the body, and the person identified with the soul ceases to exist, when he or she permanently loses the capacity for consciousness. This coincides with the permanent cessation of the functions of the cerebral cortex that generate and sustain this capacity. The soul can depart from the body even when the brainstem and other systems in the body continue to function.

The conception of the soul that I have just described seems most in line with our intuitions about what constitutes personhood and personal identity through time. In an important respect, it is more consistent with theistic religions than the whole-brain conception. These religions are based on the fundamental belief in a divine being, and the capacity to have this or any other type of belief depends on a functioning cerebral cortex. Individuals who have lost the capacity for higher brain function have also lost the capacity for religious and other forms of belief. A cortically based soul is also the most plausible conception with respect to the questions of what gives one moral status, whether one can benefit or be harmed, and whether one can value life and have an interest in continued life. I will now present reasons for accepting this fourth conception of the soul as the one that should ground our thinking about the metaphysics of death and the ethical im-plications that follow from it.

Aquinas distinguishes three phases in the organization of the human body.[42] These phases correspond to three distinct types of soul. The *nutritive* or *vegetative* soul has the lowest level of organization and is found in the human zygote and embryo. It is similar to the level of organization in plants. The *sensitive* or *animal* soul displays a higher level of organization and is manifest in the capacity for sensory experience. It is present in all sentient animals. The highest level of organization is found in the *rational soul (anima intellectiva)* and consists in the capacity for rational thought or, more generally, the capacity for mentality. Possession of this soul is what distinguishes human beings from other animals.

Unlike the first two types of soul described by Aquinas, the rational soul is not biological but psychological. Significantly, the rational soul does not begin to exist at conception but at a later stage of the biological development of a human organism. The popular belief that "ensoulment" occurs at conception can be traced to Pope Pius IX's 1869 declaration that there should be full protection of life from the moment of conception.[43] Against this view, six centuries earlier, Aquinas argued that ensoulment does not occur until 40 days after conception in males and 90 days after conception in females. Only at this point is the soul directly "infused" into the body by God. Aquinas calls this "hominization," which is when a human body becomes a human being.[44] Islam holds a similar view. The Koran states that the soul enters the body of a fetus 120 days after fertilization, when it is "blown into him by Allah."[45] Furthermore, most Jewish Talmudic scholars agree that ensoulment takes place once a human form is established 40 days or more into pregnancy. In each of these religious traditions, some biological development of a human organism already has taken place before the soul begins to exist and the human organism becomes a human being, or what many would call a person. Still, it is important to point out that Aquinas, the Koran, or the Talmud do not literally mean that humans have the *capacity* for rational thought from the time of ensoulment. Rather, from this point on, they have the *potential* for rational thought, which can become the capacity for mentality following further biological development. Humans have biological resources that may develop into a set of mental properties that they will possess and exercise in thought and action. But these properties can only emerge beyond a certain point of biological development.

If persons are defined essentially in terms of a rational soul, and they do not possess this soul until some time after conception, then persons do not exist until some time after conception. Furthermore, if the cerebral cortex is necessary to generate and sustain the rational soul, then anencephalic infants or others who fail to develop a cortex never have a rational soul and never become persons. Those who have a rational soul and who are persons can lose this soul and cease to exist when the cerebral cortex permanently ceases to function. If it is only in virtue of possessing a rational soul that individuals can have interests and moral status, then no one could be harmed by the withdrawal of life-support or similar actions if he or she lacked a rational soul. One can uphold this argument even if the individuals in question have nutritive and animal souls. Bodies that continued to have brainstem and integrated somatic functions but no higher brain function would lack rational souls, interests, and moral status. Hence individuals inhabiting these bodies could not be harmed by what others might do to them.

Some might claim that human beings have moral status and an interest in continuing to live up until the last breath of life. For this reason, human organisms with no higher brain function but with continued brainstem function should be kept alive by any means possible. Keeping a human organism alive would show respect for the sanctity of its life. This claim could justify indefinite mechanical ventilation, or artificial nutrition and hydration of what others would consider nothing more than the bodily remains of a deceased person. It suggests a vitalist view, whereby moral status can be based entirely on biological function. Yet it is difficult to defend the claim that human bodies can have value for and moral status independently of the persons who inhabit them.

McMahan's comments on this issue are instructive:

> The intrinsic or impersonal value of a human life is different from its personal value—that is, the value it has for the individual whose life it is. Even though a life may have impersonal value in part or even entirely for the same reasons that it has personal value, the two types of value are distinct. Similarly, respect for the sanctity of human life is different from respect for the worth of the person. Respect for the worth of a person is not distinct from respect for the person himself.[46]

Life has value for persons, not their bodies. Only persons have the cortically based psychological capacity to subjectively value their bodies as one biological aspect of their larger biographical lives.

Still, there is considerable disagreement about which regions of the brain we identify with the soul, when the soul leaves the body, and what this means for the permissibility or impermissibility of withdrawing life-sustaining medical treatment. This disagreement turns on the metaphysical question of whether we are essentially human organisms or persons. It also turns on the question of whether the concept of the soul we use to ground these claims corresponds to a narrow neurological criterion involving only the cerebral cortex, or a broad neurological criterion involving the brainstem. Two prominent legal cases illustrate the extent of this disagreement.

In 1990, at age 26, Terri Schiavo suffered a heart attack, probably from a potassium deficiency related to an eating disorder. This event caused a severe anoxic brain injury that deprived her brain of oxygen long enough to cause paralysis and extensive neurological damage. She gradually fell into a permanent vegetative state. Although she was able to breathe on her own and was not on a ventilator, she needed continued artificial nutrition and hydration to remain alive.

Eight years later, her husband, Michael Schiavo, asked a Florida court to permit removal of the feeding tube inserted in her stomach. Her parents, Mary and Robert Schindler, opposed this request. Many challenges and counterchallenges to withdrawing the artificial feeding were considered in numerous court proceedings.[47] In October 2003, a Florida court determined that Michael Schiavo's request to withdraw treatment should be honored, and the feeding tube was removed. But Florida Governor Jeb Bush intervened and filed an amicus curiae brief to force continuation of the feeding tube, and it was reinserted six days later. In January 2005, the U.S. Supreme Court rejected Governor Bush's appeal for continued artificial feeding. One month later, a Florida circuit court issued an order temporarily preventing the husband from stopping the life-sustaining nutrition. The feeding tube remained inserted, and both sides in the case remained at an impasse.

The case came to an end on February 26, 2005, when a Florida judge ruled that Michael Schiavo had the authority to remove the tube. Shortly after he did this, Terri Schiavo was declared dead on March 30, 2005.[48]

The main legal issue in this case was family disagreement about life-sustaining treatment for an incapacitated patient without a clear advance directive. It involved disagreement about who was the appropriate surrogate decision-maker for the patient. At a deeper metaphysical and ethical level, it involved disagreement about the value of a severely brain-damaged patient's life. Michael Schiavo believed that continued life in a permanent vegetative state could not have any value for his wife. This would have justified withdrawing all life-sustaining treatment. Although her condition, strictly speaking, was not terminal, the permanent loss of all mental capacity made it impossible for her to have any interest in continued life. Questions about whether her condition was terminal applied only to her biological organism, not to Terri the person who, from her husband's perspective, had ceased to exist.

In contrast, Terri Schiavo's parents believed that continued life had value and would have benefited her, presumably even if she remained in a vegetative state for a long period of time. Early in 2005, they argued that their daughter, a Roman Catholic, would not have wanted to violate the 2004 declaration by Pope John Paul II that individuals in a vegetative state have a right to continued nutrition and hydration. Because Terri Schiavo had lost the capacity for conscious awareness, her parents, and other right-to-life advocates insisting on continued tube feeding, seemed to base their arguments on basic biological functioning. They believed that as long as her brainstem was active and she continued to breathe and remained awake, she still existed and had moral status. This status gave Terri a right to life that would have been violated if the feeding tube were withdrawn and she had been allowed to die.

It is worth emphasizing that a permanent vegetative state must not be confused with a minimally conscious state. Brain scans and other neurological tests can provide clear and reliable clinical evidence that can distinguish one state from the other. In Terri Schiavo's case, CT scans showed massive shrinkage of her brain, with the cerebral cortex completely destroyed. The scans indicated that most of her brain contained only scar tissue and spinal fluid. The only part of her brain that remained intact was her brainstem, which continued to regulate her cardiac, circulatory, and other vital functions. In addition, the last EEG of her cortex was completely flat, with no indication of any electrical activity in this region. Most people in a permanent vegetative state show no more than 5 percent of normal brain activity. These are conclusive indications of irreversible loss of the capacity for consciousness. They are consistent with the American Academy of Neurology's statement that vegetative states are likely to become permanent after about three months.[49] After this time, it is highly unlikely that a patient in such a state could regain the capacity for consciousness. By all credible neurological accounts of her condition, Terri Schiavo was in a permanent vegetative state.

This diagnosis was confirmed by the results of the autopsy on her body on April 1, 2005. It showed massive cerebral atrophy and extensive neuronal loss in her brain, which was only half of its normal weight. These findings clearly showed that her neurological condition was irreversible. All of these considerations cast suspicion on the claim that her life could have had value for her once she fell into a permanent vegetative state. Michael Schiavo's claim that his wife's life could no longer have any value for her was based on her loss of all higher brain function. Her parents' claim that her life continued to have value for her was based on the manifestation of activity from her brainstem and ascending reticular formation that sustained her sleep-wake cycles, breathing, and circulation.

We can describe the main issues in this case in terms of the discussion at the beginning of this section. For Michael Schiavo, his wife's soul had already left her body. He identified her soul with her capacity for consciousness based on her previously functioning but now defunct cerebral cortex. From his perspective, Terri the person died long before the March 2005 declaration of her death. The artificial nutrition was only keeping her body alive. Since her body had no moral status of its own, this permitted removal of the feeding tube. For Terri Schiavo's parents, their daughter's soul continued to exist, as manifested in her continued breathing and wakefulness sustained by her functioning brainstem. These functions were enough for her to have moral status and prohibited removal of the feeding tube. From either perspective, one could say that the value or disvalue of Terri Schiavo's life and her moral status depended on the presence or absence of her soul.

The disagreement between the husband and parents about the value of her life turned on very different conceptions of the human soul. Her husband seemed to base the value of Terri's life on a conception of the rational soul, while her parents seemed to base the value of her life on some version of the hylomorphic conception of the soul. The hylomorphic conception the parents implicitly accepted was a strongly biological one. But it would not rule out an alternative interpretation. As interpreted by Aquinas, hylomorphism allows us to say that part of the form of a human being is the distinct intellective and relational functions of that being. This would intuitively offer more support for Michael Schiavo's position and the ethical justification for removing Terri Schiavo's feeding tube.

The earlier legal case of Nancy Cruzan involved a similar legal problem with the absence of an advance directive in end-of-life decision-making.[50] At a deeper level, it raised the same questions about moral status and the value of continued life for a severely brain-damaged patient. In 1983, Nancy Cruzan lost control of her car and in the accident that followed sustained brain injuries resulting in a coma. She progressed to a permanent vegetative state and was unable to take nutrition orally. Surgeons implanted a gastrostomy feeding and hydration tube in Nancy with the consent of her then husband. But her parents objected and sought a court order directing the withdrawal of the tube. The Missouri Supreme Court overruled the parents, holding that there was no clear and convincing evidence of Nancy's desire to have life-sustaining treatment withheld or withdrawn under such circumstances. In 1990, the U.S. Supreme Court upheld the right of the state of Missouri to require strict standards of evidence regarding the patient's preferences. At the same time, though, the Court affirmed the fundamental principle of the patient's right to forgo life-sustaining treatment and supported the parents by ordering the discontinuation of the artificial hydration and nutrition in 1990. This was seven years after Nancy had fallen into the vegetative state.

Like Michael Schiavo, Nancy Cruzan's parents believed that their daughter's continued biological life could not be of any value to her, since she lacked the neurologically based mental capacity necessary to have an interest in life. The family engraved the following on Nancy Cruzan's tombstone: "DEPARTED JAN. 11, 1983 / AT PEACE DEC. 26, 1990."[51] This inscription suggested that her parents believed that Nancy Cruzan the person died when she lost all higher brain function as a consequence of the 1983 accident. Identifying her (rational) soul with the cortically based capacity for mentality, they believed that her soul left her body and that she ceased to exist when her cerebral cortex ceased to function. While Nancy Cruzan's demise was based on a neurological criterion, it did not require the cessation of her brainstem and other bodily functions. The loss of higher brain function meant the loss of her soul, moral status, and her death as a person. This occurred at the time of her accident or, at the latest, when she fell into the permanent vegetative state shortly thereafter. The demise of her organism, which her parents did not identify with Nancy, occurred when all brainstem and any other remaining biological bodily functions ceased seven years later.

The parents of Terri Schiavo, on the one hand, and Michael Schiavo and the parents of Nancy Cruzan, on the other, had different convictions about when their loved ones died and on what basis life could have value for them. Terri Schiavo's parents believed that she continued to exist and that life had value for her on the basis of her breathing and other autonomic functions sustained by the brainstem. Michael Schiavo and Nancy Cruzan's parents believed that their wife and daughter ceased to exist and that life ceased to have value for them as soon as they fell into the permanent vegetative state. They had lost the neurological and psychological capacity that made them persons and gave them moral status and an interest in continuing to live. Some would argue that not withdrawing hydration and nutrition in these cases would be inhumane and violate the dignity and sanctity of the biological life embodied by the patient. United States Supreme Court justice William Brennan expressed this sentiment in his dissenting opinion in the Nancy Cruzan case. Invoking reasoning from a similar earlier case, Brennan said: "In certain, thankfully rare, circumstances, the burden of maintaining corporeal existence degrades the very humanity it was meant to serve."[52] Brennan suggested that the body has value only insofar as it is occupied by a person, by an individual with the capacity for mentality. He also alluded to some of the unpalatable consequences of life-sustaining treatment if we subscribe to a vitalist concept of life and think of ourselves as essentially human organisms rather than persons.

There has been and will continue to be public disagreement about when a person dies and whether continued biological life can have value for a patient who has lost most, or all, of his or her neurological capacities. But the mental capacity to have an interest in life, or indeed any interests, rests on the neurological functions of the cerebral cortex. In the light of this, it seems reasonable to say that a person loses his or her soul and dies once the cerebral cortex ceases to function. Moreover, if we identify personhood with the rational soul and this soul is based on cortical function, then it seems equally reasonable to say that this conception of the soul should serve as the basis for the moral status of persons. If one accepts this, then one will also accept that patients without any higher brain function cannot be harmed. They lack the neurological and psychological capacity to have interests, the violation of which is necessary for a person to be harmed. It will be helpful to further explore this idea and the ethical import of different types of action to which it can apply. I will now examine the permissibility or impermissibility of withdrawal of life-support and organ procurement from individuals with no higher brain function.

Beneficial and Harmful Acts

Mechanical ventilation and artificial hydration and nutrition can permissibly be withdrawn from patients who have lost all higher brain function. These would include patients diagnosed as permanently vegetative. Withdrawing these forms of life-support is permissable because they lack the capacity for interests and therefore cannot be harmed. Because these patients are beyond harm, after the removal of life-support viable organs or tissues could permissibly be taken from their bodies for the purpose of transplantation. But we could not make these claims in cases where patients were diagnosed as persistently vegetative until three months after an anoxic injury or twelve months after trauma. Before these times, they may progress to a minimally conscious state without becoming permanently vegetative. Removing life-support and taking organs could harm these individuals if they still have some capacity for consciousness. For a person with no cortical function, the only instance in which that person could be harmed would be if some action or omission by others failed to respect an earlier wish the person expressed regarding what should or should not be done to his or her body after his or her death.

McMahan's embodied mind account provides the theoretical basis for these claims, which have been defended by other philosophers as well. For example, Michael Tooley argues that, for a patient with no higher brain function on artificial life-support, it is "not even prima facie wrong to turn off a respirator in such a case, even though one is thereby killing a human organism."[53] The underlying rationale is that it is not wrong because the organism that remains after the cessation of cortical function has no moral status. Similarly, Peter Singer asserts that "without consciousness, continued life cannot benefit an individual. When an individual has permanently lost the capacity for consciousness, as in a permanent vegetative state or deep coma, the individual's life ceases to be worth living for him or her, and the central objections to killing cease to apply."[54] So it would be permissible to disconnect life-support and procure these patients' organs for transplantation. James Rachels defends the same position. He distinguishes between one's *biological* life and one's *biographical* life.[55] To be biologically alive is simply to be a human organism. To be alive in the biographical sense is to be the subject of a life that can be described from the inside, from the psychological point of view associated with being a person. Rachels further claims that consciousness is necessary for a biographical life, and that biological life is valuable only insofar as it supports biographical life. It follows from this that when an individual has permanently lost the capacity for consciousness, his or her biographical life has ended and any biological life that remains has no moral status. "At that point," Rachels claims, "we cannot possibly be harming him by removing his heart or kidney or whatever."[56]

For the same reason, keeping a patient with little or no brain function alive on mechanical ventilation in order to keep his or her organs perfused and viable for transplantation could not harm him or her. Even if the ventilation were used solely for this purpose, the patient could not be harmed if he or she had no higher brain function and no capacity for an interest in continued life. Such a practice could harm critically ill patients in the same ICU if there were a limited number of ventilators and using one on a brain-dead patient would deprive others of this scarce life-sustaining resource. But it could not harm a brain-dead patient. Unless killing the surviving human organism by disconnecting life-support and taking its organs violated the autonomous preferences a mentally competent person expressed prior to losing his or her capacity for consciousness, it would be permissible to perform these acts once the patient had lost all cortical function.

These claims and arguments conflict with the clinical and legal definition of death and policies for withdrawal of life-sustaining treatment and organ procurement for transplantation. This definition and these policies rest on whole-brain or brainstem criteria of death. However, these criteria do not pertain to the cerebral cortex. Because the cortex is necessary for the consciousness required for moral status, whole-brain and brainstem criteria cannot explain how a human body with no functions other than breathing and circulation could have moral status. In particular, they cannot satisfactorily explain how taking organs from an individual with no higher brain function but a functioning brainstem could harm such an individual. Although this action would mean killing the individual by taking his or her organs and would thereby violate the dead donor rule, neither whole-brain nor brainstem criteria of death could tell us in what sense the individual would be harmed.

Individuals with progressive neurological deterioration, as in Alzheimer's disease or multi-infarct dementia, are more difficult to assess. In these cases, the loss of the capacity for consciousness is gradual, and it may be difficult to determine when there is no longer any such capacity and the person has ceased to exist. It is possible that life-support could be withdrawn from these individuals when some of their cortical functions were intact. In that case, they could still have interests and could be harmed. As in the PVS cases discussed earlier, though, beyond a certain point, CT, PET, fMRI, and DTI scans and EEGs could show that there was in fact no sign of cortical activity.

Because Terri Schiavo had fallen into a permanent vegetative state, she could not have been harmed by the removal of the feeding tube that was keeping her alive. She had lost the neurological and psychological capacity to have an interest in continued life. Given her neurological condition, Terri also probably lacked the capacity to experience any pain or suffering in the period between the removal of the feeding tube and her death. She would not have been harmed by the withdrawal of nutrition in this respect either. If permanently vegetative individuals in this situation are able to experience anything, it is less likely to be pain and more likely to be a euphoric state induced by chemical imbalances in the brain resulting from starvation. Inserting or leaving a feeding tube in their bodies would be more burdensome to them than withholding or withdrawing it.

Would we make the same claims about patients who fall into and remain in a minimally conscious state? Is minimal conscious awareness enough for them to have interests, such as an interest in continued life? A patient who is only minimally conscious is not likely to have the capacity to formulate, act on, or reassess life plans or future projects. Such a patient may not be able to interact with others either. Yet he or she could have an interest in continuing to live. Although some might consider this to be a weak sense of interest, it could be enough to prohibit any action that might cause him or her to permanently lose the capacity for consciousness, however minimal this capacity might be. By defeating such a person's interest in continuing to live, such an action could harm that person. It may be possible to restore some cognitive function in these patients by using different forms of neuromodulation. This could include electrical deep-brain stimulation to the central thalamus, which has many connections with the cerebral cortex. Application of this technique could improve integration of damaged neuronal networks and restore some brain functions. Some individuals in a minimally conscious state may regain some degree of consciousness without any intervention. Withdrawing life-support in these cases would preclude these possibilities from being actualized.[57]

One might question the claim that these individuals could have an interest in *continued* life. The neurological impairment from brain injury may be significant enough to disrupt psychological continuity between their current mental states and their mental states prior to the injury. Such an individual would emerge from the minimally conscious state as *a* person, but might not survive as the *same* person he or she was before falling into this state. Personal identity involves awareness of persisting through time, and recently Terry Wallis told his parents that he has "no real sense of time."

Significantly, these claims and arguments about moral status and harm pertain not to whether a patient has a terminal condition. They pertain to how much function there is in a patient's brain. By all medical accounts, a permanent vegetative state is not a terminal condition. Many insist that a patient's condition must be terminal to justify withdrawal of life-support. Yet if decisions about withdrawing life-support are based on whether this action can harm patients, and if patients with minimal brain function but who are not terminal cannot be harmed by the withdrawal of life-support, then we should reject the claim that life-support can only be withdrawn in terminal cases. Nevertheless, because many neurodegenerative conditions involve gradual cortical deterioration, there would have to be conclusive evidence of no higher brain function before we could definitively say that these individuals were beyond harm. Some of these individuals may have an advance directive with instructions about withholding or withdrawing life-sustaining treatment at a later time. But they would have to be fully competent at the time they issued the directive for it to be morally and legally binding once they had lost the capacity for consciousness.

I have claimed that the only way a patient with no higher brain activity could be harmed would be if certain actions done to the body were contrary to preferences he or she expressed at an earlier time. This harm would be posthumous, in the sense that it would occur after the patient's death. Joel Feinberg has explained the coherence of the related ideas of surviving interests and posthumous harms.[58] He holds that the subject of a surviving interest is the living person antemortem whose interest it was. For Feinberg, the harming relation in these cases is not causal but logical. That is, if a certain fact obtains at a later time, that fact makes it true at an earlier time that that fact will obtain. Thus, if my interests in facts about the future fail to be fulfilled after I am dead, then this makes it true that these interests fail to be fulfilled while I am alive. This can be a misfortune for me, even if I could never know about it. There can be degrees of harm. Harms that befall one during conscious life are worse than harms that befall one after death because one can experience the first but not the second. Even if experienced harm is worse than posthumous harm, events that occur after we die can harm us nonetheless.

Doctors may fail to respect a patient's interest in not being sustained on life-support following an accident and the permanent loss of consciousness. If they continued to ventilate the patient, they could harm him or her posthumously. Similarly, if one's interest in bodily integrity and not having one's organs harvested for transplantation after death was not respected and organs were procured, then this would make it true that one's interest in bodily integrity while one was alive failed to be respected. On the other hand, if a family overrides a patient's expressed intent to donate organs after death and refuses to allow organ procurement for transplantation, then this, too, could harm the person posthumously.

In a different situation, a woman in the second trimester of pregnancy may lose critical brain functions as a result of a massive hemorrhagic stroke. She is put on a ventilator, which is necessary for her to remain alive and for the fetus to reach viability and be delivered as a live birth. If at an earlier time she expressed the wish that her child be born, even if she could not care for it, then removing the brain-dead woman from life-support and terminating the development of the fetus could defeat her wish and thus harm her. The harm would consist not in using her body instrumentally for the sake of the fetus and the future child, since her body would have no moral status of its own. Rather, the harm would consist in thwarting the realization of her wish that her child be born. All of these cases involve harms that can befall a person after death because of interests that are timelessly true of the person and can survive his or her death. This explains why advance directives expressing a person's wishes regarding end-of-life care can be morally and legally binding even after the person who expressed them is no longer competent or has ceased to exist. Because these wishes can extend beyond the life of the person, their realization or defeat can benefit or harm the person after his or her death.

The idea that a person's interests can survive his or her death may generate an obligation for others to respect these interests. When there is such an obligation, it involves a deontological constraint on what families, physicians, or others can or cannot do to a person's body after that person dies. So, if a person specified in an advance directive that he or she wanted his or her body to remain intact after death and objected to organ donation, family or doctors would be harming the person if they failed to act on this directive, ignored the person's wishes, and took his or her organs. This constraint would hold regardless of the potential good that might result from transplanting the organs into the bodies of dying patients. The moral weight of this constraint is based on the principle of respect for individual autonomy, as well as respect for the narrative integrity of the person's biographical life. A person's autonomy and narrative integrity may extend beyond his or her death and thus may not be limited to his or her biological life alone. Insofar as my biographical life consists of more than the biological life of my body and brain, I can have an interest in how it goes after my biological life has ended. The agency that is an essential component of my self may include intentions that extend beyond the temporal limits of my biological existence. In this regard, the realization or defeat of these intentions can make a difference in the overall value of my biographical life.

But there may be ambiguity in how a family or transplant team interprets an advance directive with an explicit reference to organ donation. This ambiguity hinges on implicit disagreement about what the different parties mean by "brain death" and "death." Suppose that a person has stipulated in his will that he would want to donate his organs and tissues after his death. Suppose further that he has an acute traumatic brain injury and permanently loses all of his higher brain functions and the capacity for consciousness. But some of his brainstem continues to function, and he remains alive with the help of drugs to sustain blood pressure and a ventilator to ensure that his breathing and circulation continue. If he believed that he was essentially a person in virtue of his capacity for consciousness from the time he spelled out his wishes in his will until the time of his injury, then by his own account this person has died. Yet the ICU physicians leave him on life-support and do not call in the organ procurement and transplant teams because the patient is still alive according to the legally and medically accepted whole-brain and brainstem criteria of death. They cannot declare the patient dead because he does not meet the standard neurological criteria of death.

Prior to a neurological determination of death in these cases, the brainstem can gradually become ischemic, which can result in an activation of the sympathetic nervous system that is unopposed by a corresponding activation of the parasympathetic nervous system. This state of imbalance is often termed "autonomic storm" and may cause a cascade of events resulting in irreversible damage to the body's organs. Organs may also be irreparably damaged by warm ischemic injury caused by lack of blood flow to organs in critically ill patients who experience a slow, progressive demise. In both instances, organs would not be viable for transplantation once the patient was declared dead by standard neurological criteria.

If this occurred in the hypothetical case at hand, and the patient's organs were no longer viable for transplantation when doctors declared the patient dead, then he would be harmed. Not declaring death sooner and not procuring the patient's still-viable organs for transplantation would defeat the patient's interest in donating his organs for transplantation. The only way the medical team could have respected the patient's interests and not caused harm would have been to withdraw life-support and remove organs earlier while there was still some brainstem function. Yet on the whole-brain and brainstem criteria of death, this would have meant removing the organs while the patient was still alive. This would have violated the DDR and would have been a case of unjustified killing. The patient's interests would be respected and realized. But it would mean performing an action that could not be justified medically or legally.

Medical staff most likely would uphold the whole-brain criterion and base the DDR and any decision about organ procurement on this criterion. Given the patient's interests, though, they could harm him by failing to withdraw life-support and take his organs or tissues once all cortical function had ceased. It is presumed that the DDR protects patients from harm. Yet basing this rule on the whole-brain criterion of death could have the opposite effect and harm the patient by failing to respect his wishes and act in his best interests.[59]

In practice, the intensive care and transplant teams would act on the default assumption that the patient is not dead until all neurological or cardiopulmonary functions have permanently ceased. This would not resolve the moral problem that I have raised, however. For if the patient believes that he or she is essentially a person rather than a human organism, and that his or her life as a person depends on the functioning of the cerebral cortex, then waiting until all activity in the brainstem stops could harm the patient in two senses. First, it would fail to respect his or her autonomy in treating him or her as an organism rather than as a person, as someone whose interest in continued life was based on the capacity for consciousness. Second, it would defeat the patient's interest in donating his or her organs for transplantation. Of course, if the patient indicated at an earlier time that he or she did not want to donate his organs, then declaring the patient dead according to whole-brain or brainstem criteria would effectively respect his or her interests. But if the patient has a different conception from that of the doctors regarding who he or she essentially is, then the patient could be harmed in the two senses I have described.

Admittedly, most of us are not likely to draw the ontological distinction between persons and human organisms when we draw up an advance directive. Nevertheless, in principle, the cases I have presented suggest that there may be different interpretations of the sort of beings we essentially are and of when we die. These differences can influence our interpretation of interests and our judgments about benefit and harm with respect to withdrawing life-support, declaring death, and possible organ procurement for transplantation.[60]

There is a sense in which individuals with advanced Alzheimer's or multi-infarct dementia could be harmed posthumously before a determination of death by whole-brain or brainstem criteria. This could occur if they distinguished their death as persons from the death of their organisms. At an earlier time, when their cognitive capacity was intact, they might have indicated in an advance directive that they would not want their bodies to be kept alive once they had lost all cortical function. At that point, they would have lost the capacity for mentality and their ontological and moral status as persons. Although they would lack any decisional capacity in the late stage of the disease, the directive they made when they had this capacity would transfer from the earlier to the later time. Unless they had indicated a change of mind along the way, there would be no moral grounds for using artificial hydration and nutrition to keep their bodies alive in what would be a vegetative state. Keeping their bodies alive would be harming them after they had ceased to exist as persons.

Although I have argued that individuals cannot be harmed if they permanently lose the capacity for consciousness because there is no longer a person with interests, this does not mean that we are morally permitted to do anything to the organisms that persons leave behind. Even if they lack *moral status*, their bodies may have *moral value*, which pertains to the objective symbolic value we attribute to human organisms.[61] Moral value can be defined as the impersonal value we attribute to different aspects of a human life. A corpse may have value because we identify it as belonging to a natural or religious order, and this may impose constraints on what we can or cannot do to it. For example, the moral value of a human corpse prohibits us from mutilating it.

We permit practices such as organ procurement on the assumption that people who leave their bodies behind at death consented to organ donation at an earlier time and that organ donation might benefit others. They are also permitted when survivors consent to them on a deceased person's behalf. Mutilating a corpse for any reason would strike most of us as morally objectionable because it would be a violation of its symbolic value. Another ethically objectionable practice would be performing brain stimulation or surgery on patients in a permanent vegetative state for the purpose of medical research. Although they would lack moral status, they would in a sense be a vulnerable population with residual moral value in the remaining functional parts of the brain that survive them.[62] Unless an individual who adhered to the higher brain criterion of death consented in advance to such a procedure, it would violate the moral value of his or her brain and thus would be a wrongful act.

Some might appeal to the concept of moral value in objecting to the use of ventilators to keep brain-dead patients alive even briefly for the purpose of keeping their organs perfused for transplantation. They might argue that this practice treats the patient's body as a mere instrument, as nothing more than a source of organs, and thereby violates the intrinsic value and sanctity of the body. Even if one accepts this point, the moral value of the body in these cases must be weighed against the moral status of patients who need organ transplants to stay alive. Assuming that consent has been given to cadaveric organ donation, it would be difficult to defend the claim that moral value outweighs moral status. Meeting the acute needs of persons seems more important morally than respecting the symbolic value of dead human bodies.

Conclusion

I have defended a neurological criterion of death based on higher brain function. We die when all activity of the cerebral cortex permanently ceases. This defense turns on the view that we are essentially persons rather than human organisms, and that what makes us persons is the capacity for consciousness, a capacity that is necessarily generated and sustained by a functioning cerebral cortex. A neurological criterion specifying that death occurs with the permanent cessation of all brain functions, including those of the brainstem, is biologically sound. But whole-brain and brainstem criteria of death do not always tell us when a person dies. A person may die before the permanent cessation of all brain functions. Neither whole-brain and brainstem criteria of death nor the metaphysical thesis that we are essentially human organisms rather than persons can explain how we can have moral status. They cannot explain how we can be harmed by actions done to us at the margin between life and death. Moral status consists in having the capacity for interests in how our biological and biographical lives go, a capacity that rests on the capacity for consciousness grounded in cortical brain function. Our capacity for conscious-ness is what makes us persons, who are benefited or harmed when our interests in what happens to our bodies and us are satisfied or defeated by what others do or fail to do.

I explored different moral implications of these neurological and metaphysical claims, examining different respects in which persons could benefit or be harmed. To illustrate these respects, I discussed two prominent legal cases concerning disputes over the withdrawal of life-support from patients in a permanent vegetative state. In addition, I presented some hypothetical cases to discuss the moral im-plications of different criteria of brain death for organ procurement. In discussing these cases, I defended an intuitive identification of the soul with the cerebral cortex and the capacity for consciousness. If the soul is what gives us moral status, then we lose this status when the rational soul leaves the body. When the cerebral cortex permanently ceases to function, we cannot benefit from or be harmed by anything done to the bodies we leave behind. The metaphysical question about the sort of beings we essentially are, the neurological question of when brain death occurs, and the ethical question of how we can benefit or be harmed are all intertwined. How we frame and respond to these questions will influence our judgments about the permissibility or impermissibility of actions done to persons and their bodies in their biological and biographical lives.

Epilogue

After moving through many different areas and techniques of clinical neuroscience and discussing some of the ethical issues they raise, it is time to take stock. Whether measures of or interventions in the brain can benefit or harm a person, and whether they are permissible or impermissible, depends on how they affect a person's mind. I defended the view that the mind emerges from the brain when it reaches a certain level of complexity, and that the brain and mind are influenced by the ways in which a human organism interacts with the environment. I considered some of the promises and pitfalls of neuroimaging for diagnosing and predicting neurological and psychiatric disorders. This included a discussion of whether brain imaging could contribute to a better understanding of such philosophical questions as free will and moral responsibility.

In addition, I explored some of the ethical implications of psychological and pharmacological interventions in the brain for both therapy and enhancement. While the potential benefits of psychopharmacology are significant, so are the potential harms, given that chronic use of psychotropic drugs can alter neural circuits in unforeseeable ways. The long-term effects of these agents are not known. This concern is more acute in neurosurgery and psychosurgery, which involve a greater risk of permanent damage to the brain. For this reason, the threshold of the competence required for informed consent to brain surgery should be higher than it is for other medical procedures. Proxy consent to neurosurgery or psychosurgery by a surrogate decision-maker is more difficult to justify, though it can be justified when certain provisos are in place. Although the risks in neurostimulation may not be as great as they are in brain lesioning, the risks of overstimulating regions of the brain are significant nonetheless, because of potentially adverse effects on thought and movement. More provocatively, I raised the question of whether forced behavior control through pharmacological or surgical intervention in the brain could ever be justified. I also explored biological, metaphysical, and ethical aspects of brain death.

Of all the points made in this book, five deserve special attention. First, no two brains are alike. No two people's brains display the same structural and functional

features, and no two people's brains respond in the same way to surgical, pharmacological, or other interventions. These differences are a reflection of the brain's
plasticity. Second, although the brain generates and sustains the mind, the mind is
not reducible to the brain. The mental states that constitute personhood, personal
identity, and the self cannot be explained entirely in terms of neurons and synapses, because these states are shaped by a tripartite interaction among the brain,
the body, and the environment. Third, before we consider manipulating the brain
to alter mental capacities, we should consider how these capacities may be adaptive. Fourth, neuroscience can inform our ethical judgments. But ethics is not just
a function of neuroscience. Normative claims about which actions are permissible
or impermissible, or about how people are expected to act, are not reducible to
empirical claims about the brain. Fifth, whole-brain death is not the same as the
death of a person. These five general points should frame any discussion of what
measures of or interventions in the brain can or cannot tell us about human
mentality, thought, and behavior, and whether or to what extent we should use
them.

Notes

Chapter 1

1. WHO World Mental Health Survey Consortium, "Prevalence, Severity, and Unmet Need for Treatment of Mental Disorders in the World Health Organization World Mental Health Surveys," *Journal of the American Medical Association* 291 (2004): 2581–2590.

2. Ronald Kessler et al., "Lifetime Prevalence and Age-of-Onset Distributions of DSM-IV Disorders in the National Comorbidity Survey Replication," *Archives of General Psychiatry* 62 (2005): 593–602. See the *Diagnostic and Statistical Manual of Mental Disorders*, 4th ed., text revision *(DSM-IV-TR)* (Washington, D.C.: American Psychiatric Association, 2002). Some would argue that what appears to be an increased incidence of mental disorders is a reflection of a broader list of such disorders in the *Diagnostic and Statistical Manual*.

3. According to Zach Hall, one of the organizers of a conference on the topic in San Francisco in May 2002, *New York Times* columnist William Safire may have coined the term "neuroethics.". But one can find citations for "neuroethics" or "neuroethical" going back to the 1970s. Speaking at the San Francisco conference, Safire noted that the first forum to discuss the general topic was held in 1816 at Lake Geneva in Switzerland. The proceedings of the San Francisco conference have been published as *Neuroethics: Mapping the Field*, ed. Steven J. Marcus (New York: Dana Press, 2002). See also Adina Roskies, "Neuroethics for the New Millennium," *Neuron* 35 (2002): 21–23, and J. Illes and T. Raffin, "Neuroethics: An Emerging New Discipline in the Study of Brain and Cognition," *Brain and Cognition* 50 (2002): 341–344.

4. Some of these issues are discussed by Robert Blank, *Brain Policy: How the New Neuroscience Will Change Our Lives and Our Politics* (Washington, D.C.: Georgetown University Press, 1999), Martha Farah, "Emerging Ethical Issues in Neuroscience," *Nature Neuroscience* 5 (2002): 1123–1129, Martha Farah and Paul Root Wolpe, "Monitoring and Manipulating Brain Function: New Neuroscience Technologies and Their Ethical Implications," *Hastings Center Report* 34 (May–June 2004): 35–45, Dai Rees and Steven Rose, eds., *The New Brain Sciences: Perils and Prospects* (Cambridge: Cambridge University Press, 2004), Steven Rose, *The Future of the Brain: The Promise and Perils of Tomorrow's Neuroscience* (Oxford: Oxford University Press, 2005), and *The Twenty-First-Century Brain: Explaining, Mending, and Manipulating the Mind* (London: Cape, 2005), and Judy Illes, ed., *Neuroethics: Defining the Issues in Theory, Practice and Policy* (Oxford: Oxford University Press, 2005).

5. Some philosophers historically have characterized ethics as grounded in the philosophy of mind, or philosophical psychology, rather than in social and political philosophy. This idea is traceable to the close connection between ethics and psychology in Plato's early and middle dialogues, where the question of how one should live is linked to the state of one's mind or soul (*psyche*). In his early work, contemporary philosopher Thomas Nagel conceived of "ethics as a branch of psychology" in *The Possibility of Altruism* (Princeton: Princeton University Press, 1970), 3. I discuss posthumous harms in chapter 6. Although these harms pertain to surviving interests the satisfaction or defeat of which cannot *directly* affect the mind, they can *indirectly* affect the mind in the sense that these interests are an extension of human agency.

6. Joel Feinberg defines benefit and harm in these terms in *Harm to Others* (New York: Oxford University Press, 1986).

7. See Shelly Kagan's discussion of moral requirements and permissions in *The Limits of Morality* (Oxford: Oxford University Press, 1989), 64–70, and in *Normative Ethics* (Boulder, Colo.: Westview Press, 1998).

8. *Reith Lectures: The Emerging Mind*, lecture 5, "Neuroscience—The New Philosophy," BBC Radio 4, April 30, 2003. Available at the website of the BBC: www.bbc.co.uk/radio4/reith2003/lecture5/transcript/html:1.

9. See Eric Kandel, "A New Intellectual Framework for Psychiatry," *American Journal of Psychiatry* 155 (1998): 457–469, and Kandel and Larry Squire, "Neuroscience: Breaking Down Scientific Barriers to the Study of the Brain and Mind," *Science* 290 (2000): 1113–1120. See also Nancy Andreasen, "Linking Mind and Brain in the Study of Mental Illnesses: A Project for Scientific Psychopathology," *Science* 275 (1997): 1586–1593, Dennis Charney and Eric Nestler, eds., *Neurobiology of Mental Illness*, 2nd ed. (Oxford: Oxford University Press, 2004), and Kenneth Heilman, *Clinical Neuropsychology*, 4th ed. (New York: Oxford University Press, 2003).

10. Many neuroscientists to whose work I refer use the term "nonconscious" to describe systems and processes that fall outside of our conscious awareness. But the meaning of this term is not fundamentally different from that of the more common term "unconscious," and thus they can be used interchangeably.

11. Michael Anderson et al., "Neural Systems Underlying the Suppression of Unwanted Memories," *Science* 303 (2004): 232–235.

12. Jean-Pierre Changeux, *Neuronal Man*, trans. Laurence Garey (Princeton: Princeton University Press, 1997), 97.

13. Wilder Penfield, "Consciousness, Memory, and Man's Conditioned Reflexes," in K. Pribram, ed., *On the Biology of Learning* (New York: Harcourt Brace, 1969), 165. See also Wilder Penfield, *The Mystery of the Mind: A Critical Study of Consciousness and the Human Brain* (Princeton: Princeton University Press, 1975).

14. For example, Colin McGinn, *The Problem of Consciousness* (Oxford: Blackwell, 1991), and *The Mysterious Flame: Conscious Minds in a Material World* (New York: Basic Books, 1999), John Searle, *The Rediscovery of the Mind* (Cambridge, Mass.: MIT Press, 1992), Jaegwon Kim, *Mind in a Physical World: An Essay on the Mind-Body Problem* (Cambridge, Mass.: MIT Press, 1998), and David Chalmers, *The Conscious Mind* (New York: Oxford University Press, 1996). Chalmers divides the problem of consciousness into "easy" and "hard" problems. The first type of problem concerns explaining mental phenomena in terms of computational or neural mechanisms. The second type of problem concerns explaining how physical events and processes in the brain can give rise to the first-person qualitative feel of conscious awareness. Among other things, this involves explaining the phenomenological nature of entertaining a mental image or experiencing an emotion.

15. See Pavel Ortinski and Kimford Meador, "Neuronal Mechanisms of Conscious Awareness," *Archives of Neurology* 61 (2004): 1017–1029, and Christof Koch, *The Quest for Consciousness: A Neurobiological Approach* (Englewood, N.J.: Roberts, 2004).

16. Among philosophers, exceptions to the view that the mind is based entirely in the brain include George Lakoff and Mark Johnson, *Philosophy in the Flesh* (New York: Basic Books, 1999), Andy Clark, *Being There: Putting Brain, Body and World Together Again* (Cambridge, Mass.: MIT Press, 1997), Marya Schechtman, "The Brain/Body Problem," *Philosophical Psychology* 10 (1997): 149–163, and Shaun Gallagher, *How the Body Shapes the Mind* (New York: Oxford University Press, 2005). Neurologist Antonio Damasio has made the most compelling case for the significance of the body to the brain and mind in *Descartes' Error: Emotion, Reason, and the Human Brain* (New York: Putnam, 1994), *The Feeling of What Happens: Body and Emotion in the Making of Consciousness* (New York: Harcourt Brace, 1999), and *Looking for Spinoza: Joy, Sorrow and the Feeling Brain* (Orlando, Fl.: Harcourt, 2003).

17. *Neurophilosophy of Free Will*, trans. Cynthia Klohr (Cambridge, Mass.: MIT Press, 2001), ix. Patricia Smith Churchland makes a similar point in *Neurophilosophy: Toward a Unified Science of the Mind/Brain* (Cambridge, Mass.: MIT Press, 1986), and *Brain-Wise: Studies in Neurophilosophy* (Cambridge, Mass.: MIT Press, 2002), chaps. 1 and 2.

18. *Neurophilosophy of Free Will*, 125. Walter notes that Nagel draws this methodological distinction in *The View from Nowhere* (New York: Oxford University Press, 1986), 5.

Chapter 2

1. Some of the more accessible books on the brain include Richard Thompson, *The Brain: An Introduction to Neuroscience* (New York: Freeman, 1985), Michael Gazzaniga, ed., *Cognitive Neuroscience: A Reader* (Malden, Mass.: Blackwell, 2000), Rhawn Joseph, *Neuropsychiatry, Neuropsychology, and Clinical Neuroscience*, 2nd ed. (Baltimore: Williams and Wilkins, 1996), J. Nolte, *The Human Brain: An Introduction to Its Functional Anatomy*, 5th ed. (St. Louis: Mosby, 2002), and Joseph LeDoux, *The Synaptic Self: How Our Brains Become Who We Are* (New York: Viking, 2002).

2. Polish neuroscientist Jerzy Konorski first coined the term "plasticity" and explained its significance in *Conditioned Reflexes and Neuron Organization* (Cambridge: Cambridge University Press, 1948).

3. See, for example, Hans Selye, *The Physiology and Pathology of Exposure to Stress* (Montreal: Acta, 1950), and *The Stress of Life* (New York: McGraw-Hill, 1956), Robert Sapolsky, *Stress, the Aging Brain, and the Mechanisms of Neuron Death* (Cambridge, Mass.: MIT Press, 1992), and Bruce McEwen, "Protective and Damaging Effects of Stress Mediators," *New England Journal of Medicine* 338 (1998): 171–179.

4. LeDoux describes the mechanisms of the body's response to stimuli in these terms in *The Emotional Brain* (New York: Simon and Schuster, 1996), chap. 4, and *The Synaptic Self*, chap. 8. LeDoux notes that his model is an adaptation from earlier models devised by William James, Walter Cannon, and Philip Bard.

5. Charles Raison and Andrew Miller describe different aspects of this phenomenon, particularly as it pertains to cortisol, in "When Not Enough Is Too Much: The Role of Insufficient Glucocorticoid Signaling in the Pathophysiology of Stress-Related Disorders," *American Journal of Psychiatry* 160 (2003): 1554–1565.

6. See, for example, Charles Janeway, *Immunobiology: The Immune System in Health and Disease*, 4th ed. (New York: Garland, 1999), and P. J. Delves and I. M. Roitt, "Advances in Immunology: The Immune System," *New England Journal of Medicine* 343 (2002): 108–117.

7. Robert Ader et al., eds., *Psychoneuroimmunology*, 3rd ed. (San Diego: Academic Press, 2001).

8. Rene Descartes, *Meditations on First Philosophy*, trans. and ed. John Cottingham (Cambridge: Cambridge University Press, 2000), especially meditations 1 and 6.

9. Karl Popper and John Eccles, *The Self and Its Brain* (New York: Springer-Verlag, 1977).

10. Representatives of this view include Daniel Dennett, *Consciousness Explained* (Boston: Little Brown, 1991), Paul Churchland, *The Engine of Reason, the Seat of the Soul* (Cambridge, Mass.: MIT Press, 1995), and Patricia Smith Churchland, *Neurophilosophy*.

11. *Altered Egos: How the Brain Creates the Self* (New York: Oxford University Press, 2001), 146.

12. *Mind in a Physical World*, 58.

13. *Mind in a Physical World*, chap. 1.

14. Damasio, for one, points this out in *The Feeling of What Happens*, chap. 2.

15. *The Synaptic Self*, 24. Steven Rose offers a similar criticism in *The Twenty-First-Century Brain*.

16. This view is defended by, among others, Alwyn Scott, *Stairway to the Mind: The Controversial New Science of Consciousness* (New York: Springer-Verlag, 1995), and Roger Sperry, "Brain Bisection and the Mechanisms of Consciousness," in J. C. Eccles, ed., *Brain and Conscious Experience* (New York: Springer-Verlag, 1966): 298–313.

17. Feinberg defends a nested hierarchy version of emergentism in *Altered Egos*, chap. 8. Damasio also defends this type of emergentism in his hierarchical model of the self, which I will discuss later in this chapter. The closest theory to emergent monism in the history of philosophy is Spinoza's monism, as discussed by Damasio in *Looking for Spinoza*.

18. *The Rediscovery of the Mind* (Cambridge, Mass.: MIT Press, 1992), and *Mind, Language and Society: Doing Philosophy in the Real World* (London: Weidenfeld and Nicolson, 1999).

19. *Altered Egos*, 128–129. See also Damasio's analogy of the tree to explain the nested hierarchy of brain and mind in *Looking for Spinoza*, 38. Kenneth Kendler defends bidirectional brain–mind and mind–brain causality in "Toward a Philosophical Structure for Psychiatry," *American Journal of Psychiatry* 162 (2005): 433–440.

20. R. C. deCharms et al., "Control over Brain Activation and Pain Learned by Using Real-Time Functional MRI," *Proceedings of the National Academy of Sciences* 102 (2005): 18626–18631.

21. E. Viding et al., "Evidence for Substantial Genetic Risk for Psychopathy in 7-Year-Olds," *Journal of Child Psychology and Psychiatry* 46 (2005): 592–597.

22. William Clark and Michael Grunstein support a similar position in *Are We Hardwired? The Role of Genes in Human Behavior* (New York: Oxford University Press, 2004). Richard Lewontin describes how the biological structures and functions of organisms are shaped by their interaction with the environment in *The Triple Helix: Gene, Organism, and Environment* (Cambridge, Mass.: Harvard University Press, 2000), chap.2.

23. *The Synaptic Self*, 8.

24. Sapolsky, *Stress, the Aging Brain, and the Mechanisms of Neuron Death*.

25. See the introduction to Daniel Schacter and Elaine Scarry, eds., *Memory, Brain, and Belief* (Cambridge, Mass.: Harvard University Press, 2000), 3. See also Daniel Schacter, *Searching for Memory: The Brain, the Mind, and the Past* (New York: Basic Books, 1996).

26. Endel Tulving and Martin Lepage, "Where in the Brain Is the Awareness of One's Past?" in Schacter and Scarry, *Memory, Brain, and Belief*, 208–228. See also Tulving, "Episodic Memory: From Mind to Brain," *Annual Review of Psychology* 53 (2002): 27–51.

I describe the other types of memory and examine their significance for agency, responsibility, and identity in chapters 3 and 4.

27. Derek Parfit gives the most well-known formulation and defense of this conception in pt. 3 of *Reasons and Persons* (Oxford: Clarendon Press, 1984). Many other philosophers have defended variations of this conception. They include Nagel, *The View from Nowhere*, chap. 4, and Peter Unger, *Identity, Consciousness, and Value* (New York: Oxford University Press, 1990). For the most recent critical discussion of identity, see David DeGrazia, *Human Identity and Bioethics* (New York: Cambridge University Press, 2005).

28. See Sapolsky et al., "Interleukin-1 Stimulates the Secretion of Hypothalamic Corticoptropin Releasing Factor," *Science* 238 (1987): 522–524, Esther Sternberg et al., "The Stress Response and the Regulation of Inflammatory Disease," *Annals of Internal Medicine* 117 (1992): 854–866, Selye, *The Stress of Life*, Frank Hucklebridge and Angela Clow, "Neuroimmune Relationships in Perspective," *International Review of Neurobiology* 52 (2002): 1–15, and Clow, "Cytokines and Depression," *International Review of Neurobiology* 52 (2002): 255–270.

29. Ziad Kronfol and Daniel Remick, "Cytokines and the Brain: Implications for Clinical Psychiatry," *American Journal of Psychiatry* 157 (2000): 683–693.

30. Robert Dantzer, "Cytokine-Induced Sickness Behavior: Where Do We Stand?" *Brain, Behavior, and Immunology* 15 (2001): 7–24.

31. Randolph Nesse argues that depression may be adaptive in "Is Depression an Adaptation?" *Archives of General Psychiatry* 57 (2000): 14–20. See Ramachandran's comments on what he calls "evolutionary neuropsychiatry" in *The Emerging Mind*, lecture 5, sec. 2.

32. Serguei Fetissov et al., "Autoantibodies against Neuropeptides Are Associated with Psychological Traits in Eating Disorders," *Proceedings of the National Academy of Sciences* 102 (2005): 14865–14870.

33. *Reasons and Persons*, 202.

34. For two philosophical accounts, see Galen Strawson, "The Self," in S. Gallagher and J. Shear, eds., *Models of the Self* (Thorverton, England: Imprint Academic, 1999), 1–24, and Charles Taylor, *Sources of the Self* (Cambridge, Mass.: Harvard University Press, 1995). From a psychiatric perspective, see Todd Feinberg, *Altered Egos*, chap. 1, and G. E. Berrios and I. S. Markova, "The Self and Psychiatry: A Conceptual History," in T. Kircher and A. David, eds., *The Self in Neuroscience and Psychiatry* (Cambridge: Cambridge University Press, 2003), 9–39. See also G. Nortoff and A. Heinzel, "The Self in Philosophy, Neuroscience, and Psychiatry: An Epistemic Approach," and D. Zahavi, "Phenomenology of Self," both in Kircher and David, *The Self in Neuroscience and Psychiatry*, 40–55, 56–75.

35. *The Emerging Mind*, lecture 2, "Synapses and The Self," and lecture 5, "Neuroscience: The New Philosophy."

36. *The Emerging Mind*, lecture 5, sec. 10.

37. *The Feeling of What Happens*, pt. 2.

38. *The Feeling of What Happens*, pt. 1.

39. *The Emerging Mind*, lecture 5, secs. 5–6. Todd Feinberg discusses these and other syndromes in *Altered Egos*, chap. 3. Many of these syndromes have been presented in the popular works of neurologist Oliver Sacks.

40. Fred Volkmar and David Pauls, "Autism," *Lancet* 326 (2003): 1133–1141.

41. See G. Rizzolatti et al., "Neurophysiological Mechanisms Underlying the Understanding and Imitation of Action," *Nature Reviews Neuroscience* 2 (2001): 661–670.

42. Michael Fitzgerald, *Autism and Creativity: Is There a Link between Autism in Men and Exceptional Ability?* (London: Brunner-Routledge, 2003). See also Uta Frith and Elisabeth Hill, eds., *Autism: Mind and Brain* (Oxford: Oxford University Press, 2003).

43. As reported by Olaf Blanke et al., "Stimulating Illusory Own-Body Perceptions," *Nature* 419 (2002): 269–270, and Olaf Blanke et al., "Out-of-Body Experiences and Auto-scopy of Neurological Origin," *Brain* 127 (2004): 243–258.

44. W. B. Britton and R. R. Bootzin, "Near-Death Experiences and the Temporal Lobe," *Psychological Science* 15 (2004): 254–258. This hypothesis is similar to that of Rhawn Joseph in *Neuropsychiatry, Neuropsychology and Clinical Neuroscience*, chap. 8, "The Limbic System and the Soul: Evolution and the Neuroanatomy of Religious Experience."

45. Harry Frankfurt, "Identification and Externality," and "Identification and Whole-heartedness," in *The Importance of What We Care About* (New York: Cambridge University Press, 1989), 58–72, 83–95. Frankfurt offers a more complete picture of his position in his 1991 presidential address to the American Philosophical Association, "The Faintest Passion," *Proceedings and Addresses of the American Philosophical Association* (1992), 5–16. Frankfurt's hierarchical account of the self, consisting of lower level and higher level desires, is an important part of his conception of free will. This is different in several critical respects from the conception of free will that I describe in chap. 3. The phrase "after a period of critical reflection" suggests that there is a historical condition to authenticity. Yet Frankfurt rejects this in his response to a collection of articles on his work. See Sarah Buss and Lee Overton, eds., *The Contours of Agency: Essays on Themes from Harry Frankfurt* (Cambridge, Mass: MIT Press, 2002).

46. Mark Salzman, *Lying Awake* (New York: Vintage Books, 2000).

47. See, for example, Norman Geschwind and S. G. Waxman, "The Interictal Behavior Syndrome in Temporal Lobe Epilepsy," *Archives of General Psychiatry* 2 (1975): 1580–1586, and Geschwind, "Behavioral Change in Temporal Lobe Epilepsy," *Psychological Medicine* 9 (1979): 217–219. Joseph offers a more recent discussion of this phenomenon in *Neuropsychiatry, Neuropsychology, and Clinical Neuroscience*, chap. 8, as do M. Jackson and K. W. M. Fulford, "Spiritual Experience and Psychopathology," *Philosophy, Psychiatry, and Psychology* 4 (1997): 41–65.

48. *Lying Awake*, 138.

49. *Lying Awake*, 120. Fyodor Dostoevsky, *Demons: A Novel in Three Parts* (1873), trans. R. Pevear and L. Volokhonsky (New York: Knopf, 1994).

50. *Lying Awake*, 121.

51. Bruce Miller et al., "Brain Damage and Compulsive Artistic Interest," *British Journal of Psychiatry* 176 (2000): 458–463.

52. Bruce Miller and Craig Hou, "Portraits of Artists: Emergence of Visual Creativity in Dementia," *Archives of Neurology* 61 (2004): 842–844.

53. There have been different formulations of these goals. Most would agree with Albert Jonsen, Mark Siegler, and William Winslade, who say that the goals of medicine minimally include "prevention, cure, and care of illness and injury," *Clinical Ethics*, 5th ed. (New York: McGraw-Hill, 2002), 13.

54. Nesse makes this point in "Is Depression an Adaptation?" See note 30.

Chapter 3

1. The authors in Illes, *Neuroethics*, address many of these questions.

2. Here I closely follow the accounts of Kenneth Hugdahl, *Psychophysiology: The Mind-Body Perspective* (Cambridge, Mass.: Harvard University Press, 2001), chap. 13, G. K. Aguirre, "Functional Neuroimaging," in Todd Feinberg and Martha Farah, eds., *Behavioral Neurology and Neuropsychology*, 2nd ed. (New York: McGraw-Hill, 2003), 363–373, and Farah and Wolpe, "Monitoring and Manipulating Brain Function," 36.

3. See, for example, Jan Panksepp, *Affective Neuroscience* (New York: Oxford University Press, 1998), and "Feeling the Pain of Social Loss," *Science* 302 (2003): 237–239. See

also Richard Lane and Lynn Nadel, eds., *Cognitive Neuroscience of Emotion* (New York: Oxford University Press, 2002), and Philippe Fossati et al., "In Search of the Emotional Self: An fMRI Study Using Positive and Negative Emotional Words," *American Journal of Psychiatry* 160 (2003): 1938–1945.

4. As noted, among others, by Ed Bullmore and Paul Fletcher, "The Eye's Mind: Brain Mapping and Psychiatry," *British Journal of Psychiatry* 182 (2003): 381–384.

5. Elizabeth Sowell et al., "Cortical Abnormalities in Children and Adolescents with Attention-Deficit Hyperactivity Disorder," *Lancet* 362 (2003): 1699–1706. George Bush et al. discuss possible future clinical uses of imaging for this condition in "Functional Neuroimaging of Attention-Deficit/Hyperactivity Disorder: A Review and Suggested Future Directions," *Biological Psychiatry* 57 (2005): 1273–1284.

6. See, for example, Richard Davidson et al., "The Neural Substrates of Affective Processing in Depressed Patients Treated with Venlafaxine," *American Journal of Psychiatry* 160 (2003): 64–75.

7. Helen Mayberg et al., "Modulation of Cortical-Limbic Pathways in Major Depression: Treatment-Specific Effects of Cognitive Behavior Therapy," *Archives of General Psychiatry* 61 (2004): 34–41. Davidson et al. have published results from a study using electroencephalography (EEG) suggesting that meditation can alter brain function, especially in the left prefrontal cortex. "Alterations in Brain and Immune Function Produced by Mindfulness Meditation," *Psychosomatic Medicine* 65 (2003): 564–570.

8. See Michael Anderson et al., "Neural Systems Underlying the Suppression of Unwanted Memories."

9. "Genetic Theorizing and Schizophrenia," *British Journal of Psychiatry* 122 (1973): 15–30.

10. "The Endophenotype Concept in Psychiatry: Etymology and Strategic Intentions," *American Journal of Psychiatry* 160 (2003): 1–10. See also Kathleen Ries Merikangas and Neil Risch, "Will the Genetics Revolution Revolutionize Psychiatry?" *American Journal of Psychiatry* 160 (2003): 625–635, Steven Hyman, "Neuroscience, Genetics, and the Future of Psychiatric Diagnosis," *Psychopathology* 35 (2002): 139–144, and Erik Parens, ed., *Genetic Differences and Human Identities: On Why Talking about Behavioral Genetics Is Important and Difficult*, special supplement, *Hastings Center Report* 34 (January–February 2004): S1–S35. Thomas Insel and Remi Quirion offer an insightful discussion of the influence of both genetics and gene–environment interactions in the development of mental disorders, in "Psychiatry as a Clinical Neuroscience Discipline," *Journal of the American Medical Association* 294 (2005): 2221–2224.

11. M. T. Tsuang et al., "Identification of the Phenotype in Psychiatric Genetics," *European Archives of Psychiatry and Clinical Neuroscience* 243 (1993): 131–142, and F. X. Castellanos and R. Tannock, "Neuroscience of Attention Deficit/Hyperactivity Disorder: The Search for Endophenotypes," *Nature Reviews Neuroscience* 3 (2002): 617–628.

12. R. Weinshilboum, "Inheritance and Drug Response," *New England Journal of Medicine* 348 (2003): 529–537, W. Evans and H. McLeod, "Pharmacogenomics: Drug Disposition, Drug Targets, and Side Effects," *New England Journal of Medicine* 348 (2003): 538–547.

13. A. Caspi et al., "Influence of Life Stress on Depression: Moderation by a Polymorphism in the 5-HTT Gene," *Science* 301 (2003): 386–389. See also Ahmad Hariri et al., "Serotonin Transporter Genetic Variation and the Response of the Human Amygdala," *Science* 297 (2002): 400–403, and Constance Holden, "Getting the Short End of the Allele," *Science* 301 (2003): 291–293.

14. R. D. Hare, *The Hare Psychopathy Checklist* (Toronto: Multi-Health Systems, 1991). See also H. Cleckley, *The Mask of Sanity* (St. Louis: Mosby, 1967).

15. Adrian Raine et al., "Reduced Prefrontal Gray Matter Volume and Reduced Autonomic Activity in Antisocial Personality Disorder," *Archives of General Psychiatry* 58 (2000): 119–127. R. Davidson et al., "Dysfunction in the Neural Circuitry of Emotion Regulation—A Possible Prelude to Violence," *Science* 289 (2000): 591–594. See also A. S. New et al., "Blunted Prefrontal Cortical 18Fluorodeoxyglucose Positron Emission Tomography Response to Meta-chlorophenylpiperazine in Impulsive Aggression," *Archives of General Psychiatry* 59 (2002): 621–629.

16. K. A. Kiel et al., "Limbic Abnormalities in Affective Processing by Criminal Psychopaths as Revealed by Functional Magnetic Resonance Imaging," *Biological Psychiatry* 50 (2001): 677–684.

17. E. Kandel and D. Freed, "Frontal Lobe Dysfunction and Antisocial Behavior: A Review," *Journal of Clinical Psychology* 45 (1989): 404–413.

18. A. Damasio et al., "Impairment of Social and Moral Behavior Related to Early Damage in Human Prefrontal Cortex," *Nature Neuroscience* 2 (1999): 1032–1037. See the accompanying editorial by R. J. Dolan, "On the Neurology of Morals," *Nature Neuroscience* 2 (1999): 927–929. See also A. R. Damasio, "A Neural Basis for Sociopathy," *Archives of General Psychiatry* 57 (2000): 128–129, W. D. Casebeer, "Moral Cognition and Its Neural Constituents," *Nature Reviews Neuroscience* 4 (2003): 840–847, R. Adolphs et al., "Neuropsychological Approaches to Reasoning and Decision-Making," in A. Damasio et al., eds., *Neurobiology of Decision-Making* (New York: Springer-Verlag, 1996), 157–178, Ekhonen Goldberg, *The Executive Brain: Frontal Lobes and the Civilized Mind* (New York: Oxford University Press, 2002), and Jeffrey Cummings and Michael Mega, *Neuropsychiatry and Behavioral Neuroscience* (Oxford: Oxford University Press, 2003).

19. R. J. R. Blair and L. Cipolotti, "Impaired Social Response Reversal: A Case of 'Acquired Sociopathy,'" *Brain* 123 (2000): 1122–1141, R. J. R. Blair, "Neurological Basis of Psychopathy," *British Journal of Psychiatry* 182 (2003): 5–7, and R. J. R. Blair et al., *The Psychopath: Emotion and the Brain* (Malden, Mass.: Blackwell, 2005). See also Nathalie Camille et al., "The Involvement of the Orbitofrontal Cortex in the Experience of Regret," *Science* 304 (2004): 1167–1170, J. D. Greene, "From Neural 'Is' to Moral 'Ought': What Are the Moral Implications of Neuroscientific Moral Psychology?" *Nature Reviews Neuroscience* 4 (2003): 847–850, J. D. Greene et al., "An fMRI Investigation of Emotional Engagement in Moral Judgment," *Science* 293 (2001): 2105–2108, and J. D. Greene et al., "The Neural Basis of Cognitive Conflict and Control in Moral Judgment," *Neuron* 44 (2004): 389–400, K. R. Ridderinkhof et al., "The Role of the Medial Frontal Cortex in Cognitive Control," *Science* 306 (2004): 443–447, and John Searle, "Free Will as a Problem in Neurobiology," *Philosophy* 76 (2001): 491–514.

20. H. Damasio et al. discuss the neurobiological significance of the Gage case in "The Return of Phineas Gage: Clues about the Brain from the Skull of a Famous Patient," *Science* 264 (1994): 1102–1105. A. Damasio discusses the cases of Gage and "Elliot" in *Descartes' Error*, chap. 6.

21. Nancy Andreasen, "Linking Mind and Brain in the Study of Mental Illnesses," 1588. Cited and elaborated by Walter in *Neurophilosophy of Free Will*, 282–283.

22. L. E. Baxter et al., "Caudate Glucose Metabolism Rate Changes with Both Drug and Behavior Therapy for Obsessive Compulsive Disorder," *Archives of General Psychiatry* 49 (1992): 687–698. Cited by Walter in *Neurophilosophy of Free Will*, 292.

23. Defenders of this view include Peter van Inwagen, *An Essay on Free Will* (Oxford: Clarendon Press, 1983), and Robert Kane, *The Significance of Free Will* (New York: Oxford University Press, 1996).

24. See, for example, John Martin Fischer, *The Metaphysics of Free Will: An Essay on Control* (Cambridge, Mass.: Blackwell, 1994), and John Martin Fischer and Mark Ravizza,

Responsibility and Control: A Theory of Moral Responsibility (New York: Cambridge University Press, 1998). Galen Strawson provides a helpful overview of the different incompatibilist and compatibilist positions on free will in *Freedom and Belief* (Oxford: Clarendon Press, 1986), chap. 1. See also Kane, *A Contemporary Introduction to Free Will* (New York: Oxford University Press, 2005).

25. *Freedom Evolves* (New York: Viking, 2003).

26. Benjamin Libet et al., "Time of Conscious Intention to Act in Relation to Onset of Cerebral Activity [Readiness Potential]," *Brain* 106 (1983): 623–642, Benjamin Libet, "Unconscious Cerebral Initiative of Conscious Will in Voluntary Action," *Behavioral and Brain Sciences* 8 (1985): 529–566, and commentaries, Benjamin Libet, "Do We Have Free Will?" in Benjamin Libet, A. Freeman, and K. Sutherland, eds., *The Volitional Brain: Towards a Neuroscience of Free Will* (Thorverton, England: Imprint Academic, 1999), 47, and Libet, *Mind Time: The Temporal Factor in Consciousness* (Cambridge, Mass.: Harvard University Press, 2004). Grant Gillett questions Libet's claims about the timing of unconscious brain events and conscious mental events and their significance for free will in *The Mind and Its Discontents: An Essay in Discursive Psychiatry* (Oxford: Oxford University Press, 1999). 284–290. In addition, A. R. Mele debunks some of the claims about free will from empirical neuroscientific studies in *Free Will and Luck* (New York: Oxford University Press, 2006).

27. Daniel Wegner, *The Illusion of Conscious Will* (Cambridge, Mass.: MIT Press, 2002). See also Sean Spence, "Free Will in the Light of Neuropsychiatry," *Philosophy, Psychiatry, and Psychology* 3 (1996): 75–100, and commentaries.

28. "New Neuroscience, Old Problems," in Brent Garland, ed., *Neuroscience and the Law: Brain, Mind, and the Scales of Justice* (New York: Dana Press, 2004), 169.

29. *The Complete Works of Aristotle*, vol. 2, bk. 3, trans. and ed. J. Barnes (Princeton: Princeton University Press, 1984). H. L. A. Hart defends a similar default position in *Punishment and Responsibility* (Oxford: Clarendon Press, 1968).

30. Fischer and Ravizza develop a theory of reasons-responsiveness in *Responsibility and Control*.

31. Patricia Churchland discusses this concept of free will in "Feeling Reasons," in Damasio et al., *Neurobiology of Decision-Making*, 181–199, and in *Brain-Wise: Studies in Neurophilosophy*, chap. 5. I do not share Churchland's reductionist view that the requisite control for moral reasoning involves only the brain and no "ectoplasmic mind-whiffle," as she claims in "Moral Decision-Making and the Brain," chap. 1 in Illes, *Neuroethics*, 5. The most persuasive accounts of control are given by Fischer, *The Metaphysics of Free Will*, and by Fischer and Ravizza, *Responsibility and Control*.

32. *Model Penal Code*, official draft and revised commentaries (Philadelphia: American Law Institute, 1985). Compare this with the *M'Naghten Rules*, 1843, 8 Eng. Rep. 718,722, cited in the *Report on the Committee on Mentally Abnormal Offenders* (London: Her Majesty's Stationery Office, 1975). For helpful discussion of the similarities and differences between philosophical and legal notions of responsibility in the light of neuroscience, see Morse, "New Neuroscience, Old Problems," and Michael Gazzaniga and Megan Steven, "Free Will in the Twenty-First Century: A Discussion of Neuroscience and the Law," in Garland, *Neuroscience and the Law*, 51–70.

33. As reported by Mary Beckman, "Crime, Culpability, and the Adolescent Brain," *Science* 305 (2004): 596–599.

34. Beckman, "Crime, Culpability, and the Adolescent Brain," 596. See also J. N. Giedd et al., "Brain Development during Childhood and Adolescence: A Longitudinal MRI Study," *Nature Neuroscience* 2 (1999): 861–865.

35. R. D. Hare, *The Hare Psychopathy Checklist*, and *Without Empathy: The Strange World of the Psychopaths among Us* (New York: Pocket Books, 1994), Cleckley, *The Mask of*

Sanity, and Carl Elliott, "Diagnosing Blame: Responsibility and the Psychopath," *Journal of Medicine and Philosophy* 17 (1992): 223–237.

36. See, for example, M. L. Platt and P. W. Glimcher, "Neural Correlates of Decision Variables in Parietal Cortex," *Nature* 400 (1999): 233–238. See also M. L. Platt, "Neural Correlates of Decisions," *Current Opinion in Neurobiology* 13 (2003): 141–148, and J. D. Schall, "Neural Correlates of Decision Processes," *Current Opinion in Neurobiology* 13 (2003): 182–186.

37. *Altered Egos*, 103.

38. See Daniel Schacter, *Searching for Memory*, 17, 134–137, 235–236.

39. Here I closely follow Schacter's account of this case in his testimony before the President's Council on Bioethics, seventh meeting, October 17, 2002, session 4: "Remembering and Forgetting: Psychological Aspects," transcript. Available at the website of the council: www.bioethics.gov/transcripts/oct02/session4/html.

40. Tulving and Lepage, "Where in the Brain Is Awareness of One's Past?" in Schacter and Scarry, *Memory, Brain, and Belief*, 208–228, and Tulving, "Episodic Memory: From Mind to Brain."

41. "Emerging Ethical Issues in Neuroscience," 1127.

42. In February 2003, the Iowa Supreme Court reversed the 1978 murder conviction of Terry Harrington on the basis of brain fingerprinting. Also in 2003, the state of Missouri used this technology to convict serial killer J. B. Grinder. It is questionable whether this technology will be used on a broader scale in the future, since it is still controversial whether it can accurately "read" people's minds.

43. National Research Council, *The Polygraph Lie Detector* (Washington: D.C.: National Academies Press, 2003). See also Jonathan Knight, "The Truth about Lying," *Nature* 428 (2004): 692–694.

44. Daniel Langleben et al., "Brain Activity during Simulated Deception: An Event-Related Functional Magnetic Resonance Study," *Neuroimage* 15 (2002): 727–732. Laurence Tancredi explores these and other possible legal applications of brain imaging in "Neuroscience Developments and the Law," in Garland, *Neuroscience and the Law*, 71–113. See also Paul Root Wolpe et al., "Emerging Neurotechnologies for Lie Detection: Promises and Perils," *American Journal of Bioethics* 5 (2005): 15–26, and Henry Greely, "Prediction, Litigation, Privacy, and Property: Some Possible Legal and Social Implications of Advances in Neuroscience," in Garland, *Neuroscience and the Law*, 114–156, and "The Social Effects of Advances in Neuroscience: Legal Problems, Legal Perspectives," chap. 17 in Illes, *Neuroethics*.

45. "Neuroscience and Neuroethics," *Science* 306 (2004): 373. Kennedy's comments, together with the cases and arguments presented in this section, should allay the fear of neurobiological determinism expressed by the main character in Don Delillo's novel *White Noise*, in the following slightly ironic passage: "They can trace everything you say, do and feel to the number of molecules in a certain region. What happens to good and evil in this system? Passion, envy and hate? Do they become a tangle of neurons? What about murderous rage? A murderer used to have a fearsome size about him. His crime was large. What happens when we reduce it to cells and molecules?" (New York: Penguin, 1986), 68. See also Clark and Grunstein, *Are We Hardwired?*, L. Tancredi, *Hardwired Behavior: What Neuroscience Reveals about Morality* (New York: Cambridge University Press, 2005), and M. Gazzaniga, *The Ethical Brain* (New York: Dana Press, 2005), chap. 6, "My Brain Made Me Do It." Curiously, Gazzaniga claims that "neuroscience can offer very little to the understanding of responsibility" (100) and that responsibility is "a social construct" (102). Yet this leaves one wondering on what basis we hold people responsible. We hold people responsible for actions and omissions on the basis of the mental states that underlie what they do or fail

to do. These mental states presuppose normal brain function. An attribution of responsibility is a social act; but the basis on which the attribution is made is not entirely a social construct. Otherwise, attributing responsibility would appear to be an arbitrary practice. Indeed, in the same chapter, Gazzaniga says "it is our brains...that ultimately enable our cognition and behavior" (91). It is in virtue of a person's cognition and behavior that we hold him or her responsible. These are not reducible to the brain; but they do depend on the brain. Just because neuroscience does not determine responsibility does not mean that it cannot contribute anything to our understanding of responsibility.

46. P. M. Thompson et al., "Mapping Adolescent Brain Change Reveals Dynamic Wave of Accelerated Gray Matter Loss in Very Early-Onset Schizophrenia," *Proceedings of the National Academy of Sciences* 98 (2001): 11650–11655.

47. C. Pantelis et al., "Neuroanatomical Abnormalities before and after Onset of Psychoses: A Cross-sectional and Longitudinal MRI Comparison," *Lancet* 361 (2003): 281–288. See also A. L. Spong et al., "Progressive Brain Volume Loss during Adolescence in Childhood-Onset Schizophrenia," *American Journal of Psychiatry* 160 (2003): 2181–2189, P. Milev et al., "Initial Magnetic Resonance Imaging Volumetric Brain Measurements and Outcomes in Schizophrenia: A Prospective Longitudinal Study with a Five-Year Follow-Up," *Biological Psychiatry* 54 (2003): 608–615, and Toshiaki Onitsuka et al., "Middle and Inferior Temporal Gyrus Gray Matter Volume Abnormalities in Chronic Schizophrenia: An MRI Study," *American Journal of Psychiatry* 161 (2004): 1603–1611.

48. J. Lieberman et al., "Effectiveness of Antipsychotic Drugs in Patients with Chronic Schizophrenia," *New England Journal of Medicine* 353 (2005): 1209–1223.

49. Sven Janno et al., "Prevalence of Neuroleptic-Induced Movement Disorders in Chronic Schizophrenia Inpatients," *American Journal of Psychiatry* 161 (2004): 160–163. See also Elizabeth Koller et al., "Pancreatitis Associated with Atypical Antipsychotics," *Pharmacotherapy* 23 (2003): 1123–1130.

50. Thomas McGlashan et al., "Randomized, Double-Blind Trial of Olanzapine Versus Placebo in Patients Prodromally Presymptomatic for Psychoses," *American Journal of Psychiatry* 163 (2006): 790–799.

51. Christopher Martyn, "Anti-inflammatory Drugs and Alzheimer's Disease: Evidence Implying a Protective Effect Is as yet Tentative," *British Medical Journal* 327 (2003): 353–354, and Lenore Launer, "Nonsteroidal Anti-inflammatory Drugs and Alzheimer's Disease: What's Next?" *Journal of the American Medical Association* 289 (2003): 2865–2867.

52. Richard Gray et al., "Long-Term Donepezil Treatment in 565 Patients with Alzheimer's Disease (AD 2000): Randomized Double-Blind Trial," *Lancet* 363 (2004): 2105–2115. However, Ben Seltzer et al. report more positive results in "Efficacy of Donepezil in Early-Stage Alzheimer Disease," *Archives of Neurology* 61 (2004): 1852–1856. See also H. Hashimoto et al., "Does Donepezil Treatment Slow the Progression of Hippocampal Atrophy in Patients with Alzheimer's Disease?" *Archives of General Psychiatry* 162 (2005): 676–686.

53. Thomas Rea et al., "Statins and the Risk of Incident Dementia," *Archives of Neurology* 62 (2005): 1047–1051.

54. S. Wiggins et al., "The Psychological Consequences of Predictive Testing for Huntington's Disease: Canadian Collaborative Study of Predictive Testing," *New England Journal of Medicine* 327 (1992): 1401–1405.

55. These and related issues are addressed by J. Illes et al., "Ethical and Practical Considerations in Managing Incidental Findings in Functional Magnetic Resonance Imaging," *Brain and Cognition* 50 (2002): 358–365, B. S. Kim et al., "Incidental Findings on Pediatric MR Images of the Brain," *American Journal of Neuroradiology* 23 (2002): 1674–1677, A. Mamourian, "Incidental Findings on Research Functional MR Images: Should

We Look?" *American Journal of Neuroradiology* 25 (2004): 520–522, and Farah and Wolpe, "Monitoring and Manipulating Brain Function." Despite some problems in interpreting ambiguous information from brain imaging, especially false-positive indications of disease, whole-body MRI scans could become helpful diagnostic tools in identifying early-stage tumors or malformations that could lead to cancer, stroke, and cardiovascular disease. The potential benefits of these scans will also have to be weighed against the risk of cancer from exposure to the radiation emitted form certain types of scans. In this regard, CT scans are of greatest concern, especially contrast CT, which involves injecting radioactive dye into the bloodstream. See D. Brenner and C. D. Elliston, "Risks of Adult Full-Body CT Scans," *Radiology* 23 (2004): 735–738. Stephen Eustace and Erik Nelson cite the uses of MRI scans for this purpose in "Whole-Body Magnetic Resonance Imaging," *British Medical Journal* 328 (2004): 1387–1388.

56. Jennifer Kulynych, "Legal and Ethical Issues in Neuroimaging Research: Human Subjects Protection, Medical Privacy, and the Public Communication of Results," *Brain and Cognition* 50 (2002): 345–375. See also S. Olson, "Brain Scans Raise Privacy Concerns," *Science* 307 (2005): 1548–1550.

57. Samuel McClure et al. report on the results of an imaging study correlating activity in certain brain regions with preferences for Coke or Pepsi between two groups of human subjects in "Neural Correlates of Behavioral Preferences for Culturally Familiar Drinks," *Neuron* 44 (2004): 379–387.

58. *The Synaptic Self*, 221.

Chapter 4

1. K.N. Botteron et al., "Volumetric Reduction in Left Subgenual Prefrontal Cortex in Early Onset Depression," *Biological Psychiatry* 15 (2002): 342–344, Yvette Sheline et al., "Untreated Depression and Hippocampal Volume Loss," *American Journal of Psychiatry* 160 (2003): 1516–1518, and Rene Hen et al., "Requirement of Hippocampal Neurogenesis for the Behavioral Effects of Antidepressants," *Science* 301 (2003): 805–809. For a general overview of these and other interventions, see Alan Schatzberg and Charles Nemeroff, eds., *Textbook of Psychopharmacology*, 3rd ed. (Washington, D.C.: American Psychiatric, 2004).

2. Christopher Varley, "Psychopharmacological Treatment of Major Depressive Disorder in Children and Adolescents," *Journal of the American Medical Association* 290 (2003): 1091–1093.

3. Varley, "Psychopharmacological Treatment of Major Depressive Disorder," 1091.

4. The message of the committee's chairman, Gordon Duff, can be found at the website of the British Medical Association: www.mca.gov.uk/julyo3.

5. A. Khan et al., "Suicide Rates in Clinical Trials of SSRIs, Other Antidepressants, and Placebo: Analysis of FDA Reports," *American Journal of Psychiatry* 160 (2003): 790–792.

6. Gregory Simon et al., "Suicide Risk during Antidepressant Treatment," *American Journal of Psychiatry* 163 (2006): 41–47. In addition, Madhukar Trivedi et al., "Evaluation of Outcomes with Citalopram for Depression Using Measurement-Based Care in STAR*D: Implications for Clinical Practice," *American Journal of Psychiatry* 163 (2006): 28–40.

7. See W. A. Carlezon et al., "Enduring Behavioral Effects of Early Exposure to Methylphenidate in Rats," *Biological Psychiatry* 16 (2003): 1330–1337. David Healy offers a more critical view in *The Antidepressant Era* (Cambridge, Mass.: Harvard University Press, 1997), and *The Creation of Psychopharmacology* (Cambridge, Mass.: Harvard University Press, 2002).

8. As Constance Holden reports in "Future Brightening for Depression Treatments," *Science* 302 (2003): 810.

9. See, for example, J. P. Antel and T. Owens, "Immune Regulation and CNS Autoimmune Disease," *Journal of Neuroimmunology* 100 (1999): 181–189.

10. See S. Hyman and W. Fenton, "What Are the Right Targets for Psychopharmacology?" *Science* 299 (2003): 350–351.

11. L. Arborelius et al., "The Role of Corticotropin-Releasing Factor in Depression and Anxiety Disorders," *Journal of Endocrinology* 160 (1999): 1–12.

12. J. K. Belanoff et al., "An Open Label Trial of C-1073 (Mifepristone) for Psychotic Major Depression," *Biological Psychiatry* 52 (2002): 386–392, and P. Gold et al., "New Insights into the Role of Cortisol and the Glucocorticoid Receptor in Severe Depression," *Biological Psychiatry* 52 (2002): 381–385.

13. B. A. Strange et al., "An Emotion-Induced Retrograde Amnesia in Humans Is Amygdala- and Beta-Adrenergic Dependent," *Proceedings of the National Academy of Sciences* 100 (2003): 13626–13631. This follows the work of Karim Nader et al., "Fear Memories Require Protein Synthesis in the Amygdala for Reconsolidation after Retrieval," *Nature* 406 (2000): 722–726. Others who have suggested the use of these drugs for this purpose include Blair, "Neurological Basis of Psychopathy," 7, and James McGaugh, in his testimony before the President's Council on Bioethics, seventh meeting, October 17, 2002, session 3, "Remembering and Forgetting: Physiological and Pharmacological Aspects," availabe at the website of the council: www.bioethics.gov/transcripts/octo2/session3.html. See also McGaugh, *Memory and Emotion: The Making of Lasting Memories* (New York: Columbia University Press, 2003).

14. J. L. C. Lee et al., "Independent Cellular Processes for Hippocampal Memory Consolidation and Reconsolidation," *Science* 304 (2004): 839–843, and M. P. Richardson et al., "Encoding of Emotional Memories Depends on Amygdala and Hippocampus and their Interactions," *Nature Neuroscience* 7 (2004): 278–285. See also Ivan Izquierdo and Martin Cammarota, "Zif and the Survival of Memory," *Science* 304 (2004): 829–830. "Zif" is short for "zif268," a gene critical for the consolidation and reconsolidation of memory.

15. Charles Hoge et al., "Combat Duty in Iraq and Afghanistan, Mental Health Problems, and Barriers to Care," *New England Journal of Medicine* 351 (2004): 13–22. For the results of the Massachusetts General Hospital Study, see R. K. Pittman et al., "Pilot Study of Secondary Prevention of Posttraumatic Stress Disorder with Propranolol," *Biological Psychiatry* 51 (2002): 189–192. Greg Miller gives a summary of Pittman's and other studies in "Learning to Forget," *Science* 302 (2004): 34–36. A more recent study indicates that memory of a traumatic event is a strong predictor and potential risk factor for subsequent development of PTSD. See Sharon Gill et al., "Does Memory of a Traumatic Event Increase the Risk for Posttraumatic Stress Disorder in Patients with Traumatic Brain Injury? A Prospective Study," *American Journal of Psychiatry* 162 (2005): 963–969.

16. K. S. LaBar et al., "Impaired Fear Conditioning Following Unilateral Temporal Lobectomy on Humans," *Journal of Neuroscience* 15 (1995): 6846–6855.

17. President's Council on Bioethics, Staff Working Paper, "Better Memories? The Promise and Perils of Pharmacological Intervention," March 2003, http://www.bioethics.gov/transcripts/mar03.html. Leon Kass, *Beyond Therapy: Biotechnology and the Pursuit of Happiness* (New York: Harper Collins, 2003).

18. "Gene Therapy for Psychiatric Disorders," *American Journal of Psychiatry* 160 (2003): 208–220.

19. G. P. Shumyatsky et al., "*Strathmin*, a Gene Enriched in the Amygdala, Controls Both Learned and Innate Fear," *Cell* 123 (2005): 697–709.

20. B. Kaspar et al., "Retrograde Viral Delivery of IGF-1 Prolongs Survival in a Mouse ALS Model," *Science* 301 (2003): 839–843.

21. For an overview of these therapies, see Jordi Cami and Magi Farre, "Drug Addiction," *New England Journal of Medicine* 349 (2003): 975–986. A. David Redish explains addiction as a form of flawed decision-making in "Addiction as a Computational Process Gone Awry," *Science* 306 (2004): 1944–1947. See also Serge Ahmed, "Addiction as Compulsive Reward Prediction," *Science* 306 (2004): 1901–1902, P. Kalivas and N. Volkow, "The Neural Basis of Addiction," *American Journal of Psychiatry* 162 (2005): 1403–1413, and Steven Hyman, "Addiction: A Disease of Learning and Memory," *American Journal of Psychiatry* 162 (2005): 1414–1422.

22. J. L. C. Lee et al., "Disrupting Reconsolidation of Drug Memories Reduces Cocaine-Seeking Behavior," *Neuron* 47 (2005): 795–801, and Courtney Miller and John Marshall, "Molecular Substrates for Retrieval and Reconsolidation of Cocaine-Associated Contextual Memory," *Neuron* 47 (2005): 873–884.

23. See, for example, Howard Brody, *Placebos and the Philosophy of Medicine* (Chicago: University of Chicago Press, 1980), and the chapters in Anne Harrington, ed., *The Placebo Effect: An Interdisciplinary Exploration* (Cambridge, Mass.: Harvard University Press, 1997).

24. Andrew Leuchter et al., "Changes in Brain Function of Depressed Subjects during Treatment with Placebo," *American Journal of Psychiatry* 159 (2002): 122–129.

25. A. Jon Stoessl et al., "Expectation and Dopamine Release: Mechanisms of the Placebo Effect in Parkinson's Disease," *Science* 293 (2001): 1164–1166.

26. F. Benedetti et al., "Conscious Expectation and Unconscious Conditioning in Analgesia, Motor, and Hormonal Placebo/Nocebo Responses," *Journal of Neuroscience* 23 (2002): 4315–4323. Howard Spiro argues that, while placebos can relieve pain, there is no conclusive scientific evidence that they can cure or control diseases, in *The Power of Hope* (New Haven: Yale University Press, 1998).

27. Arthur Shapiro and Elaine Shapiro, "The Placebo: Is It Much Ado about Nothing?" in Harrington, *The Placebo Effect*, 31.

28. Howard Brody, "The Lie That Heals: The Ethics of Giving Placebos," *Annals of Internal Medicine* 97 (1982): 112–118.

29. Several of the authors in Harrington, *The Placebo Effect*, explore the biopsychosocial aspects of the placebo response.

30. Compare psychiatrist Walter Brown's idea of offering a placebo to a patient as a third form of treatment for depression, as distinct from medication and psychotherapy: "There is a third kind of treatment, less expensive for you and less likely to cause side effects, which also helps many people with your condition. This treatment involves taking one of these pills twice a day and coming to our office every two weeks to let us know how you are doing. These pills do not contain any drug. We don't know exactly how they work; they may trigger or stimulate the body's healing process. We do know that your chances of improving with this treatment are quite good. If after six weeks of this treatment you are not feeling better, we can try one of the other treatments." "Placebo as a Treatment for Depression," *Neuropsychopharmacology* 10 (1994): 265–288.

31. Irving Kirsch, "Are Drug and Placebo Effects in Depression Additive?" *Biological Psychiatry* 47 (2000): 733–735.

32. "The Contribution of Desire and Expectation to Placebo Analgesia: Implications for New Research Strategies," in Harrington, *The Placebo Effect*, 132. See also Price and Fields, "Toward a Neurobiology of Placebo Analgesia," in Harrington, *The Placebo Effect*, 93–116. Ginger Hoffman et al. review different aspects of placebo analgesia in "Pain and the Placebo: What We Have Learned," *Perspectives in Biology and Medicine* 48 (2005): 248–265. D. A. Seminowicz offers another perspective on this phenomenon in "Believe in Your Placebo," *Journal of Neuroscience* 26 (2006): 4453–4454.

33. Tetsuo Koyama et al., "The Subjective Experience of Pain: Where Expectations Become Reality," *Proceedings of the National Academy of Sciences* 102 (2005): 12950–12955. For results of one study of behavioral intervention for pain, see Herta Flor, "Remapping Somatosensory Cortex after Injury," *Advances in Neurology* 93 (2003): 195–204. Ronald Melzack and Patrick Wall first demonstrated the connection between expectation and pain sensation. See their *Textbook of Pain*, 2nd ed. (London: Methuen, 1996).

34. Price and Fields, "The Contribution of Desire and Expectation to Placebo Analgesia," 122.

35. Tor Wager et al., "Placebo-Induced Changes in fMRI in the Anticipation and Experience of Pain," *Science* 303 (2004): 1162–1167.

36. See the letter by Wager in *Science* 304 (2004): 1110–1111. This is a response to Franklin Miller's letter, "Painful Deception," *Science* 304 (2004): 1109–1110.

37. Miller, "Painful Deception," 1110.

38. Robert Blank discusses this and other legal cases involving the involuntary use of psychosurgery and psychotropic drugs for behavioral control in *Brain Policy*, 127–131. See also Stephen Morse, "New Neuroscience, Old Problems," 187–191.

39. George Annas, "Forcible Medication for Courtroom Competence—The Case of Charles Sell," *New England Journal of Medicine* 350 (2004): 2297–2301. See also Scott Gottlieb, "Murderer Can Be Forced to Take Medication to Become Sane Enough to Be Executed," *British Medical Journal* 326 (2003): 415.

40. *Brain-Wise: Studies in Neurophilosophy*, 128. Results of empirical studies on this question have been reported by M.-T. Walsh and T. G. Dinan, "Selective Serotonin Reuptake Inhibitors and Violence: A Review of the Available Evidence," *Acta Psychiatrica Scandinavica* 104 (2001): 84–91, and by D. R. Cherek et al., "Effects of Chronic Paroxetine Administration on Measures of Aggressive and Impulsive Responses of Adult Males with a History of Conduct Disorder," *Psychopharmacology* 159 (2002): 266–274.

41. J. A. Yesavage et al., "Donepezil and Flight Simulator Performance: Effects on Retention of Complex Skills," *Neurology* 59 (2002): 123–125.

42. See, for example, Pierre Maquet, "Sleep on It!" *Nature Neuroscience* 3 (2000): 1235–1236, and Robert Stickgold et al., "Visual Discrimination Learning Requires Sleep after Training," *Nature Neuroscience* 3 (2000): 1237–1238.

43. J. M. Siegel, "The REM Sleep-Memory Consolidation Hypothesis," *Science* 294 (2001): 1058–1063. See also Robert Stickgold and M. P. Walker, "Memory Consolidation and Reconsolidation: What's the Role of Sleep?" *Trends in Neuroscience* 28 (2005): 408–415.

44. Ilana Hairston and Robert Knight, "Sleep on It," *Nature* 430 (2004): 27–28.

45. Reto Huber et al., "Local Sleep and Learning," *Nature* 430 (2004): 78–81.

46. See Miguel Nicolelis et al., "Local Forebrain Dynamics Predict Rat Behavioral States and Their Transitions," *Journal of Neuroscience* 49 (2004): 11137–11147. Gabriel Garcia Marquez's novel *One Hundred Years of Solitude*, trans. Gregory Rabassa (New York: Harper & Row, 1970), is a fictional example of the relation between sleep and memory. Early in the novel, the entire town of Macondo contracts the illness of insomnia. At first, they are quite happy about having the illness, for they believe that it will enable them to do things they previously never had time to do. But a consequence of the insomnia is a severe loss of procedural, semantic, and working memory. They try to compensate by devising an elaborate and extremely cumbersome system of written notes to remind them how to do basic daily tasks. This is similar to the system developed by the main character in the 2000 film *Memento*, who uses notes and tattoos to compensate for his anterograde amnesia in hunting down the man he believes is his wife's killer.

47. D. C. Turner et al., "Cognitive Enhancing Effects of Modafinil in Healthy Volunteers," *Psychopharmacology* 165 (2003): 260–269, and Brain Vastag, "Poised to Challenge

Need for Sleep, 'Wakefulness Enhancer' Rouses Concerns," *Journal of the American Medical Association* 291 (2004): 167–170.

48. Ulrich Muller et al., "Lack of Effects of Guanfacine on Executive and Memory Functions in Healthy Male Volunteers," *Psychopharmacology* 180 (2005): 205–213.

49. See Tim Tully et al., "Targeting the CREB Pathway for Memory Enhancers," *Nature Reviews: Drug Discovery* 2 (2003): 267–277, and G. Lynch, "Memory Enhancement: The Search for Mechanism-Based Drugs," *Nature Neuroscience* 5 (2002): 1035–1038.

50. As Dan Brock has argued in "Enhancement of Human Function: Some Distinctions for Policymakers," in Erik Parens, ed., *Enhancing Human Traits: Social and Ethical Implications* (Washington, D.C.: Georgetown University Press, 1998), 48–69.

51. Arthur Caplan argues for this position in "No Brainer: Can We Cope with the Ethical Ramifications for New Knowledge of the Human Brain?" in Marcus, *Neuroethics: Mapping the Field*, 95–106. See also Arthur Caplan and Paul McHugh, "Shall We Enhance? A Debate," *Cerebrum* 6 (2004): 13–29.

52. Francis Fukuyama makes a similar point in *Our Posthuman Future* (New York: Farrar, Straus and Giroux, 2002), chap. 6.

53. Schacter cites and discusses these cases in *Searching for Memory*, chap. 5.

54. R. Scott et al., "CREB and the Discovery of Cognitive Enhancers," *Journal of Molecular Neuroscience* 19 (2002): 171–177.

55. As Tulving argues in "Episodic Memory: From Mind to Brain." See also Larry Squire, "Declarative and Nondeclarative Memory: Multiple Brain Systems Support Learning and Memory," in Schacter and Tulving, eds., *Memory Systems* (Cambridge, Mass.: MIT Press, 1994), 203–232.

56. This view has been proposed by Ted Abel et al., "Memory Suppressor Genes: Inhibitory Constraints on the Storage of Long-Term Memory," *Science* 279 (1998): 338–341. See also John Lisman and Justin Fallon, "What Maintains Memories?" *Science* 283 (1999): 339–340.

57. "Emerging Ethical Issues in Neuroscience," 1125. See also Farah et al., "Neurocognitive Enhancement: What Can We Do and What Should We Do?" *Nature Reviews Neuroscience* 5 (2004): 421–425, Farah and Wolpe, "Monitoring and Manipulating Brain Function," Rose, *The Future of the Brain*, chaps. 10 and 12, and Peter Whitehouse et al., "Enhancing Cognition in the Intellectually Intact," *Hastings Center Report* 27 (May–June 1997): 14–22.

58. A. R. Luria, *The Mind of a Mnemonist* (London: Cape, 1969). Rose cites this case in *The Future of the Brain*, 248.

59. Jorge Luis Borges, *Ficciones*, trans. Anthony Kerrigan (New York: Grove Press, 1962), 36. Rose mentions this story in *The Future of the Brain*, 248.

60. McGaugh made this point in his testimony before the President's Council on Bioethics.

61. This possibility has been suggested by experiments on memory storage in mice conducted by Thibault Maviel et al., "Sites of Neocortical Reorganization Critical for Remote Spatial Memory," *Science* 305 (2004): 96–99. See also Rose, "'Smart Drugs': Do They Work? Are They Ethical? Will They Be Legal?" *Nature Reviews Neuroscience* 3 (2002): 975–979, S. M. Stahl, "Neurotransmission of Cognition," pt. 2, "Selective NRIs Are Smart Drugs: Exploiting Regionally Selective Actions on both Dopamine and Norepinephrine to Enhance Cognition," *Journal of Clinical Psychiatry* 64 (2003): 110–111, and Gazzaniga, *The Ethical Brain*, chap. 5.

62. Cathryn Jakobson Ramin, "In Search of Lost Time," *New York Times Magazine*, December 5, 2004, p. 15.

63. Carl Elliott, *Better Than Well: American Medicine Meets the American Dream* (New York: Norton, 2003). See also Carl Elliott and Todd Chambers, eds., *Prozac as a Way of Life* (Chapel Hill, N.C.: University of North Carolina Press, 2004).

64. Peter Kramer, *Listening to Prozac: A Psychiatrist Explores Antidepressant Drugs and the Remaking of the Self* (New York: Penguin, 1993). Kramer's *Against Depression* (New York: Viking, 2005) is a sobering antidote to the romanticized idea of depression suggested in his earlier book.

65. Cited in LeDoux, *The Synaptic Self*, 276.

66. "Emerging Ethical Issues in Neuroscience," 1125.

67. Edward Boyer and Michael Shannon, "The Serotonin Syndrome," *New England Journal of Medicine* 352 (2005): 1112–1120.

68. Anjan Chatterjee, "Cosmetic Neurology: The Controversy over Enhancing Movement, Mentation, and Mood," *Neurology* 63 (2004): 968–974, and "The Promise and Predicament of Cosmetic Neurology," *Journal of Medical Ethics* 32 (2006): 110–113. See also Richard Dees, "Slippery Slopes, Wonder Drugs, and Cosmetic Neurology; The Neuroethics of Enhancement," *Neurology* 63 (2004): 951–952. As I point out in chapter 5, drugs and different forms of neurostimulation for mental illness and movement disorders should be described as treatment rather than enhancement, given the severity of most of these conditions.

69. As suggested, for example, by the 2004 film *Eternal Sunshine of the Spotless Mind*.

70. What I have called *qualitative* identity, others have called *narrative* identity. See D. DeGrazia, *Human Identity and Bioethics* and Marya Schechtman, *The Constitution of Selves* (Ithaca: Cornell University Press, 1997).

71. Chatterjee, "The Promise and Predicament of Cosmetic Neurology," and Farah et al., "Neurocognitive Enhancement: What Can We Do and What Should We Do?"

Chapter 5

1. S. M. LaRoche and S. L. Helmers, "The New Antiepileptic Drugs," *Journal of the American Medical Association* 291 (2004): 605–614.

2. S. Wiebe, "Brain Surgery for Epilepsy," *Lancet: Extreme Medicine* 362 (2003): s48.

3. S. Wiebe et al., "A Randomized, Controlled Trial of Surgery for Temporal-Lobe Epilepsy," *New England Journal of Medicine* 345 (2001): 311–318.

4. As reported by Aaron Derfel, "Brain Surgery: A Young Girl's Courage," *Montreal Gazette*, January 25, 2003. John Broome analyzes metaphysical and ethical aspects of weighing options in high-risk brain surgery and other life-and-death choices in *Weighing Lives* (Oxford: Oxford University Press, 2004), chaps. 1, 16, and 17.

5. Paul Appelbaum, Jessica Berg, Charles Lidz, and Alan Meisel (eds.) discuss these conditions in *Informed Consent, Legal Theory, and Clinical Practice*, 2nd ed. (New York: Oxford University Press, 2001). See also L. B. McCullough, J. W. Jones, and B. A. Brody, eds., *Surgical Ethics* (New York: Oxford University Press, 1998), 16–17.

6. As reported by Denise Grady, "Two Women, Two Deaths, and an Ethical Quandary," *New York Times*, July 15, 2003.

7. T. B. Freeman et al., "Use of Placebo Surgery in Controlled Trials of a Cellular-Based Therapy for Parkinson's Disease," *New England Journal of Medicine* 341 (1999): 988–992. Ruth Macklin criticizes this and surgical trials in general in "The Ethical Problems with Sham Surgery in Clinical Research," *New England Journal of Medicine* 341 (1999): 992–996.

8. This is not to say that all drug therapy for Parkinson's is ineffective. The monoamine oxidase B inhibitor rasagaline, when used as an adjunct to levodopa, has shown benefits in

motor control for some patients in the early stages of the disease. See O. Rascol et al., "Rasa-galine as an Adjunct to Levodopa in Patients with Parkinson's Disease and Motor Fluctuations: A Randomised, Double-Blind, Parallel-Group Trial," *Lancet* 365 (2005): 947–954.

9. C. W. Olanow et al., "A Double-Blind Controlled Trial of Bilateral Fetal Nigral Transplantation in Parkinson's Disease," *Annals of Neurology* 54 (2003): 403–414. On the basis of the dyskinesias and other factors, Olanow et al. concluded that fetal-nigral trans-plantation cannot be recommended as therapy for Parkinson's.

10. R. L. Albin argues that sham surgery controls may be permitted, but only when absolutely necessary, in "Sham Surgery Controls: Intracerebral Grafting of Fetal Tissue for Parkinson's Disease and Proposed Criteria for Use of Sham Surgery Controls," *Journal of Medical Ethics* 28 (2002): 322–325. See also Franklin Miller, "Sham Surgery: An Ethical Analysis," *American Journal of Bioethics* 3 (2004): 25–35, and the commentaries by Gregory Stock, "If the Goal Is Relief, What's Wrong with a Placebo?" and John Fletcher, "Sham Neurosurgery in Parkinson's Disease: Ethical at the Time," *American Journal of Bioethics* 3 (2004): 50–51, 52–53.

11. In 1999, a Swedish team announced that in 1 out of 17 patients who had received embryonic dopamine grafts 10 years earlier, the grafts continued to release dopamine. See Roger Barker and Stephen Dunnett, "Functional Integration of Neural Grafts in Parkinson's Disease," *Nature Neuroscience* 2 (1999): 1047–1048. See also L. Melton, "Neural Trans-plantation: New Cells for Old Brains," *Lancet* 355 (2000): 2142–2143, D. Turner, "Clinical Prospects for Neural Grafting Therapy for Hippocampal Lesions and Epilepsy," *Neurosurgery* 52 (2003): 632–644, and P. Gordon et al., "Reaction Time and Movement Time after Embryonic Cell Transplantation in Parkinson Disease," *Archives of Neurology* 61 (2004): 858–861. Konrad Hochedlinger and Rudolf Jaenisch offer a more general overview of the potential of stem-cell transplantation for neurological conditions in "Nuclear Transplanta-tion, Embryonic Stem Cells, and the Potential for Cell Therapy," *New England Journal of Medicine* 349 (2003): 275–286. There has been considerable debate over whether the embryos from which embryonic stem cells are derived have moral status. I will not discuss this issue here. See Karen Lebacz et al., eds., *The Human Embryonic Stem Cell Debate* (Cambridge, Mass.: MIT Press, 2001), and Mary Mahowald, "Reflections on the Human Embryonic Stem Cell Debate," *Perspectives in Biology and Medicine* 46 (2003): 131–141.

12. Ronald Benveniste et al., "Embryonic Stem-Cell Derived Astrocytes Expressing Drug-Induced Transgenesis: Differentiation and Transplantation into the Mouse Brain," *Journal of Neurosurgery* 103 (2005): 115–123. In another experiment using a mouse model, it was found that cancer stem cells could initiate and maintain brain tumor growth. It is un-clear whether growth factors could easily separate cancerous from noncancerous stem cells. See P. B. Dirks et al., "Identification of Human Brain Tumor Initiating Cells," *Nature* 432 (2004): 396–401.

13. Susan Stagno, Martin Smith, and Samuel Hassenbusch offer a concise overview of the history of and ethical issues in psychosurgery in "Reconsidering 'Psychosurgery': Issues of Informed Consent and Physician Responsibility," *Journal of Clinical Ethics* 5 (1994): 217–223. See also J. D. Pressman, *Last Resort: Psychosurgery and the Limits of Medicine* (Cambridge: Cambridge University Press, 1998), K. R. Johnston and G. R. Cosgrove, "Psy-chosurgery: Current Status," in G. T. Tindall, ed., *Contemporary Neurosurgery* (Baltimore: Williams and Wilkins, 1997): 223–257, and R. P. Feldman and J. T. Goodrich, "Psycho-surgery: A Historical Overview," *Neurosurgery* 48 (2001): 647–659. John Kleinig was perhaps the first to raise and discuss the issue of consent to psychosurgery in *Ethical Issues in Psychosurgery* (London: Allen and Unwin, 1985), chap. 3.

14. G. S. Mahli et al., "Depression: A Role for Neurosurgery?" *British Journal of Neurosurgery* 14 (2000): 415–422.

15. As reported by G. R. Cosgrove, "Surgery for Psychiatric Disorders," *CNS Spectrums* 5 (2002): 43–52, and by D. Dougherty et al., "Prospective Long-Term Follow-up of 44 Patients Who Received Cingulotomy for Treatment-Refractory Obsessive-Compulsive Disorder," *American Journal of Psychiatry* 159 (2002): 269–275.

16. Royal College of Psychiatrists, *Neurosurgery for Mental Disorder: Report from the Neurosurgery Working Group of the Royal College of Psychiatrists* (London: Royal College of Psychiatrists, 2000). See also P. Mindus et al., "Neurosurgical Treatment of Refractory Obsessive-Compulsive Disorder: Implications for Understanding Frontal Lobe Function," *Journal of Neuropsychiatry* 6 (1994): 467–477.

17. P. Mindus and H. Nyman, "Normalization of Personality Characteristics in Patients with Incapacitating Anxiety Disorders after Capsulotomy," *Acta Psychiatrica Scandinavica* 83 (1991): 283–291.

18. J. F. Drane, "Competency to Give Informed Consent: A Model for Making Clinical Assessments," *Journal of the American Medical Association* 252 (1984): 925–927. See also Stagno, Smith, and Hassenbusch, "Reconsidering 'Psychosurgery,'" and Appelbaum et al., *Informed Consent, Legal Theory, and Clinical Practice.*

19. Keith Matthews and Muftah Eljamel, "Status of Neurosurgery for Mental Disorder in Scotland," *British Journal of Psychiatry* 56 (2003): 404–411.

20. See, for example, P. Krack et al., "Five-Year Follow-Up of Bilateral Stimulation of the Subthalamic Nucleus in Advanced Parkinson's Disease," *New England Journal of Medicine* 349 (2003): 1925–1934, and V. C. Anderson et al., "Pallidal vs. Subthalamic Nucleus Deep Brain Stimulation in Parkinson Disease," *Archives of Neurology* 62 (2005): 549–560.

21. A. Abbott, "Brain Implants Show Promise against Obsessive Disorder," *Nature* 419 (2002): 658, and S. Goodman, "France Wires Up to Treat Obsessive Disorder," *Nature* 420 (2003): 677.

22. S. D. Piasecki and J. W. Jefferson, "Psychiatric Complications of Deep-Brain Stimulation for Parkinson's Disease." *Journal of Clinical Psychiatry* 65 (2004): 845–849.

23. B. Nuttin et al., "Deep-Brain Stimulation for Psychiatric Disorders," *Neurosurgery* 51 (2002): 519. See also B. Nuttin et al., "Electrical Stimulation in Anterior Limbs of Internal Capsules in Patients with Obsessive-Compulsive Disorder," *Lancet* 354 (1999): 1526.

24. M. L. Dodd et al., "Pathological Gambling Caused by Drugs Used to Treat Parkinson Disease," *Archives of Neurology* 62 (2005): 579–583.

25. Helen Mayberg et al., "Deep-Brain Stimulation for Treatment-Resistant Depression," *Neuron* 45 (2005): 651–660.

26. Richard Abrams, *Electroconvulsive Therapy*, 4th ed. (New York: Oxford University Press, 2002). See also S. V. Eranti and D. M. McLoughlin, "Electroconvulsive Therapy—State of the Art," *British Journal of Psychiatry* 174 (2003): 8–9.

27. Alvaro Pascual-Leone et al., *Handbook of Transcranial Magnetic Stimulation* (London: Edward Arnold, 2002). See also S. Anand and J. Hotson, "Transcranial Magnetic Stimulation: Neurophysiological Applications and Safety," *Brain and Cognition* 50 (2002): 366–386. For more recent work, see Thomas Schlaepfer and Markus Kosel, "Transcranial Magnetic Stimulation in Depression," Ralph Hoffman, "Transcranial Magnetic Stimulation Studies of Schizophrenia and Other Disorders," in S. H. Lisanby, ed., *Brain Stimulation in Psychiatric Treatment* (Washington, D.C.: American Psychiatric, 2004), 1–16, 23–46, Kenneth Foster, "Engineering the Brain," chap. 13 in Illes, *Neuroethics* and Megan Steven and Alvaro Pascual-Leone, "Transcranial Magnetic Stimulation and the Human Brain: An Ethical Evaluation," chap. 14 in Illes, *Neuroethics.*

28. In depression, for example, compare A. J. Rush et al., "Vagus Nerve Stimulation for Treatment-Resistant Depression: A Multicenter Study," *Biological Psychiatry* 47 (2002):

276–285, with H. A. Sackeim et al., "Vagus Nerve Stimulation (VNS) for Treatment-Resistant Depression: Efficacy, Side Effects, and Predictors of Outcome," *Neuropsychopharmacology* 25 (2001): 713–728. See also Sackein, "Vagus Nerve Stimulation," in Lisanby, *Brain Stimulation in Psychiatric Treatment*, 99–136.

29. Y. Gidron et al., "Does the Vagus Nerve Inform the Brain about Preclinical Tumors and Modulate Them?" *Lancet Oncology* 6 (2005): 245–248.

30. Y. Z. Huang et al., "Theta Burst Stimulation of the Human Motor Cortex," *Neuron* 45 (2005): 201–206. W. Paulus presents a more critical perspective on the study of Huang et al. in "Improved Recipe for Magnetic Brain Stimulation," *Neuron* 45 (2005): 181–183.

31. Michael Rohan et al., "Low-Field Magnetic Stimulation in Bipolar Disorder Using an MRI-Based Stimulator," *American Journal of Psychiatry* 161 (2004): 93–98.

32. Miguel Nicolelis et al., "Real-Time Prediction of Hand Trajectory by Ensembles of Cortical Neurons in Primates," *Nature* 408 (2000): 361–365, and Nicolelis, "Brain-Machine Interfaces to Restore Motor Function and Probe Neural Circuits," *Nature Reviews Neuroscience* 4 (2003): 417–422. Additional studies using primates have been conducted at other research centers. Ingrid Wickelgren surveys these studies and some of the ethical issues they raise in "Tapping the Mind," *Science* 299 (2003): 496–499.

33. The company Cyberkinetics conducted this study to test its BrainGate system, as reported by Andrew Pollack, "With Tiny Brain Implants, Just Thinking May Make It So," *New York Times*, April 30, 2004. See also L. R. Hochberg et al., "Neuronal Ensemble Control of Prosthetic Devices by a Human with Tetraplegia," *Nature* 442 (2006): 164–171.

34. See, for example, Michael Bratman, *Intention, Plans, and Practical Reason* (Cambridge, Mass.: Harvard University Press, 1986), Donald Davidson, *Essays on Actions and Events*, 2nd ed. (Oxford: Clarendon Press, 2001), and Alfred Mele, *Motivation and Agency* (New York: Oxford University Press, 2005.)

35. S. Musallam et al., "Cognitive Control Signals for Neural Prosthetics," *Science* 305 (2004): 258–262.

36. See M. Persinger et al., "Enhanced Hypnotic Suggestibility Following Application of Burst-Firing Magnetic Fields over the Right Temporoparietal Lobes: A Replication," *International Journal of Neuroscience* 87 (1996): 201–207, and M. Persinger, "The Neuropsychiatry of Paranormal Experiences," *Journal of Neuropsychiatry and Clinical Neuroscience* 13 (2001): 515–524. Pehr Granqvist et al. have conducted experiments that raise questions about claims made by Blanke and Persinger and report their results in "Sensed Presence and Mystical Experience Are Predicted by Suggestibility, Not by the Application of Transcranial Weak Complex Magnetic Fields," *Neuroscience Letters* 380 (2005): 346–347.

37. The results from Beauregard's nuns' imaging study will be published in 2006 (personal correspondence). Beauregard (ed.) discusses similar types of experience in *Consciousness, Emotional Self-Regulation, and the Brain* (New York: Benjamins, 2004).

38. Radiologist Andrew Newberg and colleagues have conducted similar experiments and summarize their findings and their implications in *Why God Won't Go Away: Brain Science and the Biology of Belief* (New York: Ballantine Books, 2001).

39. Eric Cassell, *The Nature of Suffering and the Goals of Medicine*, 2nd ed. (New York: Oxford University Press, 2004), 281.

40. Antonio Damasio, *The Feeling of What Happens*, 75–76.

41. For example, Hunter Hoffman et al., "Virtual Reality May Distract the Brain from Pain," *NeuroReport* 15 (2004): 978–989.

42. See John Hick's explanation of this phenomenon in *The Fifth Dimension: An Inquiry into the Spiritual Realm*, 2nd ed. (Oxford: One World, 2004), chap. 2. Cassell discusses this as well in *The Nature of Suffering and the Goals of Medicine*, 236–240.

43. As noted in chapter 2, the study by Britton and Bootzin suggests that OBEs may be part of a similar coping mechanism that protects some people from PTSD. See "Near-Death Experience and the Temporal Lobe."

44. *Tibetan Book of the Dead*, trans. and ed. W. Y. Evans-Wentz (Oxford: Oxford University Press, 1960): 121–122, 142. This passage is cited by Joseph in *Neuropsychiatry, Neuropsychology, and Clinical Neuroscience*, chap. 8, "The Limbic System and the Soul." See also Paul Root Wolpe, "Religious Responses to Neuroscientific Questions," chap. 20 in Illes, *Neuroethics*.

Chapter 6

1. Report of the Ad Hoc Committee of the Harvard Medical School to Examine the Definition of Brain Death: "A Definition of Irreversible Coma," *Journal of the American Medical Association* 205 (1968): 337–340. For anesthesiologist Henry Beecher, the most prominent member of the Harvard committee, two main issues motivated the need for a definition of brain death. The first involved problems with defining death for the purpose of organ procurement for transplantation. The second involved the fact that patients in newly developed intensive care units could be keep alive indefinitely by mechanical ventilation, which could be very costly and an inefficient use of scarce resources.

2. President's Commission for the Study of Ethical Problems in Medicine and Biomedical and Behavioral Research, *Defining Death* (Washington, D.C.: U.S. Government Printing Office, 1981).

3. See, for example, E. F. M. Wijdicks, "Determining Brain Death in Adults," *Neurology* 45 (1995): 1003–1011, E. F. M. Wijdicks, ed., *Brain Death* (Philadelphia: Lippincott, Williams and Wilkins, 2000), E. F. M. Wijdicks, "The Diagnosis of Brain Death," *New England Journal of Medicine* 344 (2001): 1215–1221, and Stuart Youngner, Robert Arnold, and Rene Schapiro, eds., *The Definition of Death: Contemporary Controversies* (Baltimore: Johns Hopkins University Press, 2002).

4. Wijdicks, *Brain Death*, 29–43. See also D. J. Powner and J. M. Darby, "Current Considerations in the Issue of Brain Death," *Neurosurgery* 45 (1999): 1222–1226, and H. J. Gramm et al., "Acute Endocrine Failure after Brain Death?" *Transplantation* 54 (1992): 851–857.

5. D. Alan Shewmon, "Brain Stem Death, Brain Death, and Death: A Critical Evaluation of the Purported Equivalence," *Issues in Law and Medicine* 14 (1998): 125–145, "Chronic 'Brain Death': Meta-analysis and Conceptual Consequences," *Neurology* 51 (1998): 1538–1545, and "The Brain and Somatic Integration: Insights into the Standard Biological Rationale for Equating 'Brain Death' with Death," *Journal of Medicine and Philosophy* 26 (2001): 457–478.

6. James Bernat, "The Biophilosophical Basis of Whole-Brain Death," in E. F. Paul, F. D. Miller, and J. Paul, eds., *Bioethics* (New York: Cambridge University Press, 2002), 324–342, at 335. See also Bernat, "A Defense of the Whole-Brain Concept of Death," *Hastings Center Report* 28 (March–April 1998): 14–23, and *Ethical Issues in Neurology*, 2nd ed. (Boston: Butterworth-Heineman, 2002), 243–281.

7. Bernat, "The Biophilosophical Basis of Whole-Brain Death," 337.

8. Michael Green and Daniel Wikler first made this point in "Brain Death and Personal Identity," *Philosophy and Public Affairs* 9 (1980): 105–133.

9. "Recovery from 'Brain Death': A Neurologist's Apologia," *Linacre Quarterly* 64 (1997): 30–96.

10. Shewmon, "Recovery from 'Brain Death,'" 67–68.

11. Shewmon, "Recovery from 'Brain Death,'" 68.

12. See Multi-Society Task Force on the Persistent Vegetative State, "Medical Aspects of the Persistent Vegetative State," *New England Journal of Medicine* 330 (1994): 1499–1508. See also Quality Standards Committee of the American Academy of Neurology, "Practice Parameters for Determining Brain Death in Adults," *Neurology* 45 (1995): 1012–1014.

13. *In re Quinlan* (1976), 70 NJ 10.

14. These include, among others, Robert Veatch, *Death, Dying, and the Biological Revolution*, 2nd ed. (New Haven: Yale University Press, 1992), "The Impending Collapse of the Whole-Brain Definition of Death," *Hastings Center Report* 23 (July–August 1993): 18–24, and "The Death of Whole-Brain Death: The Plague of the Disaggregators, Somaticists, and Mentalists," *Journal of Medicine and Philosophy* 30 (2005): 353–378, Peter Singer, *Re-thinking Life and Death* (New York: St. Martin's Press. 1995), and Jeff McMahan, "The Metaphysics of Brain Death," *Bioethics* 9 (1995): 91–126, and *The Ethics of Killing: Problems at the Margins of Life* (New York: Oxford University Press, 2002).

15. See Wijdicks, *Brain Death*, 61–90, and "The Diagnosis of Brain Death."

16. Wijdicks, *Brain Death*, 115–134.

17. "A Defense of the Whole-Brain Concept of Death," 16. Josie Fisher defends the same position in "Re-examining Death: Against a Higher-Brain Criterion," *Journal of Medical Ethics* 25 (1999): 473–476.

18. "The Metaphysics of Brain Death."

19. "A Defense of the Whole-Brain Concept of Death," 16.

20. "Philosophical Debates about the Definition of Death: Who Cares?" *Journal of Medicine and Philosophy* 26 (2001): 527–537. See also Stuart Youngner, Robert Arnold, and Michael DeVita, "When Is 'Dead'?" *Hastings Center Report* 29 (January–February, 1999): 14–21, and Robert Truog, "Is It Time to Abandon Brain Death?" *Hastings Center Report* 27 (January–February, 1997): 29–37.

21. John Robertson, "The Dead Donor Rule," *Hastings Center Report* 29 (November–December, 1999): 6–14.

22. "Philosophical Debates about the Meaning of Death," 532–533.

23. David Wiggins, *Sameness and Substance* (Oxford: Blackwell, 1980), David Oderberg, "Modal Properties, Moral Status, and Identity," *Philosophy and Public Affairs* 15 (1997): 259–298, and McMahan, *The Ethics of Killing*, chap. 1.

24. McMahan, in *The Ethics of Killing*, offers the strongest defense of the view that we are essentially persons, while Eric Olson offers the strongest defense of the view that we are essentially human organisms, in *The Human Animal: Personal Identity without Psychology* (New York: Oxford University Press, 1997).

25. See, for example, Ingmar Persson, "Human Death—A View from the Beginning of Life," *Bioethics* 16 (2002): 20–32.

26. *Reasons and Persons*, 275. The more general point is that a person is not a separately existing entity, independent of his or her brain and body.

27. *The Ethics of Killing*, 66–94, 426–443. Although McMahan uses the term "embodied," it seems that the biological basis of mind for him does not consist in the integrated functions of the brain and body but in brain function alone. This is one respect in which his account and mine differ, since I have argued that endocrine and immune systems can influence the central nervous system and the brain. So I am proposing a thicker conception of embodied minds than McMahan does. In "The Death of Whole-Brain Death," Veatch argues that the integration of bodily and mental functions is the critical feature of human life and that death is the irreversible loss of these integrated functions.

28. *The Ethics of Killing*, chap. 5. See also Agnieszka Jaworska, "Respecting the Margins of Agency: Alzheimer's Patients and the Capacity to Value," *Philosophy and Public Affairs* 28 (1999): 105–138. David DeGrazia critically discusses these and related issues in

"Identity, Killing, and the Boundaries of Our Existence," *Philosophy and Public Affairs* 31 (2003): 413–442, and in *Human Identity and Bioethics*, chap. 4.

29. For example, Linda Emanuel, "Redefining Death: The Asymptotic Model and a Bounded Zone Definition," *Hastings Center Report* 25 (July–August, 1995): 27–35.

30. Joseph Fins spells out and discusses this threefold distinction in "Rethinking Disorders of Consciousness: New Research and Its Implications," *Hastings Center Report* 35 (March–April 2005): 22–24. See also J. T. Giacino et al., "The Minimally Conscious State: Definition and Diagnostic Criteria," *Neurology* 58 (2002): 349–353.

31. Fins cites this case in "Rethinking Disorders of Consciousness." See also N. D. Schiff and J. J. Fins, "Hope for 'Comatose' Patients," *Cerebrum* 5 (2003): 7–24, and J. J. Fins and F. Plum, "Neurological Diagnosis Is More Than a State of Mind: Diagnostic Clarity and Impaired Consciousness," *Archives of Neurology* 61 (2004): 1354–1355.

32. Steven Laureys et al., "Quantifying Consciousness," *Lancet Neurology* 4 (2005): 789–790, and Steven Laureys, "Death, Unconsciousness, and the Brain," *Nature Reviews Neuroscience* 6 (2005): 789.

33. S. Laureys et al., "Brain Function in Coma, Vegetative State, and Related Disorders," *Lancet Neurology* 3 (2004): 537–546. See also N. Schiff et al., "fMRI Reveals Large-Scale Network Activation in Minimally Conscious Patients," *Neurology* 64 (2005): 514–523, H. U. Voss et al., "Possible Axonal Regrowth in Late Recovery from the Minimally Conscious State," *Journal of Clinical Investigation* 116 (2006): 2005–2011, and Laureys et al., "Tracking the Recovery of Consciousness from Coma," *Journal of Clinical Investigation* 116 (2006): 1823–1825.

34. McMahan, *The Ethics of Killing*, 35.

35. McMahan, *The Ethics of Killing*, 35.

36. *Phaedo*, in *Plato: The Collected Dialogues*, ed. E. Hamilton and H. Cairns (Princeton: Princeton University Press, 1980), 63e–69e, 80c–84b.

37. Rene Descartes, *Meditations on First Philosophy*, meditation 6.

38. Aristotle, *De Anima* (*On the Soul*), in *The Complete Works of Aristotle*, vol. 1. See also the discussion by McMahan, *The Ethics of Killing*, 10–11.

39. For example, McMahan, *The Ethics of Killing*, chap. 1, and Bernat, "The Biophilosophical Basis of Whole-Brain Death," 326 n. 6. See also Elliot Dorff, "End-of-Life: Jewish Perspectives," *Lancet* 366 (2005): 862–865, Abdulaziz Sachedina, "End-of-Life: The Islamic View," *Lancet* 366 (2005): 774–779, and Tristram Engelhardt and A. S. Iltis, "End-of-Life: The Traditional Christian View," *Lancet* 366 (2005): 1045–1049.

40. Here I follow the interpretations of Huston Smith, *The World's Religions* (San Francisco: HarperCollins, 1991), chaps. 1 and 2, and Hick, *The Fifth Dimension*, 246–247. These interpretations draw from the *locus classicus* of Hinduism, the *Bhagavad-Gita*. See also Shirley Firth, "End-of-Life: A Hindu View," *Lancet* 366 (2005): 682–686.

41. Syogal Rinpoche gives a complete account of Buddhism in *The Tibetan Book of Living and Dying* (New York: Harper Collins, 1993).

42. Aquinas, *Summa Theologiae*, trans. Fathers of the English Dominican Province (London: Blackfriars, 1973–80), pt. 1, question 75, art. 5.

43. The Justinian Code of the sixth century said that fetuses under 40 days did not have souls. But in 1588, Pope Sixtus rejected this and declared the position that was later confirmed by Pius IX. Aquinas's view on ensoulment is consistent with the Justinian Code. David Albert Jones offers a historical account of this issue in *The Soul of the Embryo: An Inquiry into the Status of the Embryo in the Christian Tradition* (London: Continuum Press, 2004).

44. For an interpretation of Aquinas's position, see J. F. Donceel, "Immediate Animation and Delayed Hominization," *Theological Studies* 31 (1970): 76–105. See also Norman Ford, *When Did I Begin?* (Cambridge: Cambridge University Press, 1988), and Richard

Swinburne, *Is There A God?* (Oxford: Oxford University Press, 1996). Swinburne is a dualist who claims that "there could not be an explanation of soul-brain correlation" (84). But the emergent monism I defended in chapter 2 indicates that a soul–brain correlation is quite plausible.

45. Al-Mu'Minum, in Koran, trans. N. J. Dawood (London: Penguin, 1990), 12–14.

46. *The Ethics of Killing*, 331.

47. These proceedings have been summarized in *Schindler v. Schiavo*. 851 So. 2d 182, Fla. Dist. Ct. App.(2003).

48. Rebecca Dresser discusses legal and ethical issues in this case in "*Schiavo*: A Hard Case Makes Questionable Law," *Hastings Center Report* 34 (May–June 2004): 89, and in "Schiavo's Legacy: The Need for an Objective Standard," *Hastings Center Report* 35 (May–June 2005): 20–22. For other perspectives on this case, see Jay Wolfson, "Erring on the Side of Theresa Schiavo: Reflections of the Special Guardian *ad Litem*," *Hastings Center Report* 35 (May–June 2005): 16–19, Eric Cassell, "The Schiavo Case: A Medical Perspective," *Hastings Center Report* (May–June 2005): 22–23, and Carl Schneider, "Hard Cases and the Politics of Righteousness," *Hastings Center Report* 35 (May–June 2005): 24–27.

49. See Multi-Society Task Force on the Persistent Vegetative State, "Medical Aspects of the Persistent Vegetative State," and Quality Standards Committee of the American Academy of Neurology, "Practice Parameters for Determining Brain Death in Adults." Noting the widespread neuron loss, atrophy, and lack of electrical activity in Terri Schiavo's brain, Schiff and Fins support the assessment that she was in a permanent vegetative state: "In the aggregate, this evidence is as unequivocal, and lacking in reasons for hope [of recovery], as any obtainable in these circumstances" ("Hope for 'Comatose' Patients," 22).

50. *Cruzan v. Director, Missouri Department of Health* (1990).

51. Cited in McMahan, *The Ethics of Killing*, 423.

52. Brennan's comments in *Cruzan* were based on comments made in his opinion in an earlier case, *Brophy v. New England Sinai Hospital, Inc.*, 398 Mass. 417, 434, 497, NE 2d. (1986).

53. *Abortion and Infanticide* (Oxford: Clarendon Press, 1983), 65.

54. *Rethinking Life and Death*, 207.

55. *The End of Life: Euthanasia and Morality* (Oxford: Oxford University Press, 1986), 24–25. Shelly Kagan also distinguishes between biological and biographical sense of life and explains the implications of this distinction for our understanding of harm and well-being in "Me and My Life," *Proceedings of the Aristotelian Society* 94 (1994): 309–324. Similarly, DeGrazia distinguishes "numerical identity" from "narrative identity" in *Human Identity and Bioethics*, chaps. 2 and 3.

56. *The End of Life*, 42.

57. Joseph Fins, "Constructing an Ethical Stereotaxy for Severe Brain Injury: Balancing Risks, Benefits and Access," *Nature Reviews Neuroscience* 4 (2003): 323–327, and Schiff and Fins, "Hope for 'Comatose' Patients."

58. *Harm to Others* (New York: Oxford University Press, 1984), 79–95. Ronald Dworkin defends a similar view in distinguishing between "experiential interests" and "critical interests" in *Life's Dominion: An Argument about Abortion, Euthanasia, and Individual Freedom* (New York: Knopf, 1993), 63–65. Throughout this chapter and the book as a whole I have been relying on Feinberg's definition of harm as the defeat or thwarting of one's interests.

59. For helpful discussion, see Robert Veatch, "The Dead Donor Rule: True by Definition," *American Journal of Bioethics* 3 (2003): 10–11, and Norman Fost, "Reconsidering the Dead Donor Rule: Is It Important That Organ Donors Be Dead?" *Kennedy Institute of Ethics Journal* 14 (2004): 249–263. See also Truog, "Is It Time to Abandon Brain

Death?" Truog and Walter Robinson, "The Role of Brain Death and the Dead Donor Rule in the Ethics of Organ Transplantation," *Critical Care Medicine* 31 (2003): 2391–2396, Ian Kerridge et al., "Death, Dying, and Donation: Organ Transplantation and the Diagnosis of Death," *Journal of Medical Ethics* 28 92002): 89–94, and DeGrazia, *Human Identity and Bioethics*, chap. 4. Several of the authors cited here suggest that many of the ethical problems surrounding the timing of the declaration of brain death in organ procurement for transplantation can be avoided. When a patient is imminently dying and cannot benefit from continued life-support, this support can be withdrawn in a controlled manner. Cardiocirculatory and brain functions cease, and the patient is declared dead. Provided that the patient has consented to organ donation, organs can then be taken from his or her body for transplantation.

60. It is worth noting that cadaveric organ donation is consistent with the ideas of selfless giving, saving a life, relieving suffering, and compassion in all the major religions. These include Judaism, Christianity, Islam, Hinduism, Buddhism, and Sikhism. In Judaism, for example, most rabbinical interpretations say that there is a greater duty to save the life of another than to preserve the integrity of the body. Still, all of these religions accept whole-brain and cardiopulmonary criteria of death, not the higher-brain criterion. They would not permit organ procurement on the basis of the third criterion.

61. Bonnie Steinbock draws this distinction and discusses its ethical implications in *Life before Birth: The Moral and Legal Status of Embryos and Fetuses* (New York: Oxford University Press, 1992), 5–41.

62. See F. G. Miller and J. J. Fins, "Protecting Vulnerable Research Subjects without Unduly Constraining Neuropsychiatric Research," *Archives of General Psychiatry* 56 (1999): 701–702.

References

Abbot, A. 2002. "Brain Implants Show Promise against Obsessive Disorder." *Nature* 419: 658.

Abel, T., et al. 1998. "Memory Suppressor Genes: Inhibitory Constraints on the Storage of Long-Term Memory." *Science* 279: 338–341.

Abrams, R. 2002. *Electroconvulsive Therapy*. 4th ed. New York: Oxford University Press.

Ader, R., et al., eds. 2001. *Psychoneuroimmunology*. 3rd ed. San Diego: Academic Press.

Adolphs, R., et al. 1996. "Neuropsychological Approaches to Reasoning and Decision-Making." In A. Damasio et al., *Neurobiology of Decision Making*, 157–178.

Aguirre, G. K. 2003. "Functional Neuroimaging." In Feinberg and Farah, *Behavioral Neurology and Neuropsychology*, 363–373.

Ahmed, S. 2004. "Addiction as Compulsive Reward Prediction." *Science* 306: 1901–1902.

Albin, R. L. 2002. "Sham Surgery Controls: Intracerebral Grafting of Fetal Tissue for Parkinson's Disease and Proposed Criteria for Use of Sham Surgery Controls." *Journal of Medical Ethics* 28: 322–325.

American Academy of Neurology. 1995. "Practice Parameters for Determining Brain Death in Adults." *Neurology* 45: 1012–1014.

American Psychiatric Association. 2002. *Diagnostic and Statistical Manual of Mental Disorders*. 4th ed. Text revision (*DSM-IV-TR*). Washington, D.C.: American Psychiatric.

Anand, S., and Hotson, J. 2002. "Transcranial Magnetic Stimulation: Neurophysiological Applications and Safety." *Brain and Cognition* 50: 366–386.

Anderson, M., et al. 2004. "Neural Systems Underlying the Suppression of Unwanted Memories." *Science* 33: 232–235.

Anderson, V. C., et al. 2005. "Pallidal vs. Subthalamic Nucleus Deep Brain Stimulation in Parkinson Disease." *Archives of Neurology* 62: 549–560.

Andreasen, N. 1997. "Linking Mind and Brain in the Study of Mental Illnesses: A Project for Scientific Psychopathology." *Science* 275: 1586–1593.

Annas, G. 2004. "Forcible Medication for Courtroom Competence—The Case of Charles Sell." *New England Journal of Medicine* 350: 2297–2301.

Annoni, J. M., et al. 2005. "Changes in Artistic Style after Minor Posterior Stroke." *Journal of Neurology, Neurosurgery, and Psychiatry* 76: 797–803.

Antel, J. P., and Owens, T. 1999. "Immune Regulation and CNS Autoimmune Disease." *Journal of Neuroimmunology* 100: 181–189.

Appelbaum, P., et al., eds. 2001. *Informed Consent, Legal Theory, and Clinical Practice.* 2nd ed. New York: Oxford University Press.

Aquinas, T. 1973–80. *Summa Theologiae.* Translated by Fathers of the English Dominican Province. London: Blackfriars.

Arborelius, L., et al. 1999. "The Role of Corticotropin-Releasing Factor in Depression and Anxiety Disorders." *Journal of Endocrinology* 160: 1–12.

Aristotle. 1984. *De Anima* and *Nicomachean Ethics.* In *The Complete Works of Aristotle*, vols. 1 and 2, trans. J. Barnes. Princeton: Princeton University Press.

Barker, R., and Dunnett, S. 1999. "Functional Integration of Neural Grafts in Parkinson's Disease." *Nature Neuroscience* 2: 1047–1048.

Baxter, L. E., et al. 1992. "Caudate Glucose Metabolism Rate Changes with Both Drug and Behavior Therapy for Obsessive Compulsive Disorder." *Archives of General Psychiatry* 49: 687–698.

Beauregard, M., ed. 2004. *Consciousness, Emotional Self-Regulation, and the Brain.* New York: Benjamins.

Beckman, M. 2004. "Crime, Culpability, and the Adolescent Brain." *Science* 305: 596–599.

Belanoff, J. K., et al. 2002. "An Open Label Trial of C-1073 (Mifepristone) for Psychotic Major Depression." *Biological Psychiatry* 52: 386–392.

Benedetti, F., et al. 2002. "Conscious Expectation and Unconscious Conditioning in Analgesia, Motor, and Hormonal Placebo/Nocebo Responses." *Journal of Neuroscience* 23: 4315–4323.

Benveniste, R., et al. 2005. "Embryonic Stem-Cell Derived Astrocytes Expressing Drug-Induced Transgenesis: Differentiation and Transplantation into the Mouse Brain." *Journal of Neurosurgery* 103: 115–123.

Bernat, J. 1998. "A Defense of the Whole-Brain Concept of Death." *Hastings Center Report* 28 (March–April): 14–23.

———. 2002. "The Biophilosophical Basis of Whole-Brain Death." in Paul et al., *Bioethics*, 324–342.

———. 2002. *Ethical Issues in Neurology.* 2nd ed. Boston: Butterworth-Heineman.

Berrios, G. E., and Markova, I. S. 2003. "The Self and Psychiatry: A Conceptual History." In Kircher and David, *The Self in Neuroscience and Psychiatry*, 9–39.

Blair, R. J. R. 2003. "Neurological Basis of Psychopathy." *British Journal of Psychiatry* 182: 5–7.

Blair, R. J. R., and Cipolotti, L. 2000. "Impaired Social Response Reversal: A Case of 'Acquired Sociopathy.'" *Brain* 123: 1122–1141.

Blair, J., et al. 2005. *The Psychopath: Emotion and the Brain.* Malden, Mass.: Blackwell.

Blank, R. 1999. *Brain Policy: How the New Neuroscience Will Change Our Lives and Our Politics.* Washington, D. C.: Georgetown University Press.

Blanke, O. 2002. "Stimulating Illusory Own-Body Perceptions." *Nature* 419: 269–270.

———. 2004. "Out-of-Body Experiences and Autoscopy of Neurological Origin." *Brain* 127: 243–258.

Borges, J. L. 1962. *Ficciones.* Translated by A. Kerrigan. New York: Grove Press.

Botteron, K. N., et al. 2002. "Volumetric Reduction in Left Subgenual Prefrontal Cortex in Early-Onset Depression." *Biological Psychiatry* 15: 342–344.

Boyer, E., and Shannon, M. 2005. "The Serotonin Syndrome." *New England Journal of Medicine* 352: 1112–1120.

Bratman, M. 1986. *Intention, Plans, and Practical Reason.* Cambridge, Mass.: Harvard University Press.

Brenner, D., and Elliston, C. D. 2004. "Risks of Adult Full-Body CT Scans." *Radiology* 23: 735–738.

Britton, W. B., and Bootzin, R. R. 2004. "Near-Death Experiences and the Temporal Lobe." *Psychological Science* 15: 254–258.

Brock, D. 1998. "Enhancement of Human Function: Some Distinctions for Policymakers." In Parens, *Enhancing Human Traits*, 48–69.

Brody, H. 1980. *Placebos and the Philosophy of Medicine*. Chicago: University of Chicago Press.

———. 1982. "The Lie That Heals: The Ethics of Giving Placebos." *Annals of Internal Medicine* 97: 112–118.

Brophy v. New England Sinai Hospital, Inc. 1986. 398 Mass. 417, 434, 497 NE 2d 626.

Brown, W. 1994. "Placebo as a Treatment for Depression." *Neuropsychopharmacology* 10: 265–288.

Bullmore, E., and Fletcher, P. 2003. "The Eye's Mind: Brain Mapping and Psychiatry." *British Journal of Psychiatry* 182: 381–384.

Bush, G., et al. 2005. "Functional Neuroimaging of Attention-Deficit/Hyperactivity Disorder: A Review and Suggested Future Directions." *Biological Psychiatry* 57: 1273–1284.

Buss, S., and Overton, L., eds. 2002. *The Contours of Agency: Essays on Themes from Harry Frankfurt*. Cambridge, Mass.: MIT Press.

Cami, J., and Farre, M. 2003. "Drug Addiction." *New England Journal of Medicine* 349: 975–986.

Camille, N. 2004. "The Involvement of the Orbitofrontal Cortex in the Experience of Regret." *Science* 304: 1167–1170.

Caplan, A. 2002. "No Brainer: Can We Cope with the Ethical Ramifications for New Knowledge of the Human Brain?" In Marcus, *Neuroethics*, 95–106.

Caplan, A., and McHugh, P. 2004. "Shall We Enhance? A Debate." *Cerebrum* 6 (2004): 13–29.

Casebeer, W. D. 2003. "Moral Cognition and Its Neural Constituents." *Nature Reviews Neuroscience* 4: 840–847.

Caspi, A., et al. 2003. "Influence of Life Stress on Depression: Moderation by a Polymorphism in the 5-HTT Gene." *Science* 301: 386–389.

Cassell, E. 2004. *The Nature of Suffering and the Goals of Medicine*. 2nd ed. New York: Oxford University Press.

———. 2005. "The Schiavo Case: A Medical Perspective." *Hastings Center Report* 35 (May–June): 22–23.

Castellanos, F. X., and Tannock, R. 2002. "Neuroscience of Attention Deficit/Hyperactivity Disorder: The Search for Endophenotypes." *Nature Reviews Neuroscience* 3: 617–628.

Chalmers, D. 1996. *The Conscious Mind*. New York: Oxford University Press.

Changeux, J.-P. 1997. *Neuronal Man*. Translated by Laurence Garey. Princeton: Princeton University Press.

Charney, D., and Nestler, E., eds. 2004. *Neurobiology of Mental Illness*. 2nd ed. Oxford: Oxford University Press.

Chatterjee, A. 2004. "Cosmetic Neurology: The Controversy over Enhancing Movement, Mentation, and Mood." *Neurology* 63: 968–974.

———. 2006. "The Promise and Predicament of Cosmetic Neurology." *Journal of Medical Ethics* 32: 110–113.

Cherek, D. R., et al. 2002. "Effects of Chronic Paroxetine Administration on Measures of Aggressive and Impulsive Responses of Adult Males with a History of Conduct Disorder." *Psychopharmacology* 159: 266–274.

Churchland, P. 1985. *The Engine of Reason, the Seat of the Soul*. Cambridge, Mass.: MIT Press.

Churchland, P. S. 1986. *Neurophilosophy: Toward a Unified Science of the Mind/Brain*. Cambridge, Mass.: MIT Press.

————. 1996. "Feeling Reasons." In A. Damasio et al., *Neurobiology of Decision Making*, 181–199.

————. 2002. *Brain-Wise: Studies in Neurophilosophy*. Cambridge, Mass.: MIT Press.

————. 2005. "Moral Decision-Making and the Brain." In Illes, *Neuroethics*, chap. 1.

Clark, A. 1997. *Being There: Putting Brain, Body and World Together Again*. Cambridge, Mass.: MIT Press.

Clark, W., and Grunstein, M. 2004. *Are We Hardwired? The Role of Genes in Human Behavior*. New York: Oxford University Press.

Cleckley, H. 1967. *The Mask of Sanity*. St. Louis: Mosby.

Clow, A. 2002. "Cytokines and Depression." *International Review of Neurobiology* 52: 255–270.

Cosgrove, G. R. 2002. "Surgery for Psychiatric Disorders." *CNS Spectrums* 5: 43–52.

Cruzan v. Director, Missouri Department of Health. 1990.

Cummings, J., and Mega, M. 2003. *Neuropsychiatry and Behavioral Neuroscience*. New York: Oxford University Press.

Damasio, A. 1994. *Descartes' Error: Emotion, Reason, and the Human Brain*. New York: Putnam.

————. 1999. *The Feeling of What Happens: Body and Emotion in the Making of Consciousness*. New York: Harcourt Brace.

————. 2000. "A Neural Basis for Sociopathy." *Archives of General Psychiatry* 57: 128–129.

————. 2003. *Looking for Spinoza: Joy, Sorrow, and the Feeling Brain*. Orlando, Fl.: Harcourt.

Damasio, A., et al. 1999. "Impairment of Social and Moral Behavior Related to Early Damage in Human Prefrontal Cortex." *Nature Neuroscience* 2: 1032–1037.

Damasio, A., et al., eds. 1996. *Neurobiology of Decision Making*. New York: Springer-Verlag.

Damasio, H., et al. 1994. "The Return of Phineas Gage: Clues about the Brain from the Skull of a Famous Patient." *Science* 264: 1102–1105.

Dantzer, R. 2001. "Cytokine-Induced Sickness Behavior: Where Do We Stand?" *Brain, Behavior, and Immunology* 15: 7–24.

Darby, J. M. 1999. "Current Considerations on the Issue of Brain Death." *Neurosurgery* 45: 1222–1226.

Davidson, D. 2001. *Essays on Actions and Events*. 2nd ed. Oxford: Clarendon Press.

Davidson, R., et al. 2000. "Dysfunction in the Neural Circuitry of Emotion Regulation—A Possible Prelude to Violence." *Science* 289: 591–594.

Davidson, R., et al. 2003. "Alterations in Brain and Immune Function Produced by Mindfulness Meditation." *Psychosomatic Medicine* 65: 564–570.

Davidson, R., et al. 2003. "The Neural Substrates of Affective Processing in Depressed Patients Treated with Venlafaxine." *American Journal of Psychiatry* 160: 64–75.

de Charms, R. C., et al. 2005. "Control over Brain Activation and Pain Learned by Using Real-Time Functional MRI." *Proceedings of the National Academy of Sciences* 102: 18626–18631.

Dees, R. 2004. "Slippery Slopes, Wonder Drugs, and Cosmetic Neurology: The Neuroethics of Enhancement." *Neurology* 63: 951–952.

DeGrazia, D. 2003. "Identity, Killing, and the Boundaries of Our Existence." *Philosophy and Public Affairs* 31: 413–442.

————. 2005. *Human Identity and Bioethics*. New York: Cambridge University Press.

Delillo, D. 1986. *White Noise*. New York: Penguin.

Delves, P. J., and Roitt, I. M. 2002. "Advances in Immunology: The Immune System." *New England Journal of Medicine* 343: 108–117.

Dennet, D. 1991. *Consciousness Explained*. Boston: Little Brown.

————. 2003. *Freedom Evolves*. New York: Viking.

Derfel, A. 2003. "Brain Surgery: A Young Girl's Courage." *Montreal Gazette*, January 25.

Descartes, R. 2000. *Meditations on First Philosophy*. Translated and edited by J. Cottingham. Cambridge: Cambridge University Press.

Dirks, P. B., et al. 2004. "Identification of Human Brain Tumor Initiating Cells." *Nature* 432: 396–401.

Dodd, M. L., et al. 2005. "Pathological Gambling Caused by Drugs Used to Treat Parkinson Disease." *Archives of Neurology* 62: 579–583.

Dolan, R. J. 1999. "On the Neurology of Morals." *Nature Neuroscience* 2: 927–929.

Donceel, J. F. 1970. "Immediate Animation and Delayed Hominization." *Theological Studies* 31: 76–105.

Dorff, E. 2005. "End-of-Life: Jewish Perspectives." *Lancet* 366: 862–865.

Dostoevsky, F. 1994. *Demons: A Novel in Three Parts* (1873). Translated by R. Pevear nd L. Volokhonsky. New York: Knopf.

Dougherty, D., et al. 2002. "Prospective Long-Term Follow-up of 44 Patients Who Received Cingulotomy for Treatment-Refractory Obsessive-Compulsive Disorder." *American Journal of Psychiatry* 159: 269–275.

Drane, J. 1984. "Competency to Give Informed Consent: A Model for Making Clinical Assessments." *Journal of the American Medical Association* 252: 925–927.

Dresser, R. 2004. "*Schiavo*: A Hard Case Makes Questionable Law." *Hastings Center Report* 34 (May–June): 8–9.

————. 2005. "Schiavo's Legacy: The Need for an Objective Standard." *Hastings Center Report* 35 (May–June): 20–22.

Dworkin, R. 1993. *Life's Dominion: An Argument about Abortion, Euthanasia, and Individual Freedom*. New York: Vintage.

Eccles, J., ed. 1966. *Brain and Conscious Experience*. New York: Springer-Verlag.

Elliott, C. 1992. "Diagnosing Blame: Responsibility and the Psychopath." *Journal of Medicine and Philosophy* 17: 223–237.

————. 2003. *Better Than Well: American Medicine Meets the American Dream*. New York: Norton.

Elliott, C., and Chambers, T., eds. 2004. *Prozac as a Way of Life*. Chapel Hill: University of North Carolina Press.

Emanuel, L. 1995. "Redefining Death: The Asymptotic Model and a Bounded Zone Definition." *Hastings Center Report* 25 (July–August): 27–35.

Engelhardt, T., and Iltis, A. S. 2005. "End-of-Life: The Traditional Christian View." *Lancet* 366: 1045–1049.

Eranti, S. V., and McLoughlin, D. M. 2003. "Electroconvulsive Therapy — State of the Art." *British Journal of Psychiatry* 174: 8–9.

Eustace, S., and Nelson, E. 2004. "Whole-Body Magnetic Resonance Imaging." *British Medical Journal* 328: 1387–1388.

Evans, W., and McLeod, H. 2003. "Pharmacogenomics: Drug Disposition, Drug Targets, and Side Effects." *New England Journal of Medicine* 348: 538–547.

Farah, M. 2002. "Emerging Ethical Issues in Neuroscience." *Nature Neuroscience* 5: 1123–1129.

Farah, M., and Wolpe, P. R. 2004. "Monitoring and Manipulating Brain Function: New Neuroscience Technologies and Their Ethical Implications." *Hastings Center Report* 34 (May–June): 35–45.

Farah, M., et al. 2004. "Neurocognitive Enhancement: What Can We Do and What Should We Do?" *Nature Reviews Neuroscience* 5: 421–425.

Feinberg, J. 1986. *Harm to Others*. New York: Oxford University Press.

Feinberg, T. 2001. *Altered Egos: How the Brain Creates the Self.* New York: Oxford University Press.

Feinberg, T., and Farah, M., eds. 2003. *Behavioral Neurology and Neuropsychology.* 2nd ed. New York: McGraw-Hill.

Feldman, R. P., and Goodrich, J. T. 2001. "Psychosurgery: A Historical Overview." *Neurosurgery* 48: 647–659.

Fetissov, S., et al. 2005. "Autoantibodies against Neuropeptides Are Associated with Psychological Traits in Eating Disorders." *Proceedings of the National Academy of Sciences* 102: 14865–14870.

Fins, J. 2003. "Constructing an Ethical Stereotaxy for Severe Brain Injury: Balancing Risks, Benefits and Access," *Nature Reviews Neuroscience* 4: 323–327.

———. 2005. "Rethinking Disorders of Consciousness: New Research and Its Implications." *Hastings Center Report* 35 (March–April): 22–24.

Fins, J., and Plum, F. 2004. "Neurological Diagnosis Is More Than a State of Mind: Diagnostic Clarity and Impaired Consciousness." *Archives of Neurology* 61: 1354–1355.

Firth, S. 2005. "End-of-Life: A Hindu View." *Lancet* 366: 682–686.

Fischer, J. M. 1994. *The Metaphysics of Free Will: An Essay on Control.* Cambridge, Mass.: Blackwell.

Fischer, J. M., and Ravizza, M. 1998. *Responsibility and Control: A Theory of Moral Responsibility.* New York: Cambridge University Press.

Fisher, J. 1999. "Re-examining Death: Against a Higher-Brain Criterion." *Journal of Medical Ethics* 25: 473–476.

Fitzgerald, M. 2003. *Autism and Creativity: Is There a Link between Autism in Men and Exceptional Ability?* London: Brunner-Routledge.

Fletcher, J. 2004. "Sham Neurosurgery in Parkinson's Disease: Ethical at the Time." *American Journal of Bioethics* 3: 52–53.

Flor, H. 2003. "Remapping Somatosensory Cortex after Injury." *Advances in Neurology* 93 (2003): 195–204.

Ford, N. 1988. *When Did I Begin?* Cambridge: Cambridge University Press.

Fossati, P., et al. 2003. "In Search of the Emotional Self: An fMRI Study Using Positive and Negative Emotional Words." *American Journal of Psychiatry* 160: 1938–1945.

Fost, N. 2004. "Reconsidering the Dead Donor Rule: Is It Important That Organ Donors Be Dead?" *Kennedy Institute of Ethics Journal* 14: 249–263.

Foster, K. R. 2005. "Engineering the Brain." In Illes, *Neuroethics*, chap. 13.

Frankfurt, H. 1989. "Identification and Externality." In Frankfurt, *The Importance of What We Care About,* 58–72.

———. 1989. "Identification and Wholeheartedness." In Frankfurt, *The Importance of What We Care About,* 82–95.

———. 1989. *The Importance of What We Care About.* New York: Cambridge University Press.

———. 1992. "The Faintest Passion." *Proceedings and Addresses of the American Philosophical Association* 6: 5–16.

Freeman, T. B., et al. 1999. "Use of Placebo Surgery in Controlled Trials of a Cellular-Based Therapy for Parkinson's Disease." *New England Journal of Medicine* 341: 988–992.

Frith, U., and Hill, E., eds. 2003. *Autism: Mind and Brain.* Oxford: Oxford University Press.

Fukuyama, F. 2002. *Our Posthuman Future.* New York: Farrar, Strauss and Giroux.

Gallagher, S. 2005. *How the Body Shapes the Mind.* New York: Oxford University Press.

Gallagher, S., and Shear, J., eds. 1999. *Models of the Self.* Thorverton, England: Imprint Academic.

García Márquez, G. 1970. *One Hundred Years of Solitude*. Translated by G. Rabassa. New York: Harper and Row.

Garland, B., ed. 2004. *Neuroscience and the Law: Brain, Mind, and the Scales of Justice*. New York: Dana Press.

Gazzaniga, M. 2005. *The Ethical Brain*. New York: Dana Press.

Gazzaniga, M., ed. 2000. *Cognitive Neuroscience: A Reader*. Malden, Mass.: Blackwell.

Gazzaniga, M., and Steven, M. 2004. "Free Will in the Twenty-First Century: A Discussion of Neuroscience and the Law." In Garland, *Neuroscience and the Law*, 51–70.

Geschwind, N. 1979. "Behavioral Change in Temporal Lobe Epilepsy." *Psychological Medicine* 9: 217–219.

Geschwind, N., and Waxman, S. G. 1975. "The Interictal Behavior Syndrome in Temporal Lobe Epilepsy." *Archives of General Psychiatry* 32: 1580–1586.

Giacino, J. T., et al. 2002. "The Minimally Conscious State: Definition and Diagnostic Criteria." *Neurology* 58: 349–353.

Gidron, Y., et al. 2005. "Does the Vagus Nerve Inform the Brain about Preclinical Tumors and Modulate Them?" *Lancet Oncology* 6: 245–248.

Giedd, J. N., et al. 1999. "Brain Development during Childhood and Adolescence: A Longitudinal MRI Study." *Nature Neuroscience* 2: 861–865.

Giles, J. 2004. "Change of Mind." *Nature* 430: 14.

Gill, S., et al. 2005. "Does Memory of a Traumatic Event Increase the Risk for Posttraumatic Stress Disorder in Patients with Traumatic Brain Injury? A Prospective Study." *American Journal of Psychiatry* 162: 963–969.

Gillett, G. 1999. *The Mind and Its Discontents: An Essay in Discursive Psychiatry*. Oxford: Oxford University Press.

Goodman, S. 2003. "France Wires Up to Treat Obsessive Disorder." *Nature* 420: 677.

Gold, P., et al. 2002. "New Insights into the Role of Cortisol and the Glucocorticoid Receptor in Severe Depression." *Biological Psychiatry* 52: 381–385.

Goldberg, E. 2002. *The Executive Brain: Frontal Lobes and the Civilized Mind*. New York: Oxford University Press.

Gordon, P., et al. 2004. "Reaction Time and Movement Time after Embryonic Cell Transplantation in Parkinson's Disease." *Archives of Neurology* 61: 858–861.

Gottesman, I., and Gould, T. 2003. "The Endophenotype Concept in Psychiatry: Etymology and Strategic Intentions." *American Journal of Psychiatry* 160: 1–10.

Gottesman, I., and Shields, J. 1973. "Genetic Theorizing and Schizophrenia." *British Journal of Psychiatry* 122: 15–30.

Gottlieb, S. 2003. "Murderer Can Be Forced to Take Medication to Become Sane Enough to Be Executed." *British Medical Journal* 326: 415.

Grady, D. 2003. "Two Women, Two Deaths, and an Ethical Quandary." *New York Times*, July 15.

Gramm, H. J., et al. 1992. "Acute Endocrine Failure after Brain Death?" *Transplantation* 54: 851–857.

Granqvist, P. 2005. "Sensed Presence and Mystical Experience Are Predicted by Suggestibility, Not by the Application of Transcranial Weak Complex Magnetic Fields." *Neuroscience Letters* 380: 346–347.

Gray, R., et al. 2004. "Long-Term Donepezil Treatment in 565 Patients with Alzheimer's Disease (AD 2000): Randomised Double-Blind Trial." *Lancet* 363: 2105–2115.

Greely, H. 2004. "Prediction, Litigation, Privacy, and Property: Some Possible Legal and Social Implications of Advances in Neuroscience." In Garland, *Neuroscience and the Law*, 114–156.

———. 2005. "The Social Effects of Advances in Neuroscience: Legal Problems, Legal Perspectives." In Illes, *Neuroethics*, chap. 17.

Green, M., and Wikler, D. 1980. "Brain Death and Personal Identity." *Philosophy and Public Affairs* 9: 105–133.

Greene, J. D. 2003. "From Neural 'Is' to Moral 'Ought': What Are the Moral Implications of Neuroscientific Moral Psychology?" *Nature Reviews Neuroscience* 4: 847–850.

Greene, J. D., et al. 2001. "An fMRI Investigation of Emotional Engagement in Moral Judgment." *Science* 293: 2105–2108.

Greene, J. D., et al. 2004. "The Neural Basis of Cognitive Conflict and Control in Moral Judgment." *Neuron* 44: 389–400.

Hairston, I., and Knight, R. 2004. "Sleep on It." *Nature* 430: 27–28.

Hare, R. 1991. *The Hare Psychopathy Checklist*. Toronto: Multi-Health Systems.

———. 1994. *Without Empathy: The Strange World of the Psychopaths among Us*. New York: Pocket Books.

Hariri, A., et al. 2002. "Serotonin Transporter Genetic Variation and the Response of the Human Amygdala." *Science* 297: 400–403.

Harrington, A., ed. 1997. *The Placebo Effect: An Interdisciplinary Exploration*. Cambridge, Mass.: Harvard University Press.

Hart, H. L. A. 1968. *Punishment and Responsibility*. Oxford: Clarendon Press.

Harvard Medical School Ad Hoc Committee. 1968. "A Definition of Irreversible Coma." *Journal of the American Medical Association* 205: 337–340.

Hashimoto, H., et al. 2005. "Does Donepezil Treatment Slow the Progression of Hippocampal Atrophy in Patients with Alzheimer's Disease?" *Archives of General Psychiatry* 161: 676–686.

Healy, D. 1997. *The Antidepressant Era*. Cambridge, Mass.: Harvard University Press.

———. 2002. *The Creation of Psychopharmacology*. Cambridge, Mass.: Harvard University Press.

Heilman, K. 2003. *Clinical Neuropsychology*. 4th ed. New York: Oxford University Press.

Hen, R., et al. 2003. "Requirement of Hippocampal Neurogenesis for the Behavioral Effects of Antidepressants." *Science* 301: 805–809.

Hick, J. 1999. *The Fifth Dimension: An Exploration of the Spiritual Realm*. Oxford: One World.

Hochberg, L. R., et al. (2006). "Neuronal Ensemble Control of Prosethetic Devices by a Human with Tetraplegia," *Nature* 442: 164–171.

Hochedlinger, K., and Jaenisch, R. 2003. "Nuclear Transplantation, Embryonic Stem Cells, and the Potential for Cell Therapy." *New England Journal of Medicine* 349: 275–286.

Hoffman, G., et al. 2005. "Pain and the Placebo: What We Have Learned." *Perspectives in Biology and Medicine* 48: 248–265.

Hoffman, H., et al. 2004. "Virtual Reality May Distract the Brain from Pain." *NeuroReport* 15: 978–989.

Hoffman, R. 2004. "Transcranial Magnetic Stimulation Studies of Schizophrenia and Other Disorders." In Lisanby, *Brain Stimulation in Psychiatric Treatment*, 23–46.

Hoge, C., et al. 2004. "Combat Duty in Iraq and Afghanistan, Mental Health Problems, and Barriers to Care." *New England Journal of Medicine* 351: 13–22.

Holden, C. 2003. "Future Brightening for Depression Treatments." *Science* 302: 810–813.

———. 2003. "Getting the Short End of the Allele." *Science* 301: 291–293.

Huang, Y. Z., et al. 2005. "Theta Burst Stimulation of the Human Motor Cortex." *Neuron* 45: 201–206.

Huber, R., et al. 2004. "Local Sleep and Learning." *Nature* 430: 78–81.

Hucklebridge, F., and Clow, A. 2002. "Neuroimmune Relationships in Perspective." *International Review of Neurobiology* 52: 1–15.

Hugdahl, K. 2001. *Psychophysiology: The Mind-Body Perspective.* Cambridge, Mass.: Harvard University Press.

Hyman, S. 2002. "Neuroscience, Genetics, and the Future of Psychiatric Diagnosis." *Psychopathology* 35: 139–144.

———. 2005. "Addiction: A Disease of Learning and Memory." *American Journal of Psychiatry* 162: 1414–1422.

Hyman, S., and Fenton, W. 2003. "What Are the Right Targets for Psychopharmacology?" *Science* 299: 350–351.

Illes, J., ed. 2005. *Neuroethics: Defining the Issues in Theory, Practice and Policy.* Oxford: Oxford University Press.

Illes, J., and Raffin, T. 2002. "Neuroethics: An Emerging New Discipline in the Study of Brain and Cognition." *Brain and Cognition* 50: 341–344.

Illes, J., et al. 2002. "Ethical and Practical Considerations in Managing Incidental Findings in Functional Magnetic Resonance Imaging." *Brain and Cognition* 50: 358–365.

In re Quinlan. 1976. 70 NJ 10.

Insel, T., and Quirion, R. 2005. "Psychiatry as a Clinical Neuroscience Discipline." *Journal of the American Medical Association* 294: 2221–2224.

Izquierdo, I., and Cammarota, M. 2004. "Zif and the Survival of Memory." *Science* 304: 829–830.

Jackson, M., and Fulford, K. W. M. 1997. "Spiritual Experience and Psychopathology." *Philosophy, Psychiatry, and Psychology* 4: 41–65.

Jakobson Ramin, C. 2004. "In Search of Lost Time." *New York Times Magazine*, December 5, pp. 11–17.

Janeway, C. 1999. *Immunobiology: The Immune System in Health and Disease.* 4th ed. New York: Garland.

Janno, S., et al. 2004. "Prevalence of Neuroleptic-Induced Movement Disorders in Chronic Schizophrenia Inpatients." *American Journal of Psychiatry* 16: 160–163.

Jaworska, A. 1999. "Respecting the Margins of Agency: Alzheimer's Patients and the Capacity to Value." *Philosophy and Public Affairs* 28: 105–138.

Johnston, K. R., and Cosgrove, G. R. 1997. "Psychosurgery: Current Status." In Tindall, *Contemporary Neurosurgery,* 223–257.

Jones, D. A. 2004. *The Soul of the Embryo: An Inquiry into the Status of the Human Embryo in the Christian Tradition.* London: Continuum.

Jonsen, A., Siegler, M., and Winslade, W. 2002. *Clinical Ethics.* 5th ed. New York: McGraw-Hill.

Joseph, R. 1996. *Neuropsychiatry, Neuropsychology, and Clinical Neuroscience.* 2nd ed. Baltimore: Williams and Wilkins.

Kagan, S. 1989. *The Limits of Morality.* Oxford: Oxford University Press.

———. "Me and My Life." *Proceedings of the Aristotelian Society* 94: 309–324.

———. 1998. *Normative Ethics.* Boulder, Colo.: Westview Press.

Kalivas, P., and Volkow, N. 2005. "The Neural Basis of Addiction: A Pathology of Motivation and Choice." *American Journal of Psychiatry* 162: 1403–1413.

Kandel, E. 1998. "A New Intellectual Framework for Psychiatry." *American Journal of Psychiatry* 155: 457–469.

Kandel, E., and Freed, D. 1989. "Frontal Lobe Dysfunction and Antisocial Behavior: A Review." *Journal of Clinical Psychology* 45: 404–413.

Kandel, E., and Squire, L. 2000. "Neuroscience: Breaking Down Scientific Barriers to the Study of the Brain and Mind." *Science* 290: 1113–1120.

Kane, R. 1996. *The Significance of Free Will.* New York: Oxford University Press.

———. 2005. *A Contemporary Introduction to Free Will.* New York: Oxford University Press.

Kaspar, B., et al. 2003. "Retrograde Viral Delivery of IGF-1 Prolongs Survival in a Mouse ALS Model." *Science* 301: 839–843.

Kass, L. 2003. *Beyond Therapy: Biotechnology and the Pursuit of Happiness.* New York: HarperCollins.

Kendler, K. 2005. "Toward a Philosophical Structure for Psychiatry." *American Journal of Psychiatry* 162: 433–440.

Kennedy, D. 2004. "Neuroscience and Neuroethics." *Science* 306: 373.

Kerridge, I., et al. 2002. "Death, Dying, and Donation: Organ Transplantation and the Diagnosis of Death." *Journal of Medical Ethics* 28: 89–94.

Kessler, R., et al. 2005. "Lifetime Prevalence of Age-of-Onset Distributions of DSM-IV Disorders in the National Comorbidity Survey Replication." *Archives of General Psychiatry* 62: 593–602.

Khan, A., et al. 2003. "Suicide Rates in Clinical Trials of SSRIs, Other Antidepressants, and Placebo: Analysis of FDA Reports." *American Journal of Psychiatry* 160: 790–792.

Kiel, K. A., et al. 2001. "Limbic Abnormalities in Affective Processing by Criminal Psychopaths as Revealed by Functional Magnetic Resonance Imaging." *Biological Psychiatry* 50: 677–684.

Kim, B. S., et al. 2002. "Incidental Findings on Pediatric MR Images of the Brain." *American Journal of Neuroradiology* 23: 1674–1677.

Kim, J. 1998. *Mind in a Physical World: An Essay on the Mind-Body Problem.* Cambridge, Mass.: MIT Press.

Kircher, T., and David, A., eds. 2003. *The Self in Neuroscience and Psychiatry.* Cambridge: Cambridge University Press.

Kirsch, I. 2000. "Are Drug and Placebo Effects in Depression Additive?" *Biological Psychiatry* 47: 733–735.

Kleinig, J. 1985. *Ethical Issues in Psychosurgery.* London: Allen and Unwin.

Knight, J. 2004. "The Truth about Lying." *Nature* 428: 692–694.

Koch, C. 2004. *The Quest for Consciousness: A Neurobiological Approach.* Englewood, N.J.: Roberts.

Koller, E., et al. 2003. "Pancreatitis Associated with Atypical Antipsychotics." *Pharmacotherapy* 23: 1123–1130.

Konorski, J. 1948. *Conditioned Reflexes and Neuronal Organization.* Cambridge: Cambridge University Press.

Koran. 1990. Translated by N. J. Dawood. London: Penguin.

Koyama, T., et al. 2005. "The Subjective Experience of Pain: Where Expectations Become Reality." *Proceedings of the National Academy of Sciences* 102: 12950–12955.

Krack, P., et al. 2003. "Five-Year Follow-Up of Bilateral Stimulation of the Subthalamic Nucleus in Advanced Parkinson's Disease." *New England Journal of Medicine* 349: 1925–1934.

Kramer, P. 1993. *Listening to Prozac: A Psychiatrist Explores Antidepressant Drugs and the Remaking of Self.* New York: Penguin.

———. 2005. *Against Depression.* New York: Viking.

Kronfol, Z., and Remick, D. 2000. "Cytokines and the Brain: Implications for Clinical Psychiatry." *American Journal of Psychiatry* 157: 683–693.

Kulynych, J. 2002. "Legal and Ethical Issues in Neuroimaging Research: Human Subjects Protection, Medical Privacy, and the Public Communication of Research Results." *Brain and Cognition* 50: 345–357.

LaBar, K. S., et al. 1995. "Impaired Fear Conditioning Following Unilateral Temporal Lobectomy on Humans." *Journal of Neuroscience* 15: 6846–6855.

Lakoff, G., and Johnson, M. 1999. *Philosophy in the Flesh.* New York: Basic Books.

Lane, R., and Nadel, L., eds. 2002. *Cognitive Neuroscience of Emotion*. New York: Oxford University Press.

Langleben, D., et al. 2002. "Brain Activity during Simulated Deception: An Event-Related Functional Magnetic Resonance Study." *Neuroimage* 15: 727–732.

LaRoche, S. M., and Helmers, S. L. 2004. "The New Antiepileptic Drugs." *Journal of the American Medical Association* 291: 605–614.

Launer, L. 2003. "Nonsteroidal Anti-inflammatory Drugs and Alzheimer's Disease: What's Next?" *Journal of the American Medical Association* 289: 2865–2867.

Laureys, S. 2005. "Death, Unconsciousness, and the Brain." *Nature Reviews Neuroscience* 6: 789.

Laureys, S., et al. 2004. "Brain Function in Coma, Vegetative State, and Related Disorders." *Lancet Neurology* 3: 537–546.

Laureys, S., et al. 2005. "Quantifying Consciousness." *Lancet Neurology* 4: 789–790.

Laureys, S., et al. 2006. "Tracking the Recovery of Consciousness from Coma." *Journal of Clinical Investigation* 116 (2006): 1823–1825.

Lebacz, K., et al., eds. 2001. *The Human Embryonic Stem Cell Debate*. Cambridge, Mass.: MIT Press.

LeDoux, J. 1996. *The Emotional Brain*. New York: Simon and Schuster.

———. 2002. *The Synaptic Self: How Our Brains Become Who We Are*. New York: Viking.

Lee, J. L. C., et al. 2004. "Independent Cellular Processes for Hippocampal Memory Consolidation and Reconsolidation." *Science* 304: 839–843.

Lee, J. L. C., et al. 2005. "Disrupting Reconsolidation of Drug Memories Reduces Cocaine-Seeking Behavior." *Neuron* 47: 795–801.

Leuchter, A., et al. 2002. "Changes in Brain Function of Depressed Subjects during Treatment with Placebo." *American Journal of Psychiatry* 159: 122–129.

Lewontin, R. 2000. *The Triple Helix: Gene, Organism, and Environment*. Cambridge, Mass.: Harvard University Press.

Libet, B., et al. 1983. "Time of Conscious Intention to Act in Relation to Onset of Cerebral Activity (Readiness Potential)." *Brain* 106: 623–642.

Libet, B. 1985. "Unconscious Cerebral Initiative of Conscious Will in Voluntary Action." *Behavioral and Brain Sciences* 8: 529–566.

———. 1999. "Do We Have Free Will?" *Journal of Consciousness Studies* 6: 47–57.

———. 2004. *Mind Time: The Temporal Factor in Consciousness*. Cambridge, Mass.: Harvard University Press.

Lieberman, J., et al. 2005. "Effectiveness of Antipsychotic Drugs in Patients with Chronic Schizophrenia." *New England Journal of Medicine* 353: 1209–1223.

Lisanby, S. H., ed. 2004. *Brain Stimulation in Psychiatric Treatment*. Washington, D. C.: American Psychiatric.

Lisman, J., and Fallon, J. 1999. "What Maintains Memories?" *Science* 283: 339–340.

Luria, A. R. 1969. *The Mind of a Mnemonist*. London: Cape.

Lynch, G. 2002. "Memory Enhancement: The Search for Mechanism-Based Drugs." *Nature Neuroscience* 5: 1035–1038.

Macklin, R. 1999. "The Ethical Problems with Sham Surgery in Clinical Research." *New England Journal of Medicine* 341: 992–996.

Mahli, G. S., et al. 2000. "Depression: A Role for Neurosurgery?" *British Journal of Neurosurgery* 14: 415–422.

Mahowald, M. 2003. "Reflections on the Human Embryonic Stem Cell Debate." *Perspectives in Biology and Medicine* 46: 131–141.

Mamourian, A. 2004. "Incidental Findings on Research Functional MR Images: Should We Look?" *American Journal of Neuroradiology* 25: 520–522.

Maquet, P. 2000. "Sleep on It!" *Nature Neuroscience* 3: 1235–1236.

Marcus, S., ed. 2002. *Neuroethics: Mapping the Field*. New York: Dana Press.

Martyn, C. 2003. "Anti-inflammatory Drugs and Alzheimer's Disease: Evidence Implying a Protective Effect Is as yet Tentative." *British Medical Journal* 327: 353–354.

Matthews, K., and Eljamel, M. 2003. "Status of Neurosurgery for Mental Disorder in Scotland." *British Journal of Psychiatry* 56: 404–411.

Maviel, T., et al. 2004. "Sites of Neocortical Reorganization Critical for Remote Spatial Memory." *Science* 305: 96–99.

Mayberg, H., et al. 2004. "Modulation of Cortical-Limbic Pathways in Major Depression: Treatment-Specific Effects of Cognitive Behavior Therapy." *Archives of General Psychiatry* 61: 34–41.

Mayberg, H., et al. 2005. "Deep-Brain Stimulation for Treatment-Resistant Depression." *Neuron* 45: 651–660.

McClure, S., et al. 2004. "Neural Correlates of Behavioral Preferences for Culturally Familiar Drinks." *Neuron* 44: 379–387.

McCullough, L. B., et al., eds. 1998. *Surgical Ethics*. New York: Oxford University Press.

McEwen, B. 1998. "Protective and Damaging Effects of Stress Mediators." *New England Journal of Medicine* 338: 171–179.

McGaugh, J. 2002. Testimony before U. S. President's Council on Bioethics. Seventh meeting, October 17, session 3, "Remembering and Forgetting: Physiological and Pharmacological Aspects." Transcript. Available at the countil website: www.bioethics .gov/transcripts/octo2/session3/html.

———. 2003. *Memory and Emotion: The Making of Lasting Memories*. New York: Columbia University Press.

McGinn, C. 1991. *The Problem of Consciousness*. Oxford: Blackwell.

———. 1999. *The Mysterious Flame: Conscious Minds in a Material World*. New York: Basic Books.

McGlashan, T., et al. 2006. "Randomized Controlled Double-Blind Trial of Olanzapine versus Placebo in Patients Prodromally Symptomatic for Psychoses." *American Journal of Psychiatry* 163: 790–797.

McMahan, J. 1995. "The Metaphysics of Brain Death." *Bioethics* 9: 91–126.

———. 2002. *The Ethics of Killing: Problems at the Margins of Life*. New York: Oxford University Press.

Mele, A. 2005. *Motivation and Agency*. New York: Oxford University Press.

———. 2006. *Free Will and Luck*. New York: Oxford University Press.

Melton, L. 2000. "Neural Transplantation: New Cells for Old Brains." *Lancet* 355: 2142–2143.

Melzack, R., and Wall, P. 1996. *Textbook of Pain*. 2nd ed. London: Methuen.

Merikangas, K. R., and Risch, N. 2003. "Will the Genetics Revolution Revolutionize Psychiatry?" *American Journal of Psychiatry* 160: 625–635.

Milev, P., et al. 2003. "Initial Magnetic Resonance Imaging Volumetric Brain Measurements and Outcomes in Schizophrenia: A Prospective Longitudinal Study with a 5-Year Follow-Up." *Biological Psychiatry* 54: 608–615.

Miller, B., and Hou, C. 2004. "Portraits of Artists: Emergence of Visual Creativity in Dementia." *Archives of Neurology* 61: 842–844.

Miller, B., et al. 2000. "Brain Damage and Compulsive Artistic Interest." *British Journal of Psychiatry* 176: 458–463.

Miller, C., and Marshall, J. 2005. "Molecular Substrates for Retrieval and Reconsolidation of Cocaine-Associated Contextual Memory." *Neuron* 47: 873–884.

Miller, F. 2004. "Painful Deception." *Science* 304: 1109–1110.

———. 2004. "Sham Surgery: An Ethical Analysis." *American Journal of Bioethics* 3: 25–35.

Miller, F. G., and Fins, J. J. 1999. "Protecting Vulnerable Research Subjects without Unduly Constraining Neuropsychiatric Research." *Archives of General Psychiatry* 56: 701–702.

Miller, G. 2004. "Learning to Forget." *Science* 302: 34–36.

Mindus, P., and Nyman, H. 1991. "Normalization of Personality Characteristics in Patients with Incapacitation Anxiety Disorder after Capsulotomy." *Acta Psychiatrica Scandinavica* 83: 283–291.

Mindus, P., et al. 1994. "Neurosurgical Treatment of Refractory Obsessive-Compulsive Disorder: Implications for Understanding Frontal Lobe Function." *Journal of Neuropsychiatry* 6: 467–477.

M'Naghten Rules. 1843. 8 Eng. Rep. 718,722. London: Her Majesty's Stationery Office.

Model Penal Code. 1985. Official draft and revised commentaries. Philadelphia: American Law Institute.

Morse, S. 2004. "New Neuroscience, Old Problems." In Garland, *Neuroscience and the Law*, 157–198.

Muller, U., et al. 2005. "Lack of Effects of Guanfacine on Executive and Memory Functions in Healthy Male Volunteers." *Psychopharmacology* 182: 205–213.

Multi-Society Task Force on the Persistent Vegetative State. 1994. "Medical Aspects of the Persistent Vegetative State." *New England Journal of Medicine* 330: 1499–1508.

Musallam, S., et al. 2004. "Cognitive Control Signals for Neural Prosthetics." *Science* 305: 258–262.

Nader, K., et al. 2000. "Fear Memories Require Protein Synthesis in the Amygdala for Reconsolidation after Retrieval." *Nature* 406: 722–726.

Nagel, T. 1970. *The Possibility of Altruism.* Princeton: Princeton University Press.

———. 1987. *The View from Nowhere.* New York: Oxford University Press.

National Research Council. 2003. *The Polygraph Lie Detector.* Washington, D.C.: National Academies Press.

Nesse, R. 2000. "Is Depression an Adaptation?" *Archives of General Psychiatry* 57: 14–20.

New, A. S., et al. 2002. "Blunted Prefrontal Cortical 18Fluorodeoxyglucose Positron Emission Tomography Response to Meta-chlorophenylpiperazine in Impulsive Aggression." *Archives of General Psychiatry* 59: 621–629.

Newberg, A., et al. 2001. *Why God Won't Go Away: Brain Science and the Biology of Belief.* New York: Ballantine Books.

Nicolelis, M. 2003. "Brain-Machine Interfaces to Restore Motor Function and Probe Neural Circuits." *Nature Reviews Neuroscience* 4: 417–422.

Nicolelis, M., et al. 2000. "Real-Time Prediction of Hand Trajectory by Ensembles of Cortical Neurons in Primates." *Nature* 408: 361–365.

Nicolelis, M., et al. 2004. "Local Forebrain Dynamics Predict Rat Behavioral States and Their Transitions." *Journal of Neuroscience* 49: 11137–11147.

Nolte, J. 2002. *The Human Brain: An Introduction to Its Functional Anatomy.* 5th ed. St. Louis: Mosby.

Northoff, G., and Heinzel, A. 2003. "The Self in Philosophy, Neuroscience, and Psychiatry: An Epistemic Approach." In Kircher and David, *The Self in Neuroscience and Psychiatry*, 40–55.

Nuttin, B., et al. 1999. "Electrical Stimulation in Anterior Limbs of Internal Capsules in Patients with Obsessive-Compulsive Disorder." *Lancet* 354: 1526.

Nuttin, B., et al. 2002. "Deep-Brain Stimulation for Psychiatric Disorders." *Neurosurgery* 51: 519.

Oderberg, D. 1997. "Modal Properties, Moral Status, and Identity." *Philosophy and Public Affairs* 15: 259–298.

Olanow, W., et al. 2003. "A Double-Blind Controlled Trial of Bilateral Fetal Nigral Transplantation in Parkinson's Disease." *Annals of Neurology* 54: 403–414.

Olson, E. 1997. *The Human Animal: Personal Identity without Psychology.* Oxford: Oxford University Press.

Olson, S. 2005. "Brain Scans Raise Privacy Concerns." *Science* 307: 1548–1550.

Onitsuka, T., et al. 2004. "Middle and Inferior Temporal Gyrus Gray Matter Volume Abnormalities in Chronic Schizophrenia: An MRI Study." *American Journal of Psychiatry* 161: 1603–1611.

Ortinski, P., and Meador, K. 2004. "Neuronal Mechanisms of Conscious Awareness." *Archives of Neurology* 61: 1017–1029.

Panksepp, J. 1998. *Affective Neuroscience.* New York: Oxford University Press.

———. 2003. "Feeling the Pain of Social Loss." *Science* 302: 237–239.

Pantelis, C., et al. 2003. "Neuroanatomical Abnormalities before and after Onset of Psychoses: A Cross-sectional and Longitudinal MRI Comparison." *Lancet* 361: 281–288.

Parens, E., et al. 2004. "Genetic Differences and Human Identities: On Why Talking about Behavioral Genetics Is Important and Difficult." Special supplement to the *Hastings Center Report* 34 (January–February): S1–S35.

Parens, E., ed. 1998. *Enhancing Human Traits: Ethical and Social Implications.* Washington, D.C.: Georgetown University Press, 1998.

Parfit, D. 1984. *Reasons and Persons.* Oxford: Clarendon Press.

Pascual-Leone, A., et al. 2002. *Handbook of Transcranial Magnetic Stimulation.* London: Edward Arnold.

Paul, E. F., et al., eds. 2002. *Bioethics.* New York: Cambridge University Press.

Paulus, W. 2005. "Improved Recipe for Magnetic Brain Stimulation." *Neuron* 45: 181–183.

Penfield, W. 1969. "Consciousness, Memory, and Man's Conditioned Reflexes." In Pribram, *On the Biology of Learning,* 158–168.

———. 1975. *The Mystery of the Mind: A Critical Study of Consciousness and the Human Brain.* Princeton: Princeton University Press.

Persinger, M. 2001. "The Neuropsychiatry of Paranormal Experiences." *Journal of Neuropsychiatry and Clinical Neuroscience* 13: 515–524.

Persinger, M., et al. 1996. "Enhanced Hypnotic Suggestibility Following Application of Burst-Firing Magnetic Fields over the Right Temporoparietal Lobes: A Replication." *International Journal of Neuroscience* 87: 210–207.

Persson, I. 2002. "Human Death—A View from the Beginning of Life." *Bioethics* 16: 20–32.

Piasecki, S. D., and Jefferson, J. W. 2004. "Psychiatric Complications of Deep-Brain Stimulation for Parkinson's Disease." *Journal of Clinical Psychiatry* 65: 845–849.

Pittman, R. K., et al. 2002. "Pilot Study of Secondary Prevention of Posttraumatic Stress Disorder with Propranolol." *Biological Psychiatry* 51: 189–192.

Plato. 1980. *Phaedo, Phaedrus, Republic,* and *Timaeus.* In *Plato: The Collected Dialogues,* edited by E. Hamilton and H. Cairns. Princeton: Princeton University Press.

Platt, M. L. 2003. "Neural Correlates of Decisions." *Current Opinion in Neurobiology* 13: 141–148.

Platt, M. L., and Glimcher, P. W. 1999. "Neural Correlates of Decision Variables in Parietal Cortex." *Nature* 400: 233–238.

Pollack, A. 2004. "With Tiny Brain Implants, Just Thinking May Make It So." *New York Times,* April 30.

Popper, K., and Eccles, J. 1977. *The Self and Its Brain.* New York: Springer-Verlag.

President's Commission for the Study of Ethical Problems in Medicine and Biomedical and Behavioral Research. 1981. *Defining Death*. Washington, D.C.: U.S. Government Printing Office.

President's Council on Bioethics. 2002. "Remembering and Forgetting: Physiological and Pharmacological Aspects." October 17. Available online at the council's website: www.bioethics.gov/transcripts/octo2/session3.html.

———. 2003. "Better Memories? The Promise and Perils of Pharmacological Intervention." Staff Working Paper. Available online at the council's website: www.bioethics.gov/transcripts/maro3.html.

Pressman, J. D. 1998. *Last Resort: Psychosurgery and the Limits of Medicine*. Cambridge: Cambridge University Press.

Pribram, K., ed. 1969. *On the Biology of Learning*. New York: Harcourt Brace.

Price, D., and Fields, H. 1997. "The Contribution of Desire and Expectation to Placebo Analgesia: Implications for New Research Strategies." In Harrington, *The Placebo Effect*, 117–137.

———. 1997. "Toward a Neurobiology of Placebo Analgesia." In Harrington, *The Placebo Effect*, 93–116.

Rachels, J. 1986. *The End of Life: Euthanasia and Morality*. Oxford: Oxford University Press.

Raine, A., et al. 2000. "Reduced Prefrontal Gray Matter Volume and Reduced Autonomic Activity in Antisocial Personality Disorder." *Archives of General Psychiatry* 58: 119–127.

Raison, C., and Miller, A. 2003. "When Not Enough Is Too Much: The Role of Insufficient Glucocorticoid Signaling in the Pathophysiology of Stress-Related Disorders." *American Journal of Psychiatry* 160: 1554–1565.

Ramachandran, V. S. 2003. "Neuroscience—The New Philosophy." Lecture 5 in *Reith Lectures: The Emerging Mind*, BBC Radio 4, April 30. Available at the website of the BBC: www.bbc.co.uk/radio4/reith2003/lecture5/transcript/html.

Rascol, O., et al. 2005. "Rasagaline as an Adjunct to Levodopa in Patients with Parkinson's Disease and Motor Fluctuations: A Randomized, Double-Blind, Parallel-Group Trial." *Lancet* 365: 947–954.

Rea, T., et al. 2005. "Statins and the Risk of Incident Dementia." *Archives of Neurology* 62: 1047–1051.

Redish, D. 2004. "Addiction as a Computational Process Gone Awry." *Science* 306: 1944–1947.

Rees, D., and Rose, S., eds. 2004. *The New Brain Sciences: Perils and Prospects*. Cambridge: Cambridge University Press.

Richardson, M. P., et al. 2004. "Encoding of Emotional Memories Depends on Amygdala and Hippocampus and Their Interactions." *Nature Neuroscience* 7: 278–285.

Ridderinkhof, K. R., et al. 2004. "The Role of the Medial Frontal Cortex in Cognitive Control." *Science* 306: 443–447.

Rinpoche, S. 1993. *The Tibetan Book of Living and Dying*. New York: HarperCollins.

Rizzolatti, G. 2001. "Neurophysiological Mechanisms Underlying the Understanding and Imitation of Action." *Nature Reviews Neuroscience* 2: 661–670.

Robertson, J. 1999. "The Dead Donor Rule." *Hastings Center Report* 29 (November–December): 6–14.

Rohan, M., et al. 2004. "Low-Field Magnetic Stimulation in Bipolar Disorder Using an MRI-Based Stimulator." *American Journal of Psychiatry* 161: 93–98.

Roper v. Simmons. 2005. 543 U.S. 633.

Rose, S. 2002. "'Smart Drugs': Do They Work? Are They Ethical? Will They Be Legal?" *Nature Reviews Neuroscience* 3: 975–979.

————. 2005. *The Future of the Brain: The Promise and Perils of Tomorrow's Neuroscience.* Oxford: Oxford University Press.

————. 2005. *The Twenty-First-Century Brain: Explaining, Mending, and Manipulating the Mind.* London: Cape.

Rosenberg, R. 2004. "Positive Potential of Fetal Nigral Implants for Parkinson's Disease." *Archives of Neurology* 61 (2004): 837–838.

Roskies, A. 2002. "Neuroethics for the New Millennium." *Neuron* 35: 21–23.

Royal College of Psychiatrists. 2000. *Neurosurgery for Mental Disorder: Report from the Neurosurgery Working Group of the Royal College of Psychiatrists.* London: Royal College of Psychiatrists.

Rush, A. J., et al. 2002. "Vagus Nerve Stimulation for Treatment-Resistant Depression: A Multicenter Study." *Biological Psychiatry* 47: 276–285.

Sachedina, A. 2005. "End-of-Life: The Islamic View." *Lancet* 366: 774–779.

Sackeim, H. A. 2004. "Vagus Nerve Stimulation." In Lisanby, *Brain Stimulation in Psychiatric Treatment,* 99–136.

Sackeim, H. A., et al. 2001. "Vagus Nerve Stimulation (VNS) for Treatment-Resistant Depression: Efficacy, Side Effects, and Predictors of Outcome." *Neuropsychopharmacology* 25: 713–728.

Salzman, M. 2000. *Lying Awake.* New York: Vintage Books.

Sapolsky, R. 1992. *Stress, the Aging Brain, and the Mechanisms of Neuron Death.* Cambridge, Mass.: MIT Press.

————. 2003. "Gene Therapy for Psychiatric Disorders." *American Journal of Psychiatry* 160: 208–220.

Sapolsky, R., et al. 1987. "Interleukin-1 Stimulates the Secretion of Hypothalamic Corticotropin Releasing Factor." *Science* 238: 522–524.

Schacter, D. 1996. *Searching for Memory: The Brain, the Mind, and the Past.* New York: Basic Books.

————. 2002. Testimony before the U. S. President's Council on Bioethics. Seventh meeting, October 17, session 4, "Remembering and Forgetting: Psychological Aspects." Transcript. Available at the council website: www.bioethics.gov/transcripts/oct02/session4/html.

Schacter, D., and Scarry, E., eds. 2000. *Memory, Brain, and Belief.* Cambridge, Mass.: Harvard University Press.

Schacter, D., and Tulving, E., eds. 1994. *Memory Systems.* Cambridge, Mass.: MIT Press.

Schall, J. D. 2003. "Neural Correlates of Decision Processes." *Current Opinion in Neurobiology* 13: 182–186.

Schatzberg, A., and Nemeroff, C., eds. 2004. *Textbook of Psychopharmacology.* 3rd ed. Washington, D. C.: American Psychiatric.

Schechtman, M. 1997. "The Brain/Body Problem." *Philosophical Psychology* 10: 149–163.

————. 1997. *The Constitution of Selves.* Ithaca: Cornell University Press.

Schiff, N., and Fins, J. 2003. "New Hope for 'Comatose' Patients." *Cerebrum* 5: 7–24.

Schiff, N., et al. 2005. "fMRI Reveals Large-Scale Network Activation in Minimally Conscious Patients." *Neurology* 64: 514–523.

Schindler v. Schiavo. 2003. 851 So. 2d 182 Fla. Dist. Ct. App.

Schlaepfer, T., and Kosel, M. 2004. "Transcranial Magnetic Stimulation in Depression." In Lisanby, *Brain Stimulation in Psychiatric Treatment,* 1–16.

Schneider, C. 2005. "Hard Cases and the Politics of Righteousness." *Hastings Center Report* 35 (May–June): 24–27.

Scott, A. 1995. *Stairway to the Mind: The Controversial New Science of Consciousness.* New York: Springer-Verlag.

Scott, R., et al. 2002. "CREB and the Discovery of Cognitive Enhancers." *Journal of Molecular Neuroscience* 19: 171–177.

Searle, J. 1992. *The Rediscovery of the Mind*. Cambridge, Mass.: MIT Press.

———. 1999. *Mind, Language and Society: Doing Philosophy in the Real World*. London: Weidenfeld and Nicolson.

———. 2001. "Free Will as a Problem in Neurobiology." *Philosophy* 76: 491–514.

Seltzer, B., et al. 2004. "Efficacy of Donepezil in Early-Stage Alzheimer Disease." *Archives of Neurology* 61: 1852–1856.

Selye, H. 1950. *The Physiology and Pathology of Exposure to Stress*. Montreal: Acta.

———. 1956. *The Stress of Life*. New York: McGraw-Hill.

Seminowicz, D. A. 2006. "Believe in Your Placebo." *Journal of Neuroscience* 26: 4453–4454.

Shapiro, A., and Shapiro, E. 1997. "The Placebo: Is It Much Ado about Nothing?" In Harrington, *The Placebo Effect*, 12–36.

Shewmon, D. A. 1997. "Recovery from 'Brain Death': A Neurologist's Apologia." *Linacre Quarterly* 64: 30–96.

———. 1998. "Brain Stem Death, Brain Death, and Death: A Critical Evaluation of the Purported Equivalence." *Issues in Law and Medicine* 14: 125–145.

———. 1998. "Chronic 'Brain Death': Meta-analysis and Conceptual Consequences." *Neurology* 51: 1538–1545.

———. 2001. "The Brain and Somatic Integration: Insights into the Standard Biological Rationale for Equating 'Brain Death' with Death." *Journal of Medicine and Philosophy* 26: 457–478.

Shumyatsky, G. P., et al. 2005. "Strathmin, A Gene Enriched in the Amygdala, Controls Both Learned and Innate Fear." *Cell* 123: 697–709.

Siegel, J. M. 2001. "The REM Sleep-Memory Consolidation Hypothesis." *Science* 294: 1058–1063.

Simon, G., et al. 2006. "Suicide Risk during Antidepressant Treatment." *American Journal of Psychiatry* 163: 41–47.

Singer, P. 1995. *Rethinking Life and Death*. New York: St. Martin's Press.

Smith, H. 1991. *The World's Religions*. San Francisco: HarperCollins.

Sowell, E., et al. 2003. "Cortical Abnormalities in Children and Adolescents with Attention-Deficit Hyperactivity Disorder." *Lancet* 362: 1699–1706.

Spence, S. 1996. "Free Will in the Light of Neuropsychiatry." *Philosophy, Psychiatry, and Psychology* 3: 75–100.

Sperry, R. 1966. "Brain Bisection and the Mechanisms of Consciousness." In Eccles, *Brain and Conscious Experience*, 298–313.

Spiro, H. 1998. *The Power of Hope*. New Haven: Yale University Press.

Spong, A. L., et al. 2003. "Progressive Brain Volume Loss during Adolescence in Childhood-Onset Schizophrenia." *American Journal of Psychiatry* 160: 2181–2189.

Squire, L. 1994. "Declarative and Nondeclarative Memory: Multiple Brain Systems Support Learning and Memory." In Schacter and Tulving, *Memory Systems*, 203–232.

Stagno, S., et al. 1994. "Reconsidering 'Psychosurgery': Issues of Informed Consent and Physician Responsibility." *Journal of Clinical Ethics* 5: 217–223.

Stahl, S. M. 2003. "Neurotransmission of Cognition." Pt. 2. "Selective NRIs Are Smart Drugs: Exploiting Regionally Selective Actions on Both Dopamine and Norepinephrine to Enhance Cognition." *Journal of Clinical Psychiatry* 64: 110–111.

Starson v. Swayze. 2003. Supreme Court of Canada, 32.

Steinbock, B. 1992. *Life before Birth: The Moral and Legal Status of Embryos and Fetuses*. New York: Oxford University Press.

Sternberg, E., et al. 1992. "The Stress Response and the Regulation of Inflammatory Disease." *Annals of Internal Medicine* 117: 854–866.

Steven, M., and Pascual-Leone, A. 2005. "Transcranial Magnetic Stimulation and the Human Brain: An Ethical Analysis." In Illes, *Neuroethics*, chap. 14.

Stickgold, R., and Walker, M. P. 2005. "Memory Consolidation and Reconsolidation: What's the Role of Sleep?" *Trends in Neuroscience* 28: 408–415.

Stickgold, R., et al. 2000. "Visual Discrimination Learning Requires Sleep after Training." *Nature Neuroscience* 3: 1237–1238.

Stock, G. 2004. "If the Goal Is Relief, What's Wrong with a Placebo?" *American Journal of Bioethics* 4: 50–51.

Stoessl, A. J., et al. 2001. "Expectation and Dopamine Release: Mechanisms of the Placebo Effect in Parkinson's Disease." *Science* 293: 1164–1166.

Strange, B., et al. 2003. "An Emotion-Induced Retrograde Amnesia in Humans Is Amygdala- and Beta-Adrenergic Dependent." *Proceedings of the National Academy of Sciences* 100: 13626–13631.

Strawson, G. 1986. *Freedom and Belief*. Oxford: Clarendon Press.

———. 1999. "The Self." In Gallagher and Shear, *Models of the Self*, 1–24.

Swinburne, R. 1996. *Is There a God?* Oxford: Oxford University Press.

Tancredi, L. 2004. "Neuroscience Developments and the Law." In Garland, *Neuroscience and the Law*, 71–113.

———. 2005. *Hardwired Behavior: What Neuroscience Reveals about Morality*. New York: Cambridge University Press.

Taylor, C. 1995. *Sources of the Self*. Cambridge, Mass.: Harvard University Press.

Thompson, P. M., et al. 2001. "Mapping Adolescent Brain Change Reveals Dynamic Wave of Accelerated Gray Matter Loss in Very Early-Onset Schizophrenia." *Proceedings of the National Academy of Sciences* 98: 11650–11655.

Thompson, R. 1985. *The Brain: An Introduction to Neuroscience*. New York: Freeman.

Tibetan Book of the Dead. 1960. Translated and edited by W. Y. Evans-Wentz. Oxford: Oxford University Press.

Tindall, G. T., ed. 1997. *Contemporary Neurosurgery*. Baltimore: Williams and Wilkins.

Tooley, M. 1983. *Abortion and Infanticide*. Oxford: Clarendon Press.

Trivedi, M., et al. 2006. "Evaluation of Outcomes with Citalopram for Depression Using Measurement-Based Care in STAR*D: Implications for Clinical Practice." *American Journal of Psychiatry* 163: 28–40.

Truog, R. 1997. "Is It Time to Abandon Brain Death?" *Hastings Center Report* 27 (January–February): 29–37.

Truog, R., and Robinson, W. 2003. "The Role of Brain Death and the Dead Donor Rule in the Ethics of Organ Transplantation." *Critical Care Medicine* 31: 2391–2396.

Tsuang, M. T., et al. 1993. "Identification of the Phenotype in Psychiatric Genetics." *European Archives of Psychiatry and Clinical Neuroscience* 243: 131–142.

Tully, T., et al. 2003. "Targeting the CREB Pathway for Memory Enhancers." *Nature Reviews Drug Discovery* 2: 267–277.

Tulving, E. 2002. "Episodic Memory: From Mind to Brain." *Annual Review of Psychology* 53: 27–51.

Tulving, E., and Lepage, M. 2000. "Where in the Brain Is the Awareness of One's Past?" In Schacter and Scarry, *Memory, Brain, and Belief*, 208–228.

Turner, D. 2003. "Clinical Prospects for Neural Grafting Therapy for Hippocampal Lesions and Epilepsy." *Neurosurgery* 52: 632–644.

Turner, D. C., et al. 2003. "Cognitive Enhancing Effects of Modafinil in Healthy Volunteers." *Psychopharmacology* 165: 260–269.

Unger, P. 1990. *Identity, Consciousness, and Value*. New York: Oxford University Press.

United States v. Sell. 2003. 539 U. S. 166.

Van Inwagen, P. 1983. *An Essay on Free Will*. Oxford: Clarendon Press.

Varley, C. 2003. "Psychopharmacological Treatment of Major Depressive Disorder in Children and Adolescents." *Journal of the American Medical Association* 290: 1091–1093.

Vastag, B. 2004. "Poised to Challenge Need for Sleep, 'Wakefulness Enhancer' Rouses Concerns." *Journal of the American Medical Association* 291: 167–170.

Veatch, R. 1992. *Death, Dying, and the Biological Revolution*. 2nd ed. New Haven: Yale University Press.

———. 1993. "The Impending Collapse of the Whole-Brain Definition of Death." *Hastings Center Report* 23 (July–August): 18–24.

———. 2003. "The Dead Donor Rule: True by Definition." *American Journal of Bioethics* 3: 10–11.

———. 2005. "The Death of Whole-Brain Death: The Plague of the Disaggregators, Somaticists, and Mentalists." *Journal of Medicine and Philosophy* 30: 353–378.

Viding, E., et al. 2005. "Evidence for Substantial Genetic Risk for Psychopathy in 7-Year-Olds." *Journal of Child Psychology and Psychiatry* 46: 592–597.

Volkmar, F., and Pauls, D. 2003. "Autism." *Lancet* 326: 1133–1141.

Voss, H. U., et al. (2006). "Possible Axonal Regrowth in Late Recovery from the Minimally Conscious State." *Journal of Clinical Investigation* 116: 2005–2011.

Wager, T., et al. 2004. "Placebo-Induced Changes in fMRI in the Anticipation and Experience of Pain." *Science* 303: 1162–1167.

Walsh, M.-T., and Dinan, T. G. 2001. "Selective Serotonin Reuptake Inhibitors and Violence: A Review of the Available Evidence." *Acta Psychiatrica Scandinavica* 104: 84–91.

Walter, H. 2001. *Neurophilosophy of Free Will*. Translated by C. Klohr. Cambridge, Mass.: MIT Press.

Wegner, D. 2002. *The Illusion of Conscious Will*. Cambridge, Mass.: MIT Press.

Weinshilboum, R. 2003. "Inheritance and Drug Response." *New England Journal of Medicine* 348: 529–537.

Whitehouse, P., et al. 1997. "Enhancing Cognition in the Intellectually Intact." *Hastings Center Report* 27 (May–June): 14–22.

Wickelgren, I. 2003. "Tapping the Mind." *Science* 299: 496–499.

Wiebe, S. 2003. "Brain Surgery for Epilepsy." *Lancet: Extreme Medicine* 362: s48.

Wiebe, S., et al. 2001. "A Randomized Controlled Trial of Surgery for Temporal-Lobe Epilepsy." *New England Journal of Medicine* 345: 311–318.

Wiggins, D. 1980. *Sameness and Substance*. Oxford: Blackwell.

Wiggins, S., et al. 1992. "The Psychological Consequences of Predictive Testing for Huntington's Disease: Canadian Collaborative Study of Predictive Testing." *New England Journal of Medicine* 327: 1401–1405.

Wijdicks, E. F. M. 1995. "Determining Brain Death in Adults." *Neurology* 45: 1003–1011.

———. 2001. "The Diagnosis of Brain Death." *New England Journal of Medicine* 344: 1215–1221.

———, ed. 2000. *Brain Death*. Philadelphia: Lippincott, Williams, and Wilkins.

Wolfson, J. 2005. "Erring on the Side of Theresa Schiavo: Reflections of the Special Guardian *ad Litem*." *Hastings Center Report* 35 (May–June): 16–19.

Wolpe, P. R. 2005. "Religious Responses to Neuroscientific Questions." In Illes, *Neuroethics*, chap. 20.

Wolpe, P. R., et al. 2005. "Emerging Neurotechnologies for Lie Detection: Promises and Perils." *American Journal of Bioethics* 5: 15–26.

World Health Organization World Mental Health Survey Consortium. 2004. "Prevalence, Severity, and Unmet Need for Treatment of Mental Disorders in the World Health Organization World Mental Health Surveys." *Journal of the American Medical Association* 291: 2581–2590.

Yesavage, J. A., et al. 2002. "Donepezil and Flight Simulator Performance: Effects on Retention of Complex Skills." *Neurology* 59: 123–125.

Youngner, S., and Arnold, R. 2001. "Philosophical Debates about the Definition of Death: Who Cares?" *Journal of Medicine and Philosophy* 26: 527–537.

Youngner, S., et al. 1999. "When Is Dead?" *Hastings Center Report* 29 (January–February): 14–21.

Youngner, S., et al., eds. 2002. *The Definition of Death: Contemporary Controversies.* Baltimore: Johns Hopkins University Press.

Zahavi, D. 2003. "Phenomenology of Self." In Kircher and David, *The Self in Neuroscience and Psychiatry*, 56–75.

Index

Acetylcholine, 14
  in memory and Alzheimer's, 15–16, 68
  in schizophrenia, 50
Actions
  decisive reasons for or against, 4–5
  as distinct from intentions (in BCIs),
    142–143
  as obligated, 4–5, 71–74, 129, 173
  as permissible, 4–5, 170–171
  as prohibited, 4–5, 168, 172
Addiction
  brain regions involved in (mesolimbic
    dopamine system), 90
  dopamine and opiate antagonists for, 90
  environmental and psychosocial factors
    in, 91
  vaccines for, 90
Adrenaline (epinephrine)
  in pathological emotional memory and
    PTSD, 31, 84–86
  in the stress and "fight-or-flight"
    responses, 19–21, 84
Adrenocorticotropin hormone (ACTH),
  in the stress response, 20–21, 22
    (fig. 5.2), 30
Agnosia, 33
Alzheimer's disease, 3, 6, 10, 16, 35,
    48, 68–71, 91, 158, 171, 175
  amyloid plaques and neurofibrillary
    tangles in, 68, 70
  APOE4 allele in, 68–69

cholinesterase inhibitors (donepezil)
    for, 68–70
  failed vaccine for, 69
  and frontotemporal dementia, 40
  hippocampus and, 68, 86
  memantine for, 68, 70
  prefrontal cortex and, 68, 86
American Academy of Neurology
    (statement on vegetative states), 167
Amnesia
  anterograde, 30, 63, 81, 107–108, 154
  retrograde, 30, 33, 107–108, 154
Amygdala
  in anxiety, 88
  interconnection with hippocampus,
    83–85
  as part of the limbic system, 19 (fig. 2.4)
  in pathological emotional memory, 19,
    83–86
  projection to the prefrontal cortex,
    51–54, 60
  in psychopathy and violent behavior,
    51–54, 60
  in PTSD, 19, 83–86
  and strathmin, 89
  in the stress response, 19–21, 26
Amyotrophic lateral sclerosis (ALS), 4, 11,
    91, 117
  BCIs for, 142
  gene therapy for, 89
  superoxide dismutase gene (SOD1) in, 89